Recent Results in Cancer Research 100

Recent Results in Cancer Research

Volume 95: Spheroids in Cancer Research
Edited by H. Acker, J. Carlsson, R. Durand, R. M. Sutherland
1984. 83 figures, 12 tables. IX, 183. ISBN 3-540-13691-6

Volume 96: Adjuvant Chemotherapy of Breast Cancer
Edited by H. J. Senn
1984. 98 figures, 91 tables. X, 243. ISBN 3-540-13738-6

Volume 97: Small Cell Lung Cancer
Edited by S. Seeber
1985. 44 figures, 47 tables. VII, 166. ISBN 3-540-13798-X

Volume 98: Perioperative Chemotherapy
Edited by U. Metzger, F. Largiadèr, H. J. Senn
1985. 48 figures, 45 tables. XII, 157. ISBN 3-540-15124-9

Volume 99: Peptide Hormones in Lung Cancer
Edited by K. Havemann, G. Sorenson, C. Gropp
1985. 100 figures, 63 tables. XII, 248. ISBN 3-540-15504-X

Therapeutic Strategies in Primary and Metastatic Liver Cancer

Edited by
Ch. Herfarth, P. Schlag, and P. Hohenberger

With 164 Figures and 97 Tables

Springer-Verlag
Berlin Heidelberg New York Tokyo

Professor Dr. Christian Herfarth
Professor Dr. Peter Schlag
Dr. Peter Hohenberger

Chirurgische Klinik, Klinikum der Universität Heidelberg
Im Neuenheimer Feld 110, 6900 Heidelberg 1, FRG

ISBN-13:978-3-642-82637-5 e-ISBN-13:978-3-642-82635-1
DOI: 10.1007/978-3-642-82635-1

Library of Congress Cataloging-in-Publication Data. Main entry under title: Therapeutic strategies in primary and metastatic liver cancer. (Recent results in cancer research; 100) Includes bibliographies and index. 1. Liver-Cancer-Treatment. 2. Metastasis-Treatment. I. Herfarth, Christian, 1933-. II. Schlag, P. (Peter), 1948-. III. Hohenberger, P. (Peter), 1953-. IV. Series. [DNLM: 1. Liver Neoplasms-therapy. W1 RE106P v. 100/WI 735 T398] RC261.R35 vol. 100 616.99'4s [616.99'43606] 85-27746 [RC280.L5]

2125/3140-543210

The Publisher and Editors of the series *Recent Results in Cancer Research* would like to express their thanks to the Swiss Cancer League, on the occasion of its 75th anniversary in 1985, for providing extensive support to the series from 1965 through 1985. Without this support, it would not have been possible to develop and maintain the high scientific standard of the series, and thereby its present reputation.

This series demonstrates that the financial support awarded to publications can have a lasting, positive effect extending far beyond the duration of that support. We are hopeful that the Swiss Cancer League is able, for the next quarter of a century and longer, to continue its fruitful work for the benefit of patients.

Heidelberg, St. Gallen
March 1986

Springer-Verlag
Ch. Herfarth
H. J. Senn

The Swiss Cancer League has sponsored *Recent Results in Cancer Research* during the last 20 years. Right from the beginning the League was convinced that this publication was a very valuable tool for continuous information on latest advances in the field of basic and clinical cancer research. The League is highly satisfied to notice that these periodical publications have won an increasing audience - thus showing that this initiative has finally reached its initial goal.

The Swiss Cancer League wishes to express its gratitude to the editor for publishing volume 100 in honour of it's 75th anniversary.

Bern, March 1986

P. Siegenthaler
Scientific Secretary
Swiss Cancer League

Preface

Primary and metastasizing malignant carcinoma of the liver represent a challenge to both the diagnostician and the therapist. For this reason, it appears a worthwhile task to review the current status of knowledge about the treatment of primary and metastasizing tumors of the liver. The question is whether modern diagnostic methods and new therapeutic concepts can help to improve the prospects of treatment. Of particular interest is the role played by therapeutic procedures directly involving the liver. Thus, it is equally important to discuss the pathophysiological and pharmacological bases for a modern therapy concept as it is to consider diagnostic issues and possible definitions of stages of progression. Therapeutic concepts comprise systemic therapy and organ-related therapeutic methods, including surgical resection, changes in the blood supply, regional selective chemotherapy, and other localized or regional, highly specialized forms of therapy.

This survey of the various possibilities in the field is meant too to stimulate further scientific research, given that methods of treatment are as yet by no means standardized, but are still in the stage of clinical research, where experimental models can find an application. The only well-established operative procedure is surgery on the isolated liver tumor. In this area, specialized techniques and various intraoperative procedures are discussed.

There is a wealth of information available on all the topics covered. The aim of the editors in compiling this multitude of results and experiences has been to define the current status of research, thus opening the door to further clinical and research activity as well as having a direct influence on therapy.

All methods of treatment - systemic therapy, selective localized application of cytostatics, various procedures involving the vascular system, surgery - cannot be standardized and are applicable only to the individual liver tumor in question. Highly stimulating are therapeutic procedures using polyclonal and monoclonal antibodies.

It is to be hoped that the wide range of experiences covered in this volume will serve as a stimulus to further experimental, randomized studies and clinical or research activity.

Contents

List of Contributors*

* The address of the principal author is given on the first page of each contribution

[1] Page on which contribution begins

Pathogenesis of Primary Liver Tumors Induced by Chemicals

P. Bannasch and H. Zerban

Institut für Experimentelle Pathologie, Deutsches Krebsforschungszentrum,
Im Neuenheimer Feld 280, 6900 Heidelberg, FRG

Our knowledge on the pathogenesis of primary liver tumors induced by chemicals is mainly based on investigations of experimental models, especially the rat liver treated with various carcinogens. It is evident from these studies that hepatocarcinogens may have at least four different types of target cells in the liver, namely, the hepatocytes, the bile ductular epithelia, and the sinusoidal and perisinusoidal cells (Fig. 1). All of these cell types may be specifically altered by the carcinogen and give rise to tumors or tumor-like lesions [7]. According to the similarity of the neoplastic cells to their normal counterparts, the liver tumors of the rat may be classified as neoplastic hepatic nodules (corresponding to human hepatic adenomas), hepatocellular carcinomas, cholangiofibromas, cholangiocarcinomas, benign hemangioendotheliomas, angiosarcomas, and pericytomas. Sequential cellular changes have been observed during the development of most of these tumor types. Detailed analysis of the different steps of tumorigenesis has considerably improved our understanding of the pathogenesis of primary liver tumors.

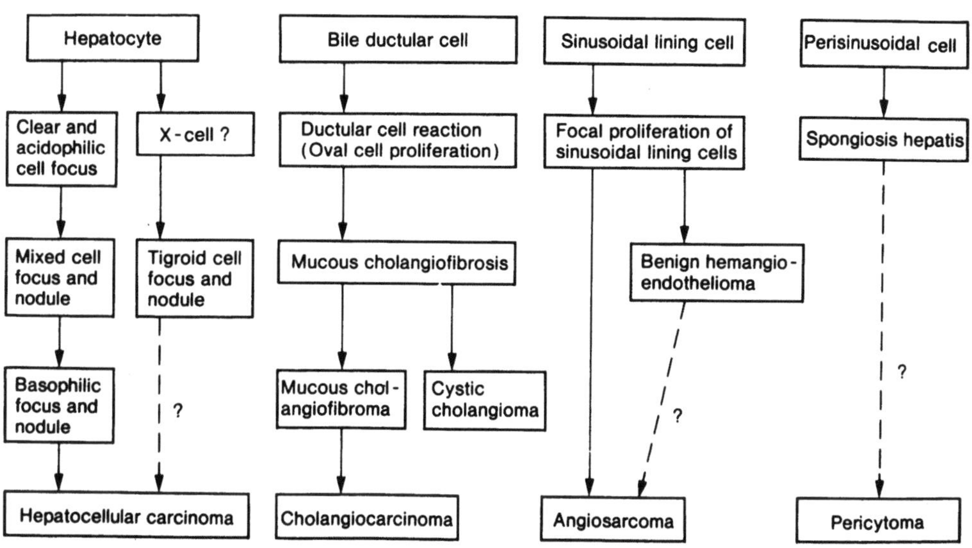

Fig. 1. Schematic presentation of sequential cellular changes in the development of epithelial and mesenchymal liver tumors

Recent Results in Cancer Research. Vol 100

Hepatocellular Tumors

Hepatocellular carcinomas induced in rats by chemical carcinogens show fundamentally the same histology and cytology as the corresponding human tumors [6]. They are usually composed of basophilic cells which are poor in glycogen. The tumors grow in trabecular, adenoid, or solid formations, and they may be combined with liver cirrhosis.

For more than 100 years, the association between liver cirrhosis and carcinoma dominated the discussion on the pathogenesis of this tumor type [2, 29] although it had been known for a long time that human hepatic tumors may occur without any concomitant cirrhosis [30, 35, 45, 55]. A number of experiments in rats have clearly shown that the combination of cirrhosis and carcinoma as induced by chemicals depends on the dose and duration of treatment [3, 27, 50]. Fibrosis and cirrhosis develop in addition to hepatocellular carcinomas only after continuous application of high doses which induce considerable necrotic parenchymal change, predominantly in acinuscentral parts of the liver lobule. After administration of low doses that do not produce significant liver cell necrosis, hepatocellular tumors develop independently of liver fibrosis and cirrhosis. While there seems to be no direct causal relationship between liver cirrhosis and liver carcinoma, cirrhosis might certainly modify the action of oncogenic agents on the liver parenchyma (e.g., by eliciting DNA synthesis in hepatocytes by regenerative stimuli). Some authors have speculated that liver cirrhosis might be especially important in the frequent association of chronic liver disease due to viral hepatitis B with hepatocarcinomas in humans. However, Okuda et al. [40] concluded from a comparative study of the histopathology and frequency of hepatitis B markers that the generally held view that hepatocarcinoma in a noncirrhotic liver is caused by nonviral carcinogens and that hepatocarcinoma arising from a background of cirrhosis is due to hepatitis B virus seems untenable. Chemicals for which epidemiological studies suggested an involvement in the development of human hepatic tumors are the aflatoxins, arsenic, and combined oral contraceptives [51]. The possible interaction between chemicals and viruses in the neoplastic transformation of hepatocytes will be discussed in the following chapter (zur Hausen, this volume).

During the past 20 years, putative preneoplastic foci of altered hepatocytes have been described in different species after administration of various chemical carcinogens (for review see [12, 14, 23, 24, 26, 41, 44, 56]. From our own experimental experience and observations in other laboratories, we inferred that an ordered pattern of sequential metabolic and morphological cellular changes is followed during hepatocarcinogenesis [3, 4, 12, 18]. When we detected years ago in rat liver treated with nitrosomorpholine that the low-glycogen hepatocellular carcinomas originated from foci storing glycogen in excess this appeared to be a paradox [10]. In the meantime, many findings have been reported which are in favor of a sequence of cellular changes leading from the glycogenotic cells to hepatoma cells poor in glycogen, but rich in ribosomes (Fig. 1). As demonstrated only recently by microdissection and biochemical microanalysis, the early preneoplastic foci contain on average 100% more glycogen than the normal liver parenchyma [32]. In tissue sections stained with H & E, the glycogen storage cells appear clear or acidophilic (Fig. 2a, b). The acidophilia is due to an additional proliferation of the smooth endoplasmic reticulum. The preneoplastic clear or acidophilic glycogen storage foci persist even after withdrawal of the carcinogen for weeks and months, and may progress through mixed and basophilic cell foci to neoplastic nodules and carcinomas (Figs. 2c, d and 3). This sequence has been adopted for the classification of preneoplastic lesions of the rat [47] and appears to be applicable to other species, too [7]. It is important to realize, however, that under certain conditions, especially after repeated administration of high doses of one or several hepatocar-

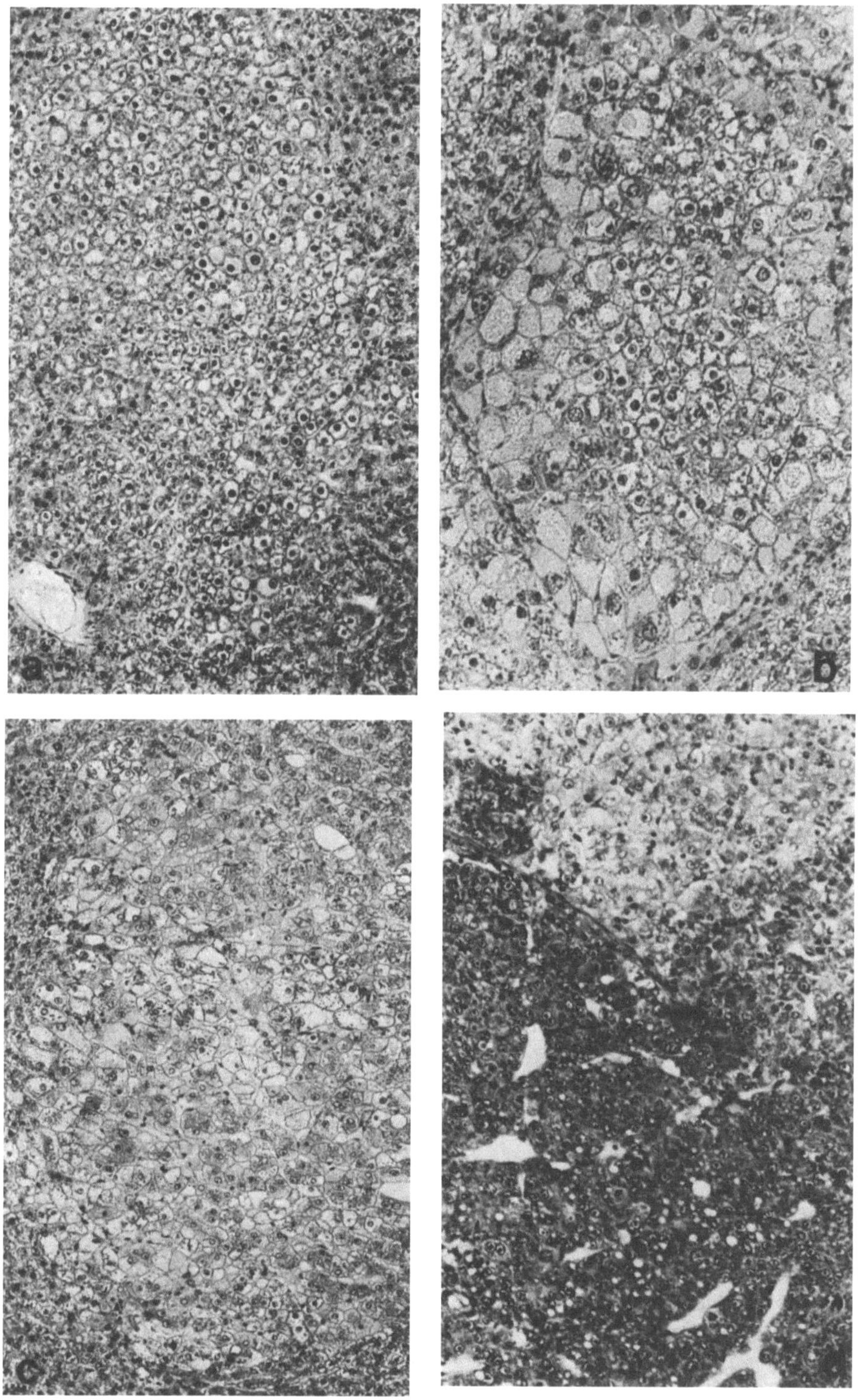

Fig. 2 a–d. Preneoplastic and neoplastic lesions induced in rat liver by *N*-nitrosomorpholine. **a** Clear cell glycogen storage focus, H & E, × 270. **b** Acidophilic glycogen storage focus, H & E, × 120. **c** Neoplastic nodule composed of a mixed cell population, H & E, × 110. **d** Hepatocellular carcinoma predominantly composed of glycogen-poor basophilic cells. Note transition from glycogen-rich clear cells into glycogen-poor basophilic cells *at the top*, H & E, × 135

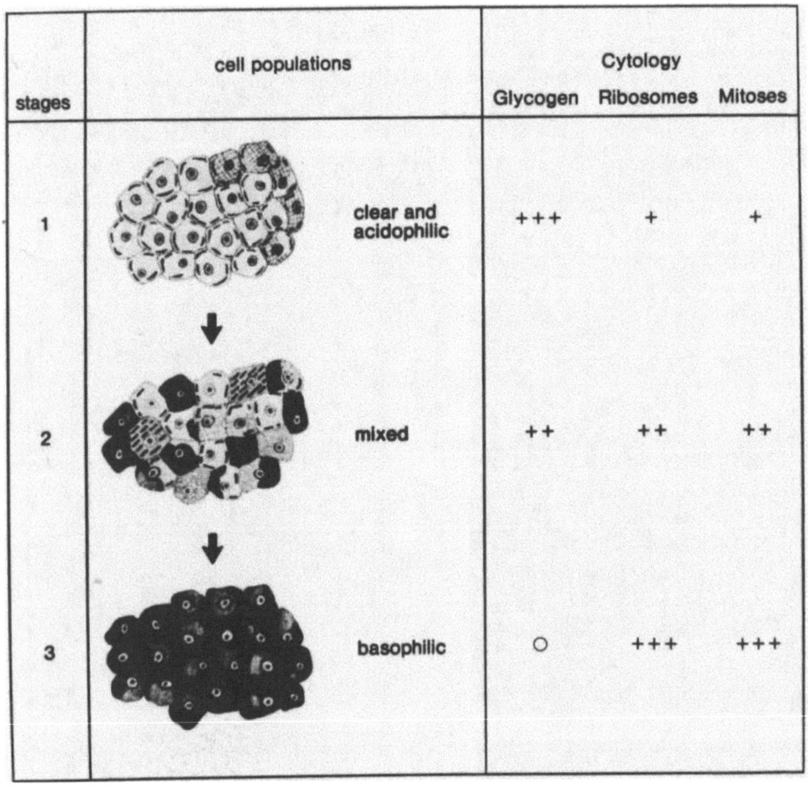

Fig. 3. Schematic presentation of the sequential cellular changes during hepatocarcinogenesis induced in rats by stop experiments with *N*-nitrosomorpholine

cionogens, reversible foci and nodules may develop which resemble the persistent lesions in their cytology and cytochemical pattern [31, 37, 39, 48]. Confusion with these hitherto poorly understood lesions can be avoided by using "stop experiments" in which the behavior of the preneoplastic cell populations and their progression toward neoplasms is followed after withdrawal of the carcinogen. We used this experimental approach to study the dose dependence and sequential development of the different cell populations morphometrically in rats treated for 7 weeks with *N*-nitrosomorpholine (NNM) given in the drinking water in concentrations of 80, 120, 160, and 200 mg/liter [36]. The majority of the foci emerged after cessation of the carcinogenic treatment. The sequence of cellular changes outlined was confirmed at all dose levels. The first appearance and the frequency of the different lesions proved to depend on the dose of the carcinogen in a similar way to the hepatic tumors developing later on. There was no indication of any reversibility under these experimental conditions. On the contrary, the foci became larger and acquired phenotypic markers closer to neoplasia without further action of the carcinogen.

The cytomorphological and cytochemical changes described are usually closely related to a great variety of alterations in the activity of enzymes, including those of the carbohydrate metabolism (see [12, 23, 24, 41, 56]. We were especially interested in the enzymes of the alternative pathways of carbohydrate metabolism and investigated by enzyme histochemistry and biochemical microanalysis some important enzymes in glycogen storage foci, neoplastic nodules, and hepatocellular carcinomas in rats treated with NNM [28, 32].

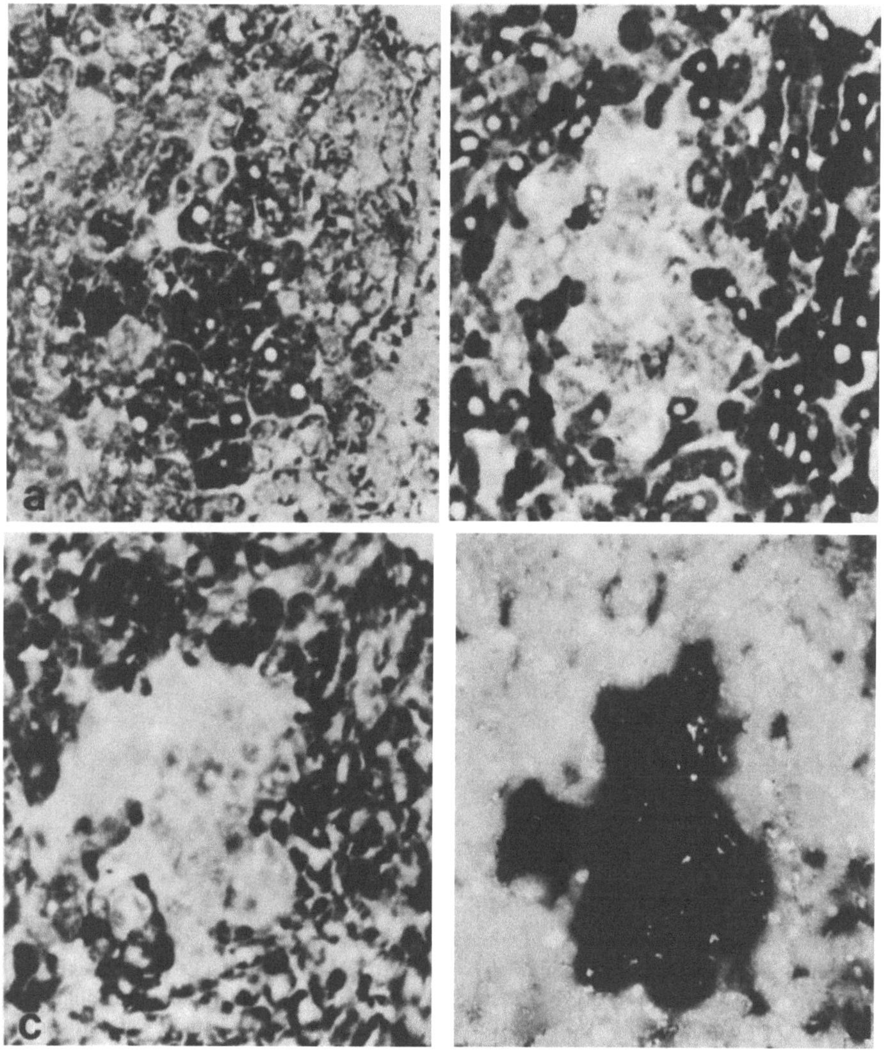

Fig. 4a–d. Serial sections through an enzyme-altered glycogen storage focus induced in rat liver by *N*-nitrosomorpholine. **a** Demonstration of glycogen by the PAS reaction. **b** Decreased activity of glucose-6-phosphatase (lead salt method). **c** Decreased activity of glycogen phosphorylase (iodine staining of newly synthesized glycogen). **d** Increased activity of glucose-6-phosphate dehydrogenase (tetrazolium salt method). All figures: ×200

Unfortunately, we have so far been unable to define the cause of carcinogen-induced hepatocellular glycogenosis, but it may be speculated that a still-unexplained excess of glucose-6-phosphate plays a key role. Some weeks after the appearance of the first glycogen storage cells, the majority of the pronounced glycogen storage foci show a decreased activity of glycogen phosphorylase and of glucose-6-phosphatase, while the activity of glucose-6-phosphate dehydrogenase, the key enzyme of the pentose phosphate pathway, increases (Fig. 4a–d). More detailed quantitative studies of the glucose-6-phosphate dehydrogenase revealed that there is a gradual increase in enzyme activity from the small gly-

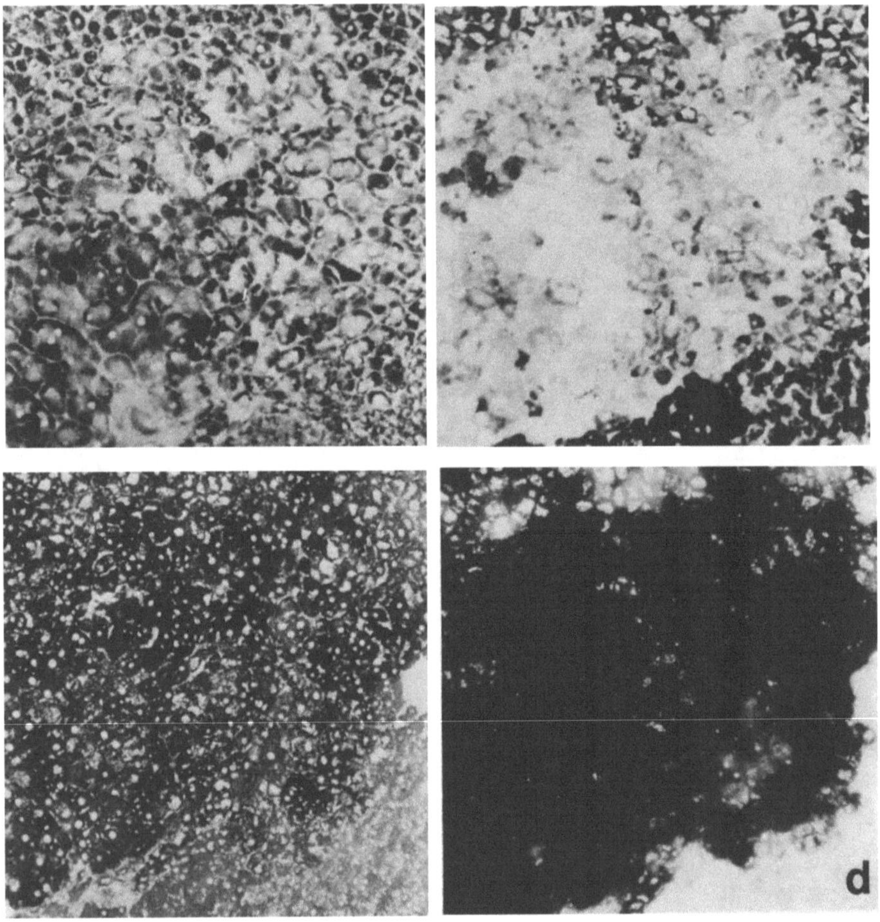

Fig. 5 a–d. Serial sections through an enzyme-altered neoplastic nodule induced in rat liver by *N*-nitrosomorpholine. **a** Demonstration of glycogen by the PAS reaction. **b** Decreased activity of glucose-6-phosphatase (lead salt method). **c** Increased activity of glyceraldehyde-3-phosphate dehydrogenase (tetrazolium salt method). **d** Increased activity of glucose-6-phosphate dehydrogenase (tetrazolium salt method). All figures: ×70

cogenotic foci, which show only a tendency to higher values, over the large glycogenotic to the mixed cell foci [32]. The development of neoplastic nodules and hepatocellular carcinomas from the foci is associated with additional enzyme histochemical changes (Fig. 5 a–d): the reduction of the glycogen initially stored in excess is usually correlated with an increase in the activity of the glycolytic enzyme glyceraldehyde-3-phosphate dehydrogenase, while that of the glucose-6-phosphate dehydrogenase remains high [28]. These results agree with the hypothesis that the molecular changes underlying the glycogenosis might trigger an adaptation of cellular enzymes which could gradually redirect the carbohydrate metabolism toward other metabolic pathways, such as glycolysis and the pentose phosphate pathway [12, 18]. The results of the cytochemical investigations in situ are also in line with many earlier biochemical findings in transplantable hepatomas, especially with the molecular correlation concept of Weber [54]. The tigroid cell foci (Fig. 1) which have been described as a prestage of benign hepatic tumors in rats recently [17] are not preceded by an obvious hepatocellular glycogenosis, but they show enzymatic changes in the alternative pathways of carbohydrate metabolism similar to the other types of preneoplastic liver lesions.

Some observations in humans suggest that the sequence of cellular changes in man and experimental animals is in principle identical [6]. Thus, foci of clear or acidophilic (ground glass) cells storing glycogen in excess have occasionally been found in the livers of patients bearing multicentric hepatocellular carcinomas [1]. The predominance of glycogen-rich cells in many adenomas and in clear cell carcinomas of the liver is well known [1, 8, 57]. According to Wu and colleagues, the clear cell variety of hepatocarcinoma may also develop in patients with persistent hepatitis B virus infection. An even more interesting aspect of human pathology pertinent to our experimental results is the appearance of hepatic tumors increasingly reported in patients suffering from inborn hepatic glycogenosis, mostly that of the von Gierke type (see [18] for literature). Liver tumors could be detected by scintigrams, sonograms, biopsies, or autopsies in many patients with this genetically fixed disease. Whereas the tumors were relatively rate in the 1st decade of life, they appeared in all patients who survived adolescence. Histologically, both adenomas and carcinomas were diagnosed, and in some cases the clinical course of the disease suggested transformation from adenomas into carcinomas. The observations in humans lend further support to the hypothesis that the metabolic disturbance leading to the hepatocellular glycogenosis, which is probably fixed at the genetic level in both humans and experimental animals, might also be causally related to the neoplastic transformation of the hepatocytes [3, 12].

Cholangiocellular Tumors

In addition to hepatocellular tumors, virtually all types of cholangiocellular tumors known from human pathology may be induced in rats by chemical carcinogens [4, 7, 22]. The tumors develop in particular after application of high doses of carcinogens such as NNM, which produce pronounced necrotic alterations of the liver parenchyma. Under these experimental conditions, a very complex sequence of cellular changes occurs in which four distinct stages can be identified (Fig. 1). The changes of the bile duct epithelia start with a ductular (oval) cell reaction, which may progress to cholangiofibrotic areas, benign cystic cholangiomas, cholangiofibromas, and eventually also cholangiocarcinomas [9, 11]. I do not wish to go into details of the controversial discussion of the fate of the oval cell (see [5, 25, 49]), but shall stick to the well-documented relation of this cell type to the development of the cholangiocellular tumors.

During the second stage of tumorigenesis, the ductular cell reaction proceeds to a mucous cholangiofibrosis (Fig. 6a) looking like a scar at both the macroscopic and the microscopic level. Many ductular cells are converted into goblet cells storing and secreting abundant mucus substances which contain PAS-positive neutral glycoproteins and alcianophilic acid components. The production of mucopolysaccharides in proliferated bile ducts appears to be specific for carcinogenic liver intoxications [11, 20] and might be a phenomenon analogous to hepatocellular glycogenosis. According to Chou and Gibson [19] an accumulation of mucopolysaccharides might also play an important role in the development of human cholangiocellular tumors.

In rat liver, expansively growing tumors may originate from the mucous cholangiofibrosis after long lag periods. There are two possibilities: either benign cystic cholangiomas (Fig. 6b) develop which no longer synthesize mucous substances, or the cholangiofi-

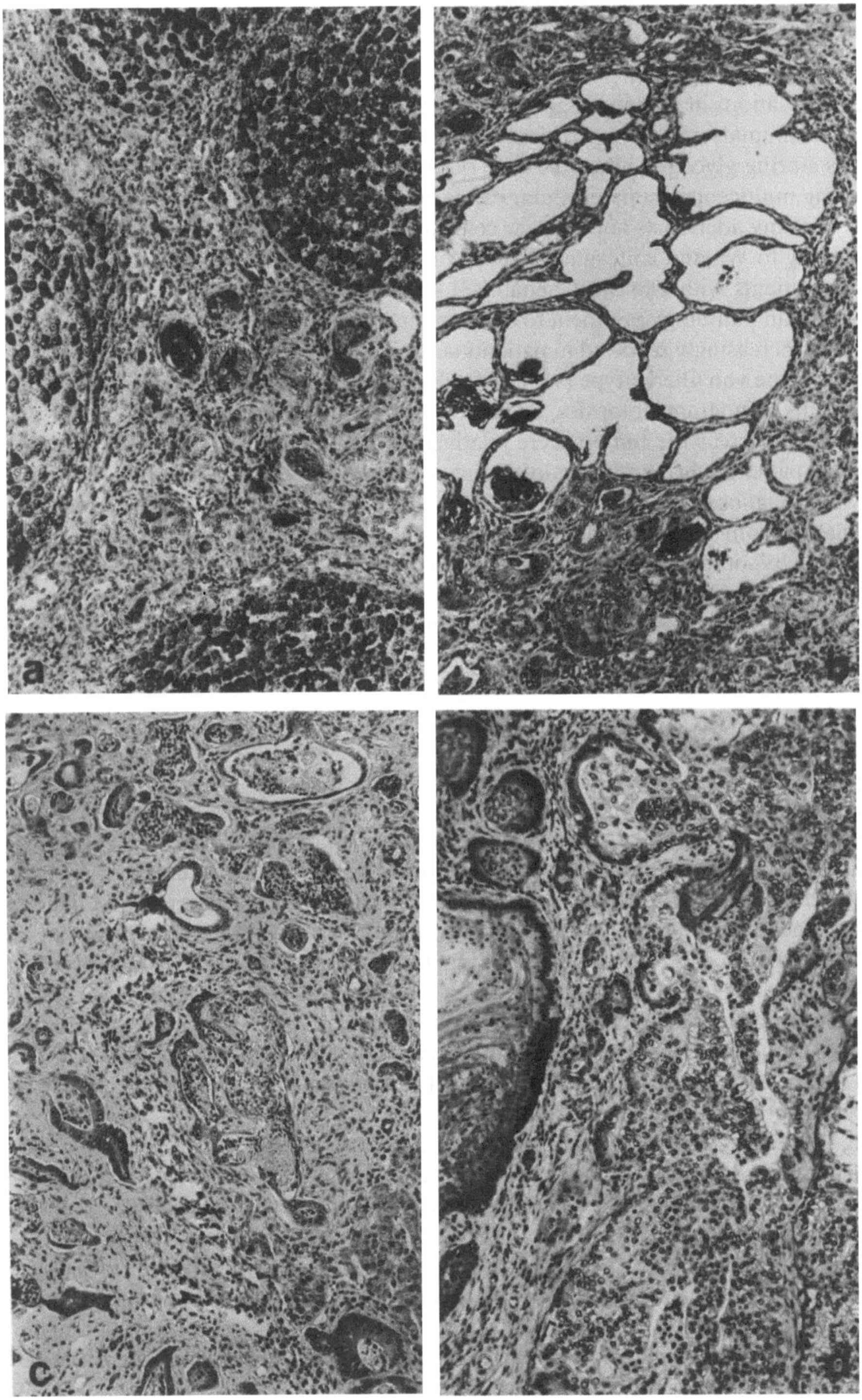

Fig. 6a–d. Preneoplastic and neoplastic cholangiocellular lesions induced in rat liver by *N*-nitrosomorpholine. **a** Cholangiofibrosis, PAS. **b** Benign cystic cholangioma, PAS. **c** Cholangiofibroma, H & E. **d** Cholangiocarcinoma. Note transition from component rich in mucopolysaccharides *(to the left)* into mucus-free carcinoma. Alcian blue. All figures: ×110

brosis progresses to a cholangiofibroma (Fig. 6 c) which is characterized by an especially pronounced production of collagenous fibers and mucopolysaccharides. The cholangiofibroma does not metastasize, but it is potentially malignant and may transform into a cholangiocarcinoma (Fig. 6 d). During this process, the excessive production of mucopolysaccharides gradually disappears again. While the pathogenesis of human polycystic disease of the liver shows many similarities to that of benign cystic cholangiomas in rodents [4, 11], little is known about possible early stages of cholangiocarcinoma in man [55].

Vascular Liver Tumors

Vascular liver tumors are attracting considerable interest in view of their recently increased incidence in man. They arise from the sinusoidal lining cells - most probably the endothelial cells - and can be induced by chemical carcinogens in various animal species (for literature see [7, 42, 46]. Maltoni [34] produced angiosarcomas in rodent liver by exposure to vinyl chloride shortly before the association of this chemical with liver angiosarcomas was recognized in man [21, 33]. Thus, vinyl chloride represents an excellent example of a chemical that not only induces malignant tumors in both animals and man, but also acts at the same site and hits the same type of target cells [42].

During the development of vascular liver tumors, no aberrations in carbohydrate metabolism comparable to those in preneoplastic hepatocytes or bile duct epithelia have been detected in the sinusoidal lining cells up to the present. However, the pathogenesis of

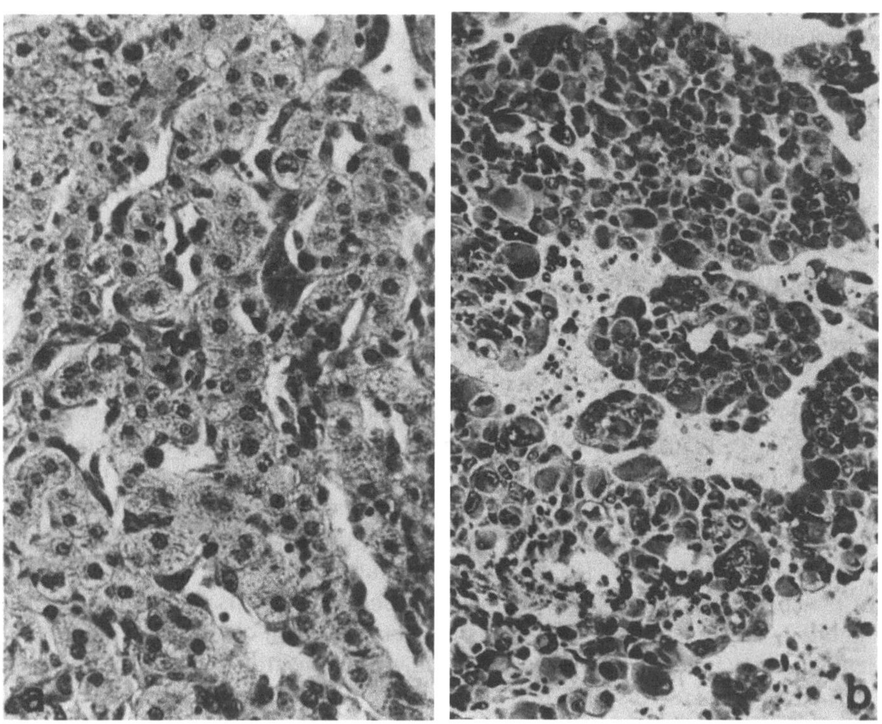

Fig. 7 a, b. Early **a** and fully developed **b** angiosarcoma induced in rat liver by *N*-nitrosomorpholine. Both figures H & E; **a** × 280; **b** × 180

vascular liver tumors is also linked with characteristic cellular changes. The sequential histological alterations that occur during the morphogenesis of angiosarcomas in rodents and man show many similarities [42], but the antecedent fibrosis seen in human liver does not seem to play an important role in rodents.

The sinusoidal lining cells may give rise to three types of vascular lesions occurring after treatment with chemical carcinogens, namely peliosis hepatis, benign angiomas, and angiosarcomas. Peliosis hepatis is characterized by an irregular focal dilatation of the sinuses. The classification of this lesion as a neoplastic disease or a preneoplastic condition is controversial. The lining sinusoidal cells may at best show some minor alterations such as nuclear enlargement. However, in *Mastomys* given single or twofold intraperitoneal injections of 10 or 5 mg/kg body wt. *N*-nitrosodimethylamine [53], we were able to observe all transitions to unequivocal angiomas. Especially interesting is that anabolic androgenic steroids, which have been related to the liver-cell adenomas frequently developing in association with peliosis hepatis in man, may induce this lesion in rats, too [37 a]. In the nitrosamine-treated rodents, we observed transitions from benign angiomas to angiosarcomas after very long lag periods, but this seems to be the exception rather than the rule. Angiosarcomas induced in rat liver by NNM usually develop without a preceding benign prestage. The first sign of tumorigenesis observed in this case is a proliferation of highly atypical mesenchymal cells along the liver cell plates (Fig. 7 a). These cells can be nicely demonstrated by antibodies to vimentin, the intermediate filaments characteristic for normal and neoplastic mesenchymal cells. This immunocytochemical method is not only very helpful in the sometimes difficult differential diagnosis of angiosarcomas and anaplastic hepatocellular carcinomas, but it also reveals that many cells of the angiosarcomas (Fig. 6 b) accumulate excessive amounts of vimentin filaments [13, 16]. These vimentin storage cells (Fig. 8) most probably correspond to the polyhedral cells (Fig. 7, inset) described in human angiosarcomas by Popper and colleagues [43] and are pathognomonic for malignant mesenchymal liver tumors, especially the angiosarcomas. The cause of the accumulation of the intermediate filaments in sarcoma cells is not known. However, it may be speculated that similar metabolic aberrations to those which lead to the storage of polysaccharides or lipids in epithelial cells hit by the chemical carcinogens might be responsible [16].

Spongiosis Hepatis and Pericytoma

Finally, the perisinusoidal cells may be the target of chemical carcinogens (Fig. 1). This cell type has only been clearly identified during the past 20 years and variously called Ito cell, lipocyte, or fat-storing cell [52]. The perisinusoidal cells are located between the sinusoidal lining cells and the hepatocytes, and have been shown to be involved in the metabolism of vitamin A and most probably also in the production of collagen. In rat liver treated with hepatocarcinogens, these cells are considered to be the site of origin of a peculiar, hitherto largely neglected cyst-like lesion (Fig. 9 a) for which we proposed the descriptive term "spongiosis hepatis" [15, 58]. Under the light microscope, it is evident that the holes of the sponge are not lined by epithelial or endothelial cells. In contrast to peliosis, the multilocular formations of spongiosis are not filled with blood, but with a finely flocculent material rich in acid mucopolysaccharides. Electron microscopic analysis of the spongiotic areas reveals that they are composed of cells which are very similar to fibroblasts and sometimes even to typical fat-storing cells (Fig. 9 b). The fibroblast-like cells possess extremely elongated cytoplasmic processes which form the walls of the spongy lesions and are usually observed in close association with a thick coat resembling a base-

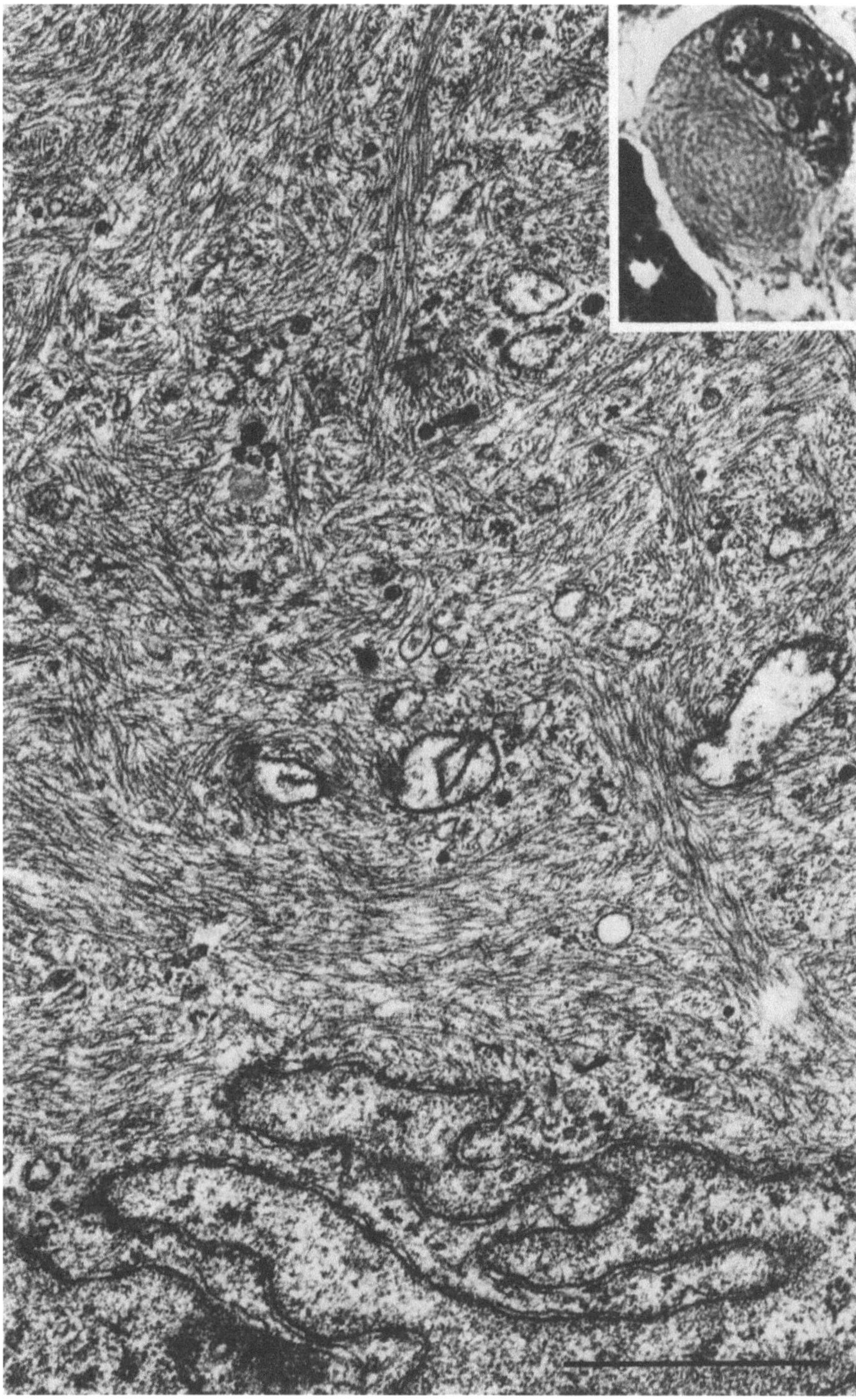

Fig. 8. Electron microscopic demonstration of accumulation of intermediate filaments (vimentin) in angiosarcoma cell. Uranyl acetate and lead citrate, × 36000. *Inset:* Vimentin storage cell as seen under the light microscope. *Bar* = 1 μm. H & E, × 1100

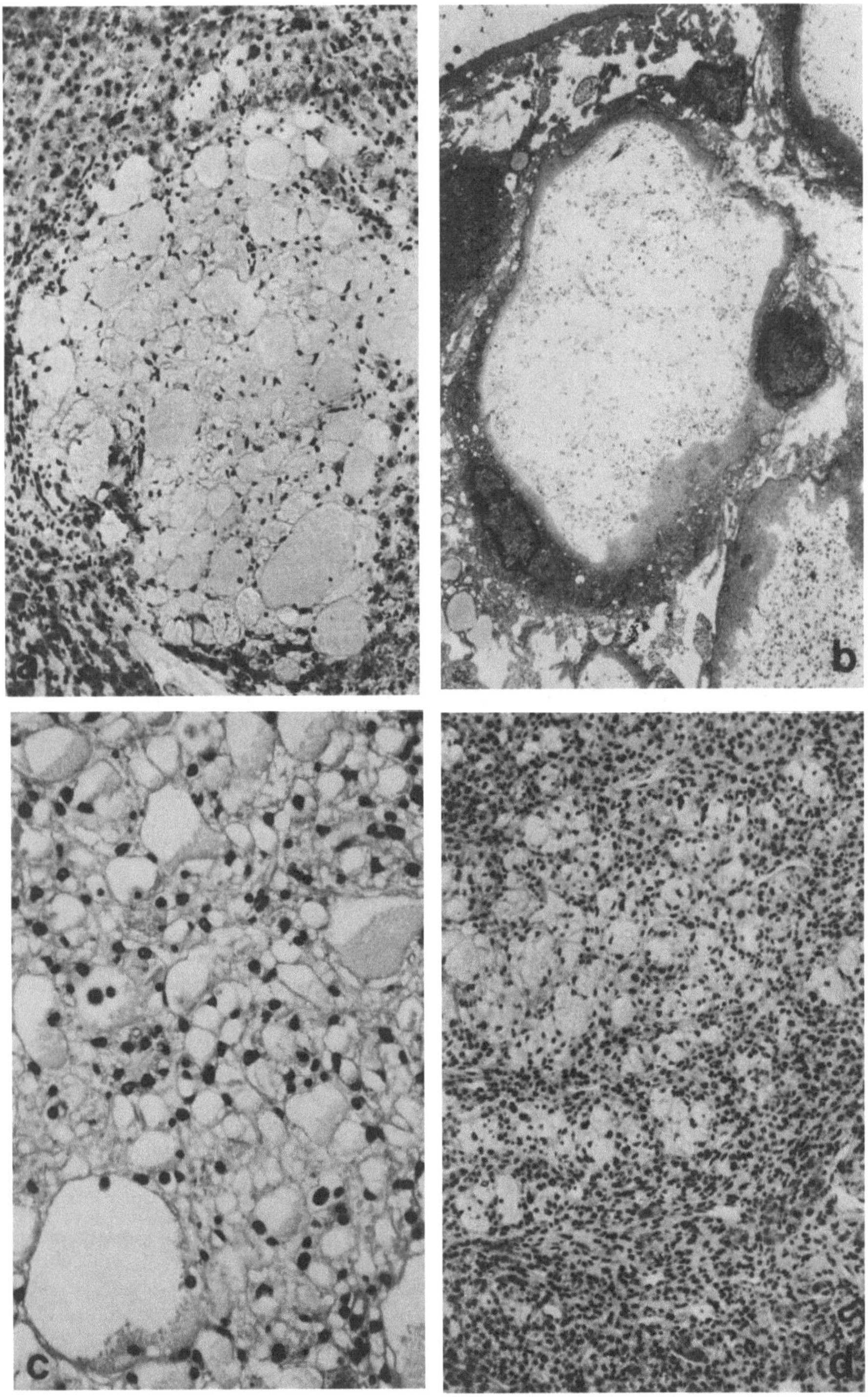

Fig. 9 a–d. Spongiosis hepatis (**a–c**) and pericytoma (**d**) induced in rat liver by *N*-nitrosomorpholine. **a** Spongiosis hepatis as seen under the light microscope, H&E, × 120. **b** Portion of spongiosis hepatis as seen under the electron microscope. Uranyl acetate and lead citrate, × 1760. **c** Spongiosis hepatis showing considerable proliferation, H&E, × 70. **d** Pericytoma, H&E, × 120 ment membrane. To my knowledge, spongiosis hepatis has not been recognized as a pathomorphological entity in other species. Only in a report of human hepatic adenomas that appeared in users of oral contraceptives has a picture been published showing spongiosis-like changes within an adenoma [38]. It is still unclear whether spongiosis hepatis should be considered as a preneoplastic or as a neoplastic liver lesion. However, during the last few weeks we observed a considerable cell proliferation within spongiotic areas in some rats treated with NNM after long lag periods (Fig. 9c). There were apparently also transitions into malignant mesenchymal tumors which we classified as pericytomas (Fig. 9d). With respect to the pathogenesis of this tumor type, it is of particular interest that our preliminary results suggest that the accumulation of acid mucopolysaccharides within the spongiotic formations seems to disappear during transformation of spongiosis into the pericytoma. If this surmise can be confirmed, the analogy between sequential alterations of carbohydrate metabolism during neoplastic transformation of epithelial liver cells and at least one type of mesenchymal liver cell should occasion more detailed studies of these metabolic aberrations.

References

1. Altmann HW (1978) Pathology of human liver tumors. In: Remmer H, Bolt HM, Bannasch P, Popper H (eds). Primary liver tumors. MTP Press, Lancaster, pp 53-71
2. Anthony PP (1976) Precursor lesions for liver cancer in humans. Cancer Res 36: 2579-2583
3. Bannasch P (1968) The cytoplasm of hepatocytes during carcinogenesis. Recent Results Cancer Res 19: 1-100
4. Bannasch P (1975) Die Cytologie der Hepatocarcinogenese. In: Altmann HW et al. (eds) Handbuch der Allgemeinen Pathologie, vol 7. Springer, Berlin Heidelberg New York, pp 123-276
5. Bannasch P (1978) Cellular and subcellular pathology of liver carcinogenesis. In: Remmer H, Bolt P, Bannasch P, Popper H (eds). Primary liver tumors. MTP Press, Lancaster, pp 87-111
6. Bannasch P (1979) Morphologie und Pathogenese der Lebertumoren. In: Kühn HA, Wernze H (eds) Klinische Hepatologie. Thieme, Stuttgart, pp 6386-6403
7. Bannasch P (1983) Strain and species differences in the susceptibility to liver tumor induction. IARC Sci Publ 51: 9-38
8. Bannasch P, Klinge O (1971) Hepatocelluläre Glykogenose und Hepatombildung beim Menschen. Virchows Arch [A] 352: 157-164
9. Bannasch P, Massner B (1976) Histogenese und Cytogenese von Cholangiofibromen und Cholangiocarcinomen bei Nitrosomorpholin-vergifteten Ratten. Z Krebsforsch 87: 239-255
10. Bannasch P, Müller HA (1964) Lichtmikroskopische Untersuchungen über die Wirkung von *N*-nitrosomorpholin auf die Leber von Ratte und Maus. Arzneimittelforsch 14: 805-814
11. Bannasch P, Reiss W (1971) Histogenese und Cytogenese cholangiocellulärer Tumoren bei Nitrosomorpholin-vergifteten Ratten. Zugleich ein Beitrag zur Morphogenese der Cystenleber. Z Krebsforsch 77: 108-133
12. Bannasch P, Mayer D, Hacker HJ (1980a) Hepatocellular glycogenosis and hepatocarcinogenesis. Biochim Biophys Acta 605: 217-245
13. Bannasch P, Zerban H, Schmid E, Franke WW (1980b) Liver tumors distinguished by immunofluorescence microscopy with antibodies to proteins of intermediate-sized filaments. Proc Natl Acad Sci USA 77: 4948-4952
14. Bannasch P, Benner U, Hacker HJ, Klimek F, Mayer D, Moore, M, Zerban H (1981a) Cytochemical and biochemical microanalysis of carcinogenesis. Histochem J 13: 799-820
15. Bannasch P, Bloch M, Zerban H (1981b) Spongiosis hepatis. Specific changes of the perisinusoidal liver cells induced in rats by *N*-nitrosomorpholine. Lab Invest 44: 252-264
16. Bannasch P, Zerban H, Schmid E, Franke WW (1981c) Characterization of cytoskeletal compo-

nents in epithelial and mesenchymal liver tumors by electron and immunofluorescence microscopy. Virchows Arch [Cell Pathol] 36: 139-158
17. Bannasch P, Benner U, Hacker HJ (1984a) Tigroid cell foci and their possible relation to hepatic tumors. In: Bezooijen van CFA (ed) Pharmacological, morphological and physiological aspects of liver aging, EURAGE, Rijswijk, pp 195-204
18. Bannasch P, Hacker HJ, Klimek F, Mayer D (1984b) Hepatocellular glycogenosis and related pattern of enzymatic changes during hepatocarcinogenesis. Adv Enzyme Regul 22: 97-121
19. Chou ST, Gibson JB (1970) The histochemistry of biliary mucins and the changes caused by *Clonorchis sinensis*. J Pathol 101: 185-197
20. Chou ST, Gibson JB (1972) A comparative histochemical study of rat livers in alpha-naphthyl-iso-thiocyanate (ANIT) and DL-ethionine intoxication. J Pathol 108: 73-83
21. Creech JL, Johnson MN (1974) Angiosarcoma of liver in the manufacture of polyvinyl chloride. J Occup Med 16: 150-151
22. Dominis M, Damjanov L (1977) Cystic cholangiofibrosis of the liver. Arch Geschwulstforsch 47: 661-669
23. Emmelot P, Scherer E (1980) The first relevant stage in rat liver carcinogenesis. A quantitative approach. Biochim Biophys Acta 605: 247-304
24. Farber E (1980) The sequential analysis of liver cancer induction. Biochim Biophys Acta 605: 149-166
25. Farber E, Cameron R (1980) The sequential analysis of cancer development. Adv Cancer Res 31: 125-226
26. Goldfarb St, Pugh ThD, Koen H, He Y-Z (1983) Preneoplastic and neoplastic progression during hepatocarcinogenesis in mice injected with diethylnitrosamine in infancy. Environ Health Perspect 50: 149-161
27. Grundmann E, Sieburg H (1962) Die Histogenese und Cytogenese des Lebercarcinoms der Ratte durch Diäthylnitrosamin im lichtmikroskopischen Bild. Beitr Pathol Anat 126: 57-90
28. Hacker HJ, Moore MA, Mayer D, Bannasch P (1982) Correlative histochemistry of some enzymes of carbohydrate metabolism in preneoplastic and neoplastic lesions in the rat liver. Carcinogenesis 3: 1265-1272
29. Higgins GK (1970) The pathologic anatomy of primary hepatic tumors. Recent Results Cancer Res 26: 15-37
30. Higginson J, Svoboda DS (1970) Primary carcinoma of the liver as a pathologist's problem. Pathol Annu 5: 61-89
31. Kitagawa T (1971) Histochemical analysis of hyperplastic lesions and hepatomas of the liver of rats fed 2-fluorenylacetamide. Gann 62: 207-216
32. Klimek F, Mayer D, Bannasch P (1984) Biochemical microanalysis of glycogen content and glucose-6-phosphate dehydrogenase activity in focal lesions of rat liver induced by *N*-nitrosomorpholine. Carcinogenesis 5: 265-268
33. Lloyd JW (1975) Angiosarcoma of the liver in vinyl chloride/polyvinyl chloride workers. J Occup Med 17, 333-334
34. Maltoni C (1974) Occupational carcinogenesis. In: Maltoni C (ed). Cancer detection and prevention, Proceedings of the 2nd International Symposium on Cancer Detection and Prevention, Bologna 1973, Excerpta Medica, Amsterdam, pp 19-26
35. Miyai K, Ruebner B (1963) Acute yellow atrophy, cirrhosis and hepatoma. Arch Pathol 75: 609-617
36. Moore MA, Mayer D, Bannasch P (1982) The dose-dependence and sequential appearance of putative preneoplastic populations induced in the rat liver by stop experiments with *N*-nitrosomorpholine. Carcinogenesis 3: 1429-1436
37. Moore MA, Hacker HJ, Bannasch P (1983) Phenotypic instability in focal and nodular lesions induced in a short term system in the rat liver. Carcinogenesis 4: 595-603
38. Nadell J, Kosek J (1977) Peliosis hepatis. Arch Pathol Lab Med 101: 405-410
39. Nime F, Pickren JW, Vana J, Aronoff BL, Baker HW, Murphy GP (1979) The histology of liver tumors in oral contraceptive users observed during a national survey by the American College of Surgeons Commission on Cancer. Cancer 44: 1481-1489

40. Ogawa K, Medline A, Farber E (1979) Sequential analysis of hepatic carcinogenesis. A comparative study of the ultrastructure of preneoplastic, malignant, prenatal, postnatal, and regenerating liver. Lab Invest 41: 22-35
41. Okuda K, Nakashima T, Sakamoto K, Ikari T, Hidaka H, Kubo Y, Sakuma K, Motioke Y, Okuda H, Obata H (1982) Hepatocellular carcinoma arising in noncirrhotic and highly cirrhotic livers: a comparative study of histopathology and frequency of hepatitis B markers. Cancer 49: 450-455
42. Pitot HC, Sirica AE (1980) The stages of initiation and promotion in hepatocarcinogenesis. Biochim Biophys Acta 605: 191-215
43. Popper H, Maltoni C, Selikoff IJ, Squire RA, Thomas LB (1977) Comparison of neoplastic hepatic lesions in man and experimental animals. In: Hiatt HH, Watson JD, Winsten JA (eds) Origin of human cancer, book C. Human risk assessment. Cold Spring Harbor Conferences on Cell Proliferation, vol 4, Cold Spring Harbor, pp 1359-1382
44. Popper H, Thomas LB, Telles LC, Falk H, Selikoff IJ (1978) Development of hepatic angiosarcoma in man induced by vinyl chloride, thorotrast and arsenic. Am J Pathol 92: 349-370
45. Rabes HM (1983) Development and growth of early preneoplastic lesions induced in the liver by chemical carcinogens. J Cancer Res Clin Oncol 106: 85-92
46. Steiner PE (1960) Cancer of the liver and cirrhosis in Trans-Saharan Africa and the United States of America. Cancer 13: 1085-1166
47. Stewart HL (1975) Comparative aspects of certain cancers. In: Becker FF (ed) Cancer. A comprehensive treatise, vol 4. Plenum, New York, pp 303-374
48. Stewart HL, Williams G, Keysser CH, Lombard LS, Montali RJ (1980) Histologic typing of liver tumors of the rat. J Natl Cancer Inst 65: 179-206
49. Tatematsu M, Ho RH, Kaku T, Ekem JK, Farber E (1984) Studies on the proliferation and fate of oval cells in the liver of rats treated with 2-acetylaminofluorene and partial hepatectomy. Am J Pathol 114: 418-430
50. Tatematsu M, Takano T, Hasegawa R, Imaida K, Nakanowatari J, Ito N (1980) A sequential quantitative study of the reversibility or irreversibility of liver hyperplastic nodules in rats exposed to hepatocarcinogens. Gann 71: 843-855
51. Thomas C (1961) Zur Morphologie der durch Diäthylnitrosamin erzeugten Leberveränderungen und Tumoren bei der Ratte. Z Krebsforsch 64: 224-233
52. Tomatis L (1984) Exposures associated with cancer in humans. J Cancer Res Clin Oncol 108: 6-10
53. Wake K (1980) Perisinusoidal stellate cells (fat-storing cells, interstitial cells, lipocytes), their related structure in and around the liver sinusoids, and vitamin A-storing cells in extrahepatic organs. Int Rev Cytol 66: 303-353
54. Wayss K, Bannasch P, Mattern J, Volm M (1979) Vascular liver tumors in *Mastomys* induced by single or twofold administration of dimethylnitrosamine. J Natl Cancer Inst 62: 1199-1207
55. Weber G (1982) Differential carbohydrate metabolism in tumor and host. In: Arnott MS, Van Eys J, Wang Y-M (eds) Molecular interrelations of nutrition and cancer. Raven, New York, pp 191-208
56. Weinbren K (1984) Precancerous states in the liver. In: Carter RL (ed) Precancerous states. Oxford Medical, London, pp 254-277
57. Williams GM (1980) The pathogenesis of rat liver cancer caused by chemical carcinogens. Biochim Biophys Acta 605: 167-189
58. Wu PC, Lai CL, Lam KC, Lok ASF, Lin HJ (1983) Clear cell carcinoma of liver. An ultrastructural study. Cancer 52: 504-507
59. Zerban H, Bannasch P (1983) Spongiosis hepatis in rats treated with low doses of hepatotropic nitrosamines. Cancer Lett 19: 247-252

Radiation-Induced Primary Liver Tumors in "Thorotrast Patients"

G. van Kaick, H. Wesch, H. Lührs, and D. Liebermann

Institut für Nuklearmedizin, Deutsches Krebsforschungszentrum,
Im Neuenheimer Feld 280, 6900 Heidelberg, FRG

Introduction

For more than 30 years it has been known that radiation-induced cancer can occur in almost every type of tissue. The scientific question that concerns us is the evaluation of dose-effect relationships especially with regard to radiation protection. Tissue doses used in animal experiments, however, cannot be transferred to human beings for the calculation of radiation late effects. Therefore all data obtained from epidemiological studies of radiation-exposed persons are extremely important. The so-called Thorotrast patients have given us the most useful information of radiation-induced liver cancers.

Biophysical Data

Thorotrast was the trade name of an X-ray contrast medium used in Germany and other countries from 1930 to 1951. The predominant form of application was an intravascular injection, especially for cerebral angiography. Thorotrast consists of a 25% colloidal solution of thorium dioxide. It was sold in 12-ml ampoules. After intravascular injection the ThO_2 aggregates accumulate in the reticuloendothelial system and are stored for life. Thorium has natural radioactivity; the half-life is more than 10^{10} years and 95% of the radiation is alpha particles. The typical distribution of thorium-232 described by Kaul and Noffz [2] is shown in Table 1.

The tissue dose depends on the total injected volume of Thorotrast. Mean tissue dose rates based on a 25-ml intravascular Thorotrast injection are summarized in Table 2 (Kaul and Noffz, 1978).

Table 1. Distribution of thorium-232 in a standard patient (%). Kaul and Noffz [2]

Liver	59
Spleen	29
Red bone marrow	9
Calcified bone	2
Kidney	0.1

Recent Results in Cancer Research. Vol 100

Table 2. Mean tissue dose rates. (25-ml Thorotrast injections). Kaul and Noffz [2]

Organ	Dose rate (rad/year)
Liver	25
Spleen	70
Red bone marrow	9
Bone surface	15
Main bronchi	13
Kidney	0.4

Table 3. German Thorotrast Study

Patient status	Thorotrast	Control
Examined	894	662
Not examined		
Survival time >3 years	1440	1250
Survival time <3 years	1829	533
Did not respond	80	1473
Not traced	916	1233
Total	5159	5151

The history of the Thorotrast tragedy cannot be presented here. It should, however, be noted that the former director of the University Hospital of Surgery and founder of the German Cancer Research Center, Heidelberg, Prof. K. H. Bauer, was the first scientist in Germany to recognize the potential danger of Thorotrast. He banned its use in his hospital after being appointed director of surgery [1].

The German Thorotrast Study

The German Thorotrast Study was started in 1968. Names and addresses of more than 5000 patients who received angiography with Thorotrast - 70% for cerebral angiography - were obtained from hospital records in the Federal Republic of Germany. The control group was selected from patients who were treated at the same time in the same hospital, but failed to receive Thorotrast. Patients have been divided in two subgroups: (1) the group of Thorotrast patients who were located and examined and are invited for reexamination every 2 years and (2) the group of nonexamined patients, whose cause of death was established from medical records [5, 6].

Patients who died within the first 3 years after Thorotrast injection or hospitalization in controls were excluded from the study. Other patients, especially from the control group, did not reply to the letters of enquiry. A large number of patients could not be traced as a result of the general circumstances of World War II (Table 3).

Table 4. Final fate of the patients

Diagnosis	Thorotrast (n=1964 of 2334)	Control (n=1409 of 1912)
Liver cancer	347 (18)	2 (0.14)
Cancer of extrahepatic bile ducts	14 (0.7)	6 (0.4)
Liver cirrhosis	292 (15)	42 (3)
Myeloproliferative disease	35 (1.8)	3 (0.2)
Chronic lymphatic leukemia	3 (0.15)	2 (0.14)
Bone marrow failure	20 (1.0)	1 (0.07)

( ) = percentage related to n (deceased, examined, and nonexamined patients, survival time > 3 years)

Results

Some important causes of death in the groups of examined and nonexamined patients are listed in Table 4.

The most important observation is the extremely high number of cases of liver cancer in the Thorotrast group. Furthermore, liver cirrhosis occurred five times as often in the Thorotrast group as in the controls. There was a clear excess rate with a factor of 10 in the group of myeloproliferative diseases, mostly classified as acute myeloid leukemia. However, chronic lymphatic leukemia occurred in both populations equally often. The incidence of bone marrow failure (aplastic anemia, agranulocytosis, and fatal thrombocytopenia) was also about ten times higher than in the control group.

Attention is focused on the problem of Thorotrast-induced liver tumors. The complete results of the study were presented by van Kaick et al. [7].

The shortest latency period for liver tumor development was 16 years (Fig. 1). After this time the liver tumor incidence increases rapidly. In comparison leukemias appeared after only 5 years following injection and continued to increase slowly.

The mean age at which Thorotrast was given to those patients who developed liver tumors was 29 years, while other Thorotrast carriers were 36 years old at the time of injection of the contrast material. An explanation of this phenomenon could be that the younger patients had a longer exposure time and therefore had a greater opportunity of developing liver cancer. This is probable in view of the increasing frequency of liver tumors after 20 years of exposure.

Sixty-five percent of the liver tumors were classified as hepatocellular or cholangiocellular carcinomas, and 35% of the tumors as hemangiosarcomas. Pathologists also described four patients with simultaneous occurrence of sarcoma and carcinoma in the liver.

Cirrhosis was present in 30% of the liver tumor patients and in less than 10% of the nontumor patients. That means that the incidence of liver cirrhosis was found to be three times greater in the liver cancer group than in the other Thorotrast patients.

There was a statistically significant higher frequency of liver tumors in male patients than in female patients. This could be sex dependent since there was no difference with respect to age at the time of injection, age at death, mean amount of Thorotrast injected, or the latency period of the tumors.

An important task of the study was the calculation of dose-effect relationships. Exact information on the injected volume of Thorotrast was obtained with whole body countermeasurements by analysis of the X-ray plain films. Accordingly, the calculation of the dose-effect relationship was only obtained in the group of examined patients.

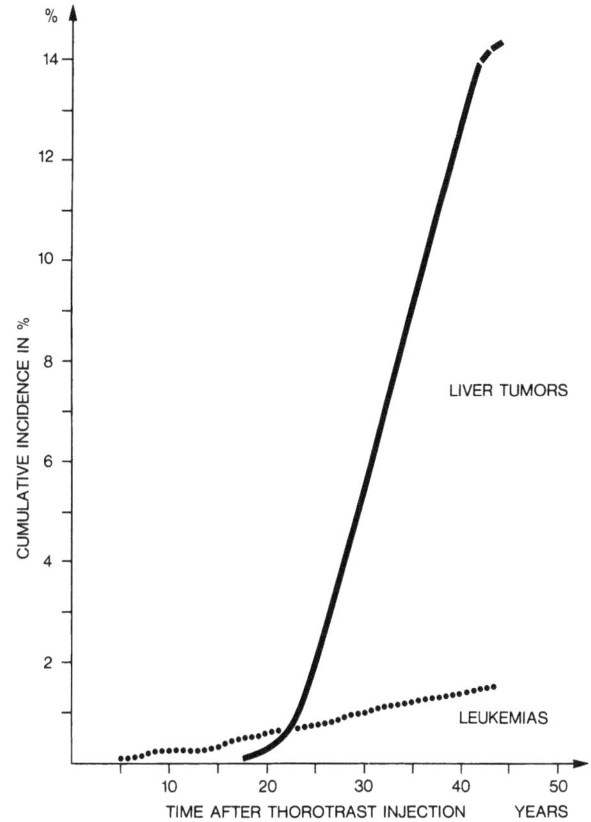

Fig. 1. Cumulative incidence of primary liver tumors and leukemias of German Thorotrast Study patients (examined and non-examined group, $n = 2334$)

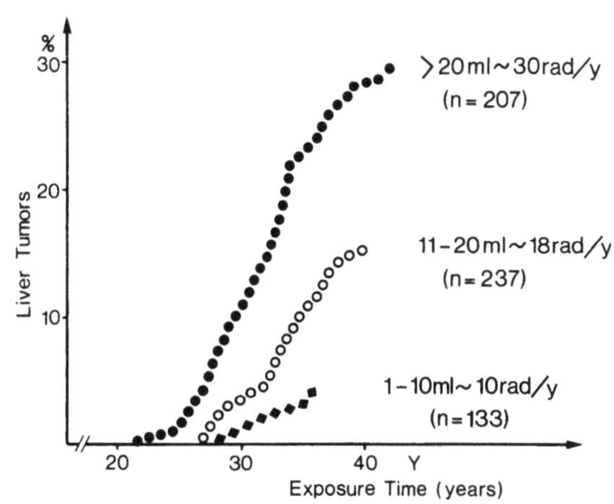

Fig. 2. Cumulative incidence of liver tumors of different dose rate groups (examined patients)

The Thorotrast patients were divided into three subgroups according to the measured radioactivity and the mean dose rate to the liver. The cumulative incidence of liver tumors of each group is presented (Fig. 2). Note that the different tumor incidence expressed as steepness of the curves depends on the dose rate to the liver. It is quite evident that there is a dose-effect relationship.

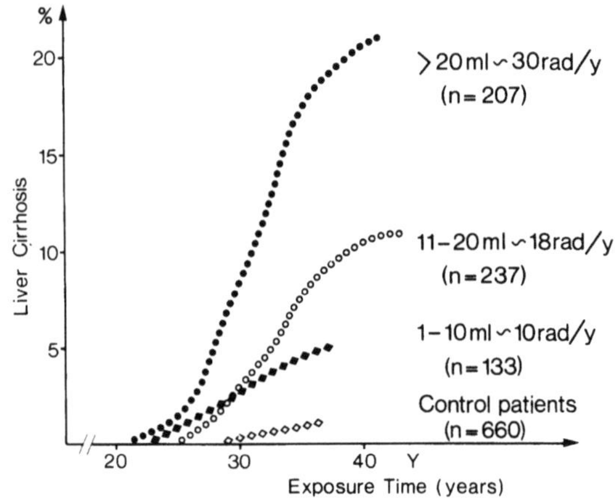

Fig. 3. Cumulative incidence of liver cirrhosis of different dose rate groups (examined patients)

Figure 3 shows that there is also a good correlation between dose rate of the liver and cirrhosis incidence in the Thorotrast patients. The cirrhosis incidence of the control group is presented for comparison.

Calculations of a dose-effect relationship in Thorotrast patients cannot be made without considering a concomitant nonradiation effect. We therefore carried out experiments on 1920 Wistar rats. Twenty groups, each containing 96 animals, were intravascularly injected different volumes and dosages of Thorotrast, enriched with various amounts of thorium-232. The total alpha-energy emission rate varied from 1 to 50. The results reported by Wesch et al. [8] demonstrated a linear correlation between the dose rate and the number of primary hepatic and splenic tumors (Fig. 4).

To evaluate the foreign body effect, the number of particles was also varied by a factor of 50 (Fig. 5). This failed to influence the number of tumors as long as the dose rate was kept constant. However, groups injected with larger numbers of particles had tumors appear earlier than groups of the same dose rate but having fewer Thorotrast particles. This experiment demonstrated that the tumor incidence depends primarily on the dose rate, while the foreign body effect may influence the appearance time of the tumors.

Epidemiological studies have demonstrated a close correlation between the incidence of hepatocellular carcinoma and the hepatitis-B virus (HBV). The hepatitis-B virus surface antigen marker for chronic HBV infection is found with a significantly higher frequency in patients with hepatocellular carcinoma than in tumor-negative controls. A high frequency of integration of viral DNA into the cellular genome of hepatomas has been found. Roggendorf et al. sought to determine whether Thorotrast patients with liver tumors might have a higher incidence of chronic HBV infection compared with Thorotrast patients without tumors or with controls [3]. The results of the serological study indicate that chronic HBV infections fail to contribute to the development of liver tumors in Thorotrast carriers.

Comparing radiation and chemical induction of liver tumors, Spirtas pooled data of patients with vinyl chloride- and Thorotrast-induced angiosarcomas of the liver. The minimal latent periods were shorter for vinyl chloride tumor induction than for Thorotrast [4]. This is in agreement with animal experimental data, suggesting that radiation-induced tumors have longer latency periods than chemically induced malignancies.

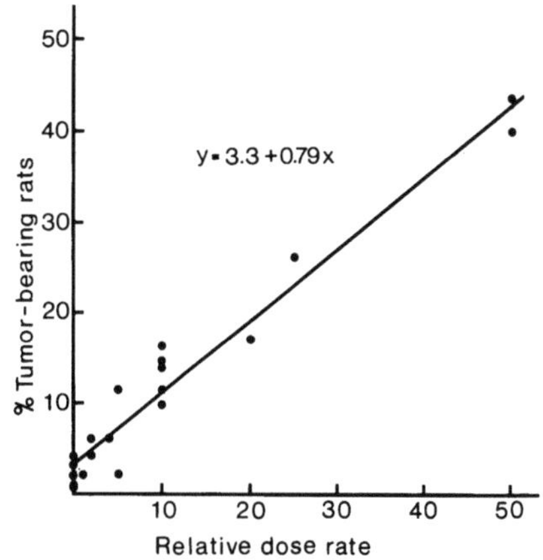

Fig. 4. Percentage of experimental animals with primary liver and spleen tumors as a function of relative dose rate

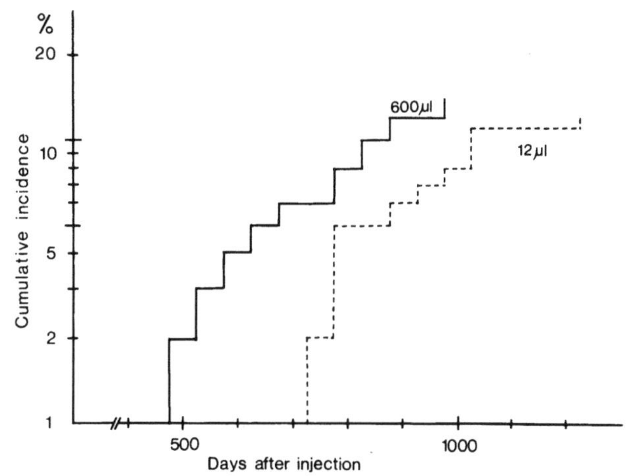

Fig. 5. Cumulative incidence of primary liver or spleen tumors in experimental animals at a constant relative dose rate of 10, as a function of the volume injected or number of particles, respectively

Concluding Remarks

The extremely high incidence of liver tumors in Thorotrast patients gives rise to severe clinical problems. We made available modern diagnostic methods to the patients to aid in the early detection of liver tumors. This was possible in 15 patients in recent years due to the use of computed tomography and ultrasonography (Fig. 6 a, b).

Acknowledgment. The authors are indebted to Mrs. R. Strulik and Mr. D. Millenet for their assistance in the follow-up of the patients. This research has been supported by the Federal Ministries of Research and Technology and of the Interior (FRG) and by the Commission of the European Communities (Directorate General of Science, Research and Development).

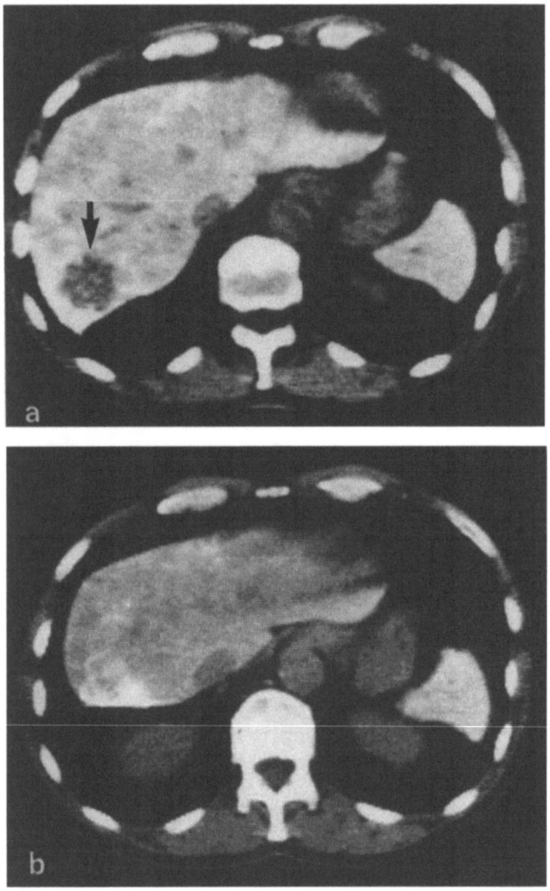

Fig. 6. **a** Computed tomography picture of a 3.5-cm cholangiocellular carcinoma in the right lobe of the liver *(arrow)*. **b** Status 1 year after surgical removal of the tumor

References

1. Bauer KH (1943) Thorotrast und Krebsgefahr. Chirurg 15: 204-207
2. Kaul A, Noffz W (1978) Tissue dose in Thorotrast patients. Health Phys 35: 113-121
3. Roggendorf M, van Kaick G (1985) Epidemiological studies on hepatitis B markers in Thorotrast patients (to be published)
4. Spirtas R, Beebe G, Baxter P, Dacey E, Faber M, Falk H, van Kaick G, Stafford J (1983) Angiosarcoma as a model for comparative carcinogenesis. (Letter to the editor). Lancet II: 456
5. van Kaick G, Lorenz D, Muth H, Kaul A (1978) Malignancies in German Thorotrast patients and estimated tissue dose. Health Phys 35: 127-136
6. van Kaick, G, Muth H, Kaul A, Immich H, Liebermann D, Lorenz D, Lorenz WJ, Lührs H, Scheer KE, Wagner G, Wegener K, Wesch H (1983) Recent Results of the German Thorotrast Study - epidemiological results and dose effect relationships in Thorotrast patients. Health Phys 44: 299-306
7. van Kaick G, Muth H, Kaul A, Immich H, Liebermann D, Lorenz D, Lorenz WJ, Lührs H, Scheer KE, Wagner G, Wegener K, Wesch H (1984) Results of the German Thorotrast Study. In: Boice JD, Fraumeni JF Jr. (ed) Radiation carcinogenesis: epidemiology and biological significance. Raven, New York, pp 253-262
8. Wesch H, Riedel W, Wegener K, Kaul A, Immich H, Hasenöhrl K, Muth H, van Kaick G (1983) Recent Results of the German Thorotrast Study - statistical evaluation of animal experiments with regard to the nonradiation effect in human Thorotrastosis. Health Phys 44: 317-321

Mechanisms of Metastatic Spread to Liver

V. Schirrmacher

Abteilung zelluläre Immunologie, Institut für Immunologie und Genetik,
Deutsches Krebsforschungszentrum, Im Neuenheimer Feld 280, 6900 Heidelberg, FRG

The ability of malignant cells to disseminate from a locally growing tumor mass to visceral organs such as lung or liver to form there secondary lesions (metastases) is known to be the most life threatening aspect of cancer. In spite of much effort devoted to metastasis research, particularly in recent years, we still do not know why tumors metastasize and how they do it. Differences between metastatic and nonmetastatic tumor cell lines are beginning to emerge, however, and in the cascade theory the complex overall process of metastasis formation has been subdivided into sequential steps.

Since this volume is devoted to liver cancer, in this contribution I would like to focus on liver metastases and to ask questions concerned with basic mechanisms. I shall subdivide the discussion into the following parts:

1. Anatomical factors
2. Tumor cell properties (the "seed")
3. Specific cell interactions
4. Liver-determined modulation of tumor growth (liver as proper "soil")
5. Liver as a tumor-cell-killing organ

Anatomical Factors

The locations of most initial metastases, at least of cancers with moderate metastatic potential, appear to be determined simply by regional anatomy [7]. Cancer cells frequently travel from the primary lesion to regional nodes and from nodes to veins via lymphaticovenous communications. Colorectal carcinomas for instance tend to metastasize via the mesenteric lymphatics and portal venous system into the liver as the initial resting place. From the liver these tumors can metastasize to the lungs via the inferior vena cava, the right ventricle, and the pulmonary artery. Although anatomical and hemodynamic factors appear to be able to explain some of the metastatic patterns seen, they do not provide a reasonable explanation for others.

Tumor Cell Properties (the "Seed")

It has been shown that only 1% or less of the millions of tumor cells which may escape from the primary tumor into the circulation survive to become viable metastases, while the majority of cells die [13]. The primary tumor must therefore reach a critical population size and/or growth rate to deliver sufficient cells into the circulation in order to succeed in homing into internal organs. The high rate of cell death in the circulation has been suggested to be due to mechanical shear forces, loss of attachment substrate, or destruction by host defense mechanisms. The few cells which eventually survive may either represent a random fraction of the whole population or a specialized subpopulation thereof. Many experimental data suggest the latter, namely, that survival in the circulation and ability to metastasize are dependent upon properties unique to the tumor cells (for reviews see [9, 16]). In some tumor systems no selection of high metastatic subpopulations was seen [10], however, and therefore random processes are not excluded [33].

A systematic analysis of the colonization potential of spontaneous mouse mammary tumors inoculated via different routes revealed that each tumor line had its intrinsic colonization potential [29]. The expression of this, however, was influenced by the microenvironment of an organ, for instance, its circulatory anatomy. The degree and sites of colonization were thus the results of interactions between tumor- and organ-specific factors.

Organ Site Predilection and Specific Adhesive Cell Interactions

The selective involvement of certain organs in certain types of cancer has long been recognized and several theories have been proposed as explanation, for instance, the "seed and soil" hypothesis [19], the "mechanistic theory" [7], and the "theory of specific cell interactions" [11, 8]. A theoretical analysis was performed by Weiss [31], who suggested that the phenomenon of organ preference is due to the ability of tumor cells to discriminate between various vascular beds during their travel in the circulation. Evidence for specific aggregation of organ-selected tumor lines with cell suspensions of the target organ, be they lung, liver, or ovary, has been presented [17], but it could not be established which cells the tumor cells were interacting with.

Dingemans et al. [6] performed a detailed ultrastructural analysis of the mode of invasion of mouse liver tissue by different types of tumor cells, based on serial sections. One of their conclusions was that the tumor cells migrated through, rather than between, the sinusoidal endothelial cells. The lymphosarcoma cells studied initiated their invasion by extending large numbers of thin processes, many of which completely traversed the endothelium while others merely indented its surface. Migration probably came about by retraction of the endothelial cells so that the invading cells came gradually into contact with the neighbouring hepatocytes. After the migration, the invading cells deeply invaginated the adjacent hepatocytes but without becoming fully intracellular.

The interactions of liver-metastasizing tumor cells with hepatocytes have been analyzed in vitro using either isolated single cells [23] or hepatocyte monolayer cultures [21]. In the latter system, different types of antisera raised against either liver or tumor tissue were used to inhibit the respective tumor cell adhesion. It was suggested from these studies that different types of hepatocyte molecules were involved in tumor cell adhesion, one type exposed on the hepatocyte surface, the other at the contiguous face leading to infiltration by the tumor cells [14].

We recently reported on a mouse hepatocyte carbohydrate-specific receptor and its interaction with liver-metastasizing tumor cells [23]. Spontaneous high-metastatic variants (ESb) of the DBA/2 mouse lymphoma L5178Y which show heavy liver involvement were found to form rosettes in vitro with isolated autologous hepatocytes, while low-metastatic sublines of the same tumor (Eb) did not. An analysis of the molecules involved in the hepatocyte-tumor cell interaction was performed by affinity adsorption and sodium dodecyl sulfate (SDS) polyacrylamide gel electrophoresis of ^{125}I-labeled membrane components from either the hepatocytes or the tumor cells. The hepatocytes were found to bind ESb tumor cells through lectin-like hepatic-binding proteins (HBP) with molecular weights of 52, 56, and 110 kd and specificity for D-galactosyl and *N*-acetyl-D-galactosaminyl residues [4]. Thompson-Friedenreich (T) antigen, which expresses immunodominant Gal-β 1-3 GalNac determinants, was found to be present on our tumor cells [28] and, in soluble form, this T-antigen was a powerful inhibitor of the spontaneous hepatocyte rosettes [27].

More than ten different cell surface glycoproteins of ESb tumor cells and none of the Eb-type tumor cells served as ligands in the hepatocyte interaction. The low-metastatic subline Eb formed hepatocyte rosettes only after neuraminidase pretreatment, indicating that lectin-binding carbohydrate structures existed in a cryptic form masked on these cells by sialic acid. Although lectin-carbohydrate interactions have been found to play a crucial role in many intercellular recognition processes, this apparently is the first molecular description of such an interaction between organ-derived normal parenchymal cells and tumor cells. The possible relevance of such an interaction for cancer metastasis is suggested by the finding that spleen-selected ESb sublines differed from liver-selected ones in their organotropism as well as in their ability to form hepatocyte rosettes [4].

From these and other studies [26] it appears that tumor cell recognition via organ-specific receptors could be an important factor in the organotropism of certain cancers. Since lectin-like receptors have been detected not only on organ-derived cells but also on tumor cell surfaces [20], it is possible that the homing of metastatic cells to certain organs could involve lectin-carbohydrate interactions in both directions.

It was apparent from our studies that expression of D-galactosyl and *N*-acetyl-D-galactosaminyl residues was essential for hepatocyte-tumor cell binding. Such residues were blocked on Eb cells by sialic acid. Although the low and high metastatic tumor lines Eb and ESb expressed similar amounts of neuraminidase releasable sialic acid, the site-specific positioning of sialic acid at the cell surface was different as shown by lectin-binding studies [1]. We have thus put forward the hypothesis that via changes in positioning sialic acid could play an important role in metastasis, because it could lead to either blocking or unblocking of cellular adhesion sites or antigenic determinants [24].

It is thus possible that cell surface carbohydrate changes which may occur randomly in a heterogeneous tumor cell population can give rise to variants which are selected out during metastasis because of their better organ-homing properties.

Although in the Eb/ESb tumor system the selective adhesion observed was with hepatocytes, we do not suggest that hepatocytes are the only cells in the liver for selective adhesion. There is some evidence that liver endothelial cells as well as Kupffer cells also possess lectin-like receptors ([25]; H. Kolb, personal communication) which could also play a role in liver metastases. Differential binding of various high and low metastatic tumor lines to liver endothelial cells has indeed been recently reported [5, 22].

It can thus be assumed that the organotropic distribution of metastases might be due to or influenced by the recognition via organ-characteristic lectin receptors of tumor cell exposed cryptic carbohydrate structures as suggested by Uhlenbruck [30]. Since the first discovery of β-galactosyl-specific hepatocyte lectins by Ashwell and his group [2], several other lectin receptors of the liver have been characterized. They have specificities, respectively, for *N*-acetylglucosamine, fucose, and phosphomannose (for review see [2]).

It is interesting in this context that a study involving more than 1500 cancer patients revealed that those with damaged liver function due to cirrhosis had a greatly reduced incidence in liver metastases (G. Uhlenbruck, personal communication). It remains to be seen, of course, whether this phenomenon is due to a malfunction of lectin-like hepatocyte receptors.

Liver-Determined Modulation of Tumor Growth

Once tumor cells have entered a target organ it is by no means decided that they will grow into metastases. The organ microenvironment could exert modulatory effects by inhibition or stimulation of tumor growth. Certain tissues may release factors that either inhibit or stimulate tumor cell proliferation [12]. Cell-cell or cell-matrix contacts could also play an important role. The asialoglycoprotein receptor of hepatocytes, for instance, has been shown to have mitogenic properties [18]. It may thus not only play a role in the trapping of circulating cancer cells but may also stimulate their growth.

Passage of B16 melanoma cells through liver vasculature has been reported to have a traumatic effect on the cells so that their implantation capacity for a second organ (i.e., the lung) is greatly reduced [34]. Similarly, analysis of Walker-256 cancer cell traffic from lungs to liver showed that the failure of tumors to develop in the liver was not due to inherent unsuitability of liver as "soil," but appeared due to the cancer cells having been processed while in the pulmonary circulation so that the majority arrived in the liver either moribund or dead [32]. As possible mechanisms for this phenomenon have been suggested mechanical trauma, attack by NK-cells, or damage subsequent to the cellular and humoral inflammatory responses to interactions of the cancer cells with vascular endothelium.

Tumor Defense Mechanisms of the Liver

The liver is well equipped with Kupffer cells having a scavenger function. Furthermore, this organ receives with the blood circulatory cells of the host defense system and should therefore be potentially capable of destroying tumor cells. Such a destruction could indeed be documented with some tumor cells both in vivo and in vitro [3, 5]. In one such study high metastatic ESb variant cells were found to be more resistant to liver destruction after mesenteric vein inoculation than the low metastatic parental line Eb. In vitro studies suggested that this effect was mostly due to natural killer (NK) activity of nonparenchymal cells isolated from the liver [3].

It is obvious from this overview that liver metastasis formation depends on and is influenced at various steps by intimate tumor-host interactions. The outcome of such tumor-host interactions seems to depend on intrinsic properties of the tumor cells themselves as well as on the responsiveness of the host.

References

1. Altevogt P, Fogel M, Cheingsong-Popov R, Dennis J, Robinson P, Schirrmacher V (1983) Different patterns of lectin binding and cell surface sialylation detected on related high- and low-metastatic tumor lines. Cancer Res 43: 5138–5144
2. Ashwell G, Harford J (1982) Carbohydrate-specific receptors of the liver. Ann Rev Biochem 51: 531–554
3. Burkart V, Malter M, Süss R, Friedrich EA (1984) Liver as a tumor cell killing organ. Immun Commun 13: 77–81
4. Cheingsong-Popov R, Robinson P, Altevogt P, Schirrmacher V (1983) A mouse hepatocyte carbohydrate-specific receptor and its interaction with liver-metastasizing tumor cells. Int J Cancer 32: 359–366

5. Cohen SA, Salazar D, Nolan JP (1982) Natural cytotoxicity of isolated rat liver cells. J Immunol 129: 495-501
6. Dingemans KP, Roos E, van den Bergh Weerman MA, van de Pavert IV (1978) Invasion of liver tissue by tumor cells and leukocytes: comparative ultrastructure. J Natl Cancer Inst 60: 583-598
7. Ewing J (1928) Neoplastic diseases, 3rd edn. Saunders, Philadelphia
8. Fidler IJ, Nicolson GL (1977) Fate of recirculating B16 melanoma metastatic variant cells in parabiotic syngeneic recipients: brief communication. J Natl Cancer Inst 58: 1867-1872
9. Fidler IJ, Gersten DM, Hart IR (1978) The biology of cancer invasion and metastasis. Adv Cancer Res 28: 149-250
10. Giavazzi R, Allessandri G, Spreafico F, Garattini S, Mantovani A (1980) Metastasizing capacity of tumour cells from spontaneous metastases of transplanted murine tumours. Br J Cancer 42: 462-472
11. Hagmar B (1972) Cell surface charge and metastasis formation. Acta Pathol Microbiol Scand [A] Pathol 80: 357-366
12. Klein K, Coetzee ML, Madhav R, Ove P (1979) Inhibition of tritiated thymidine incorporation in cultured cells by rat kidney extract. J Natl Cancer Inst 62: 1557-1564
13. Liotta LA, Kleinerman J, Saidel GM (1974) Quantitative relationships of intravascular tumor cells, tumor vessels, and pulmonary metastases following tumor implanation. Cancer Res 34: 997-1004
14. Middelkoop OP, Roos E, van de Pavert IV (1982) Infiltration of lymphosarcoma cells into hepatocyte cultures: inhibition by univalent antibodies against liver plasma membranes and lymphosarcoma cells. J Cell Sci 56: 461-470
15. Nicolson G (1982a) Organ specificity of blood-borne tumour metastasis determined by cell adhesion? Biochim Biophys Acta 695: 113-176
16. Nicolson GL (1982b) Cell surface properties of metastatic tumor cells. In: Liotta LA, Hart JR (eds) Tumor invasion and metastasis. Nijhoff, The Hague, pp 57-79
17. Nicolson GL, Winkelhake JL (1975) Cancer metastasis. Organ colonization and the cell-surface properties of malignant cells. Nature 255: 230-232
18. Novogrodsky A, Ashwell G (1977) Lymphocyte mitogenesis induced by a mammalian liver protein that specifically binds desialylated aglycoproteins. Proc Natl Acad Sci USA 74: 676-678
19. Paget S (1889) The distribution of secondary growth in cancer of the breast. Lancet 1: 571-573
20. Raz A, Lotan R (1981) Lectin-like activities associated with human and murine neoplastic cells. Cancer Res 41: 3642-3647
21. Roos E, van de Pavert IV (1982) Effect of tubulin-binding agents on the infiltration of tumour cells into primary hepatocyte cultures. J Cell Sci 55: 233-245
22. Roos E, Tulp A, Middelkoop OP, van de Pavert IV (1984) Interactions between lymphoid tumor cells and isolated liver endothelial cells. J Natl Cancer Inst 72: 1173-1180
23. Schirrmacher V, Cheingsong-Popov R, Arnheiter H (1980) Hepatocyte-tumor cell interaction in vitro. I. Conditions for rosette formation and inhibition by anti H-2 antibody. J Exp Med 151: 984-989
24. Schirrmacher V, Altevogt P, Fogel M, Dennis J, Waller CA, Barz D, Schwartz R, Cheingsong-Popov R, Springer GF, Robinson PJ, Nebe T, Brossmer R, Vlodavsky I, Paweletz N, Zimmermann H-P, Uhlenbruck G (1982) Importance of cell surface carbohydrates in cancer cell adhesion, invasion and metastasis. Does sialic acid direct metastatic behavior? Inv Met 2: 313-360
25. Schlepper-Schäfer J, Friedrich E, Kolb H (1981) Galactosyl specific receptor on liver cells: binding site for tumor cells. Eur J Cell Biol 25: 95-102
26. Shearman PJ, Gallatin WM, Longenecker BM (1980) Detection of a cell-surface antigen correlated with organ-specific metastasis. Nature 286: 267-269
27. Springer GF, Cheingsong-Popov R, Schirrmacher V, Desai PR, Tegtmeyer H (1983) Proposed molecular basis of murine tumor cell-hepatocyte interaction. J Biol Chem 258: 5702-5706
28. Springer GF, Desai PR, Tegtmeyer H, Schirrmacher V, Cheingsong-Popov R (1983) Murine lymphoma cells possess blood group Tn-, T-, N-, M- and S-active substances. Naturwissenschaften 70 (2): 98

29. Tarin D, Price JE (1981) Influence of microenvironment and vascular anatomy on "metastatic" colonization potential of mammary tumors. Cancer Res 41: 3604-3609
30. Uhlenbruck G (1981) The Thomson-Friedenreich (TF) receptor: an old history with new mystery. Immunol Commun 10: 251-264
31. Weiss L (1975) In: Rubin P (ed) Current concepts in cancer. Pergamon, New York, pp 97-99
32. Weiss L (1980) Cancer cell traffic from the lungs to the liver: an example of metastatic inefficiency. Int J Cancer 25: 385-392
33. Weiss L (1983) Random and nonrandom processes in metastasis, and metastatic inefficiency. Inv Met 3: 193-207
34. Weiss L, Ward PM, Holmes JC (1983) Liver-to-lung traffic of cancer cells. Int J Cancer 32: 79-83

Prevention of Liver Metastases of Colorectal Carcinoma

U. Metzger

Chirurgische Klinik, Universitätsspital, 8091 Zürich, Switzerland

Introduction

Liver metastases are present on initial diagnosis of large-bowel cancer in 25%-30% of patients [2]. After curative resection of colorectal primary tumors, the liver again is the most frequent site of relapse in 40%-50% [4, 18]. Once liver metastases have developed, the prognosis is poor, with an expected median survival time of 6-9 months [2, 14], the extent of the tumor being the most important prognostic factor [22]. A great deal of work has been done to determine the factors that influence development of liver metastases. There is evidence that tumor cells embolize into the portal venous system via the invaded mesenteric veins and enter the liver. In 1957, Dukes [7] found evidence of venous spread in 17% of operative rectal cancer specimens. Fisher and Turnbull [8] discovered tumor cells in the mesenteric venous blood of 32% of colorectal carcinoma patients at surgery. They suggested that manipulation of the tumor may force malignant cells into the circulation and they initiated the so-called "no touch-isolation" technique. This led to a significant reduction of the incidence of liver metastases at 2 years and an increased survival at 5 years, compared with historical controls [21]. In a recently closed prospective randomized trial on 231 patients, Wiggers et al. [23] found 19 recurrences and 8 tumor-related deaths in the conventionally resected group. Of the recurrences, 12 were liver metastases, 6 were recurrences elsewhere, and 1 was a new colon carcinoma. In the no-touch isolation group 13 recurrences and 4 tumor-related deaths were observed. Seven recurrences were liver metastases; 6 were recurrences elsewhere. The average time of discovering liver metastases was 8 months (range 6-18 months) in the conventional group and 15 months (range 6-28 months) in the no-touch group. The recurrence rate in this trial is relatively low and the follow-up too short for definitive conclusions.

However, not all circulating cancer cells give rise to metastases. Several reports have shown that patients with malignant cells in the venous blood fare not worse than those without [15, 17].

Metachronous liver metastases may originate from microscopic deposits not visible at surgery for the primary tumor. These micrometastases are the most important target for adjuvant systemic therapy [5, 16]. Since systemic chemotherapy is of limited value in large-bowel cancer [6, 9, 10, 13], numerous studies have approached the issue of hepatic artery or portal venous infusion of fluorinated pyrimidines. Almersjö et al. [1] have shown the safety of portal venous infusion in man. They found that during continuous portal infusion of 15 mg 5-FU/kg for 24 h, systemic serum concentrations were generally below

Recent Results in Cancer Research. Vol 100

100 μg/ml and no side effects were noticed. It is generally accepted that adjuvant therapy should be started as soon as possible after surgery when the tumor burden is minimal [3, 16]. Morales et al. [12] advocated intraportal injection of cytotoxic agents at the time of surgery for colorectal cancer in an attempt to prevent liver metastases by diminishing the number of circulating tumor cells.

In 1979, Taylor et al. [19] reported on a randomized study evaluating adjuvant cytotoxic liver perfusion for colorectal cancer. After a mean follow-up of 26–28 months, 23 patients died in the control group and 7 patients in the perfusion group. In the control group, five had multiple liver metastases alone, eight had generalized metastases as well as liver metastases, and seven had local recurrence only. One patient in the perfusion group had liver metastases alone, one had liver metastases as well as metastases elsewhere, and four had local recurrence. The incidence of liver metastases in the two groups (13 control, 2 perfusion) was statistically significantly different. After a median follow-up of 4 years, 53 patients died with recurrent disease in the control group and 25 patients in the perfusion group. In the control group, 22 patients developed liver metastases and in the perfusion group 5 developed liver deposits as the predominant site of recurrence. The patients in the perfusion group appeared to have an improved overall survival. However, when individual groups are analyzed, only patients with Dukes B colon tumors have a significant improvement in overall survival [20]. In 1981, thc Swiss Group for Clinical Cancer Research (SAKK) initiated a similar prospective randomized study of adjuvant portal liver infusion to evaluate Taylor's data in a multicenter trial [11].

Patients and Methods

Two hundred and forty-seven patients were admitted to the trial from July 1981 to February 1984 with primary adenocarcinoma of either the colon or rectum. By preoperative randomization the patients were assigned to no adjuvant treatment or to liver infusion through the portal vein with 5-fluorouracil (5-FU) (500 mg/m^2 daily × 7, continuous infusion during the first seven postoperative days) and mitomycin C (10 mg/m^2, 24 h postoperatively as a 2-h infusion). A portal venous catheter was placed through any side branch of the mesenteric venous system during laparotomy. All patients had normal blood counts and normal renal/liver function tests before surgery. Preoperative carcinoembryonic antigen (CEA) and liver scan or ultrasound scanning was carried out. Thirty-eight patients were randomized but were subsequently excluded from the study because of the discovery of unexpected liver metastases at the operation in 15, incomplete resection in 9, treatment refusal in 5, and various reasons in 14 patients. It is too early for a valid evaluation in 31 patients, leaving a total of 173 patients (85 infusions and 88 controls) for analysis of peri- and postoperative morbidity, mortality, and initial follow-up.

Standard surgical techniques of resection were adhered to, the actual procedure to be performed being left to the discretion of the surgeon. Postoperative blood counts and liver function tests were performed every other day until day 10, then on days 14, 28, and 42. A portal venogram was performed during the operation to ensure that the catheter was well positioned and was equally infusing both main portal branches. If not, the catheter was manipulated under the image intensifier until adequate infusion was achieved. At day 7, after a final angiography, the catheter was pulled out percutaneously.

The operative specimens were histologically examined and classified according to Duke's (Astler-Coller modification) categorization. The degree of differentiation was also noted. All patients were followed at 3-monthly intervals for 1 year, then at 6-monthly intervals by the participating institutions. Again, blood counts, liver/renal function tests, liver scan or liver ultrasound, chest X-rays, and colonoscopic examination were carried out according to the protocol.

Results

Age and Sex

The mean age of the patients in the control group was 62.6 (36–75) years and that of the patients in the infusion group was 60.6 (31–75) years. There were 53 males in the control group and 49 in the infusion group.

Site and Stage

The site and stage of each tumor are shown in Table 1. There are no statistically significant differences between the Duke's categorization and the degree of differentiation of the tumors in each group.

Table 1. Site, stage, and degree of differentiation (SAKK 40/81)

Stage	Control			Infusion		
	A	B	C	A	B	C
Right colon	–	9	9	–	11	8
Transverse colon	–	2	3	–	2	2
Left colon	2	11	14	3	11	12
Rectum	2	22	14	2	18	16
Total	4	44	40	5	42	38
Degree of differentiation						
Well		36			30	
Moderately		50			54	
Poorly		2			1	

Table 2. Postoperative morbidity

SAKK 40/81	Control ($n=88$)	Infusion ($n=85$)
Wound infection	6	9
Anastomotic leakage	4	4
Bowel obstruction	2	3
Hemorrhage	2	3
Thrombosis/embolism	2	1
Mean hospital stay (days)	18.5 ± 10.1	22.9 ± 16.7

Postoperative Morbidity

Twenty out of 85 (24%) in the infusion group and 16 out of 88 (18%) patients in the control group experienced a moderate or more severe complication using the WHO code. The complications are listed in Table 2. The mean postoperative hospital stay was 22.9 ± 16.7 days in the infusion group and 18.5 ± 10.1 days in the control group. These differences were not statistically significant.

Postoperative Mortality

In the immediate 30-day postoperative period, there were four deaths, three in the control and one in the infusion group. One patient died of irreversible cardiac arrest during surgery; the others died of therapy-resistant gram-negative septicemia on day 15, 17, and 21. It was considered that the cytotoxic infusion was a contributory factor in one of these patients. This 72-year-old diabetic male had a persistent purulent secretion following right hemicolectomy. On the 11th postoperative day he developed necrotizing fasciitis of the abdominal wall with bronchopneumonia and irreversible gram-negative septicemia. At this time, he had marked leukopenia of $2200/mm^3$.

Hematologic Toxicity

Six patients developed transient leukopenia of below $3000/mm^3$ during infusion. The white cell count was statistically significantly lower at day 7 and 10 in the infusion group compared with the control group. With one exception (see above) the values returned toward normal upon completion of hospitalization. There were only two thrombocytopenias of 56000 and $71000/mm^3$ in the infusion group. Bilirubin and other liver function tests (SGOT, SGPT, alkaline phosphatase) were not significantly influenced by the infusion treatment.

Follow-up Data

Twenty-two recurrences have been observed so far in a median follow-up period of 18 months. There were 14 recurrences in the control group, 8 in the infusion group, 6 and 4 local failures respectively, 8 distant failures in the control group, and 4 in the infusion group. Seven patients of the control group had already developed liver metastases, whereas three patients of the infusion group had liver involvement.

There were eight deaths in the control group, five due to recurrence, one to myocardial infarction, one to small-bowel obstruction, and one to suicide, compared with five deaths in the infusion group, one due to myocardial infarction, one to local recurrent cancer, and three to disseminated malignant disease.

Discussion

The primary aim of this study is to confirm the results of Taylor and coworkers [19, 20] and to assess the possible benefit of the 5-FU/mitomycin C combination in portal infusion. The actual method of liver infusion through any side branch of the mesenteric veins according to the surgeon's preference was easy to perform; cannulation proved to be technically impossible in two patients only, which seems to be superior to a 10% failure rate in cannulating the umbilical vein [19]. Using the transabdominal route, there have been no direct catheter-related complications with therapeutic consequences.

Despite a large cumulative dose of 5-FU given during the immediate postoperative period, the systemic side effects were minimal and morbidity of large-bowel surgery was not significantly increased nor was the hospital stay significantly prolonged by the adjuvant treatment.

Interestingly, the overall operative mortality rate of below 2% in this study is considerably lower than that reported by previous multicenter trials. This indicates a possible advance in surgical techniques and pre-/postoperative patient management in this type of elective surgery. Only one patient in the infusion group experienced lethal septic complications. It was thought that cytotoxic infusion contributed to this death of a 72-year-old diabetic male and accordingly patients with insulin-dependent diabetes are no longer included in the study.

During the follow-up period eight patients have died in the control group, compared with five in the infusion group; seven of the control patients have developed multiple liver metastases compared with three patients in the infusion group. Eighteen of the 22 relapsing patients were initially staged as Duke's C lesions, indicating the high risk of early recurrence for this subgroup. There is recent evidence that Duke's B patients are more likely to profit from adjuvant therapy possibly due to lower tumor burden [20].

Prolonged follow-up and continuous patient entry in the study is needed for drawing definitive statistical conclusions.

In summary, our data appear encouraging and tend to support the data of Taylor [20]; they confirm the feasibility of locoregional adjuvant portal chemotherapy in the immediate postoperative period. They also demonstrated that the combination of 5-fluorouracil with mitomycin C does not significantly increase surgical morbidity, mortality, or duration of hospitalization. Further patient entry and prolonged follow-up is needed for definitive conclusions.

References

1. Almersjö O, Brandberg A, Gustavsson B (1975) Concentration of biologically active 5-fluorouracil in general circulation during continuous portal infusion in man. Cancer Lett 1: 113-118
2. Bengmark S, Hafström L (1969) The natural history of primary and secondary malignant tumours of the liver. 1. The prognosis for patients with hepatic metastases from colonic and rectal carcinoma by laparotomy. Cancer 23: 198-202
3. Burchenal JH (1976) Adjuvant therapy - theory, practice, and potential. The James Ewing Lecture. Cancer 37: 46-57
4. Cedermark BJ, Schultz SS, Bakshi S, Parthasarathy KL, Mittelman A, Evans TJ (1977) Value of liver scan in the follow-up study of patients with adenocarcinoma of the colon and rectum. Surg Gynecol Obstet 144: 745-748
5. DeVita VT (1983) The relationship between tumor mass and resistance to chemotherapy. Implications for surgical adjuvant treatment of cancer. The James Ewing Lecture. Cancer 51: 1209-1220
6. Dwight RW, Humphrey WE, Higgins GA, Keehn RJ (1973) FUdR as an adjuvant to surgery in cancer of the large bowel. J Surg Oncol 5: 243-249
7. Dukes CE (1957) Discussion on major surgery in carcinoma of the rectum, with or without colostomy, excluding the anal canal and including the rectosigmoid. Proc R Soc Med 50: 1031-1052

8. Fisher ER, Turnbull RB (1955) The cytological demonstration and significance of tumor cells in the mesenteric venous blood in patients with colorectal cancer. Surg Gynecol Obstet 100: 102-106
9. Higgins GA, Amadeo JH, McElhinney J, McCaughan JJ, Keehn RJ (1984) Efficacy of prolonged intermittent therapy with combined 5-fluorouracil and methyl-CCNU following resection for carcinoma of the large bowel. Cancer 53: 1-8
10. Lawrence W, Terz JJ, Horsley S, Donaldson M, Lovett WL, Brown PW, Ruffner BW, Regelson W (1975) Chemotherapy as an adjuvant to surgery for colorectal cancer. Ann Surg 616-623
11. Metzger U, Aeberhard P, Egeli R, Harder F, Largiader F, Muller W, Pettavel J, Weber W, Cavalli F (1982) Adjuvante portale Leberperfusion beim kolorektalen Karzinom. Helv Chir Acta 49: 175-178
12. Morales F, Bell M, McDonald GD, Cole WH (1957) The prophylactic treatment of cancer at the time of operation. Ann Surg 146: 588-595, 1957
13. Gastrointestinal Tumor Study Group (1984) Adjuvant therapy of colon cancer - results of a prospectively randomized trial. N Engl J Med 310: 737-743
14. Pestana C, Reitemeier RJ, Moertel CG, Judd ES, Dockerty MB (1964) The natural history of carcinoma of the colon and rectum. Am J Surg 108: 826-829
15. Roberts S, Jonasson O, Long L, McGrath R, McGrew EA, Cole WH (1961) Clinical significance of cancer cells in the circulating blood: two- to five-year survivals. Ann Surg 154: 362-371
16. Schabel FM (1975) Concepts for systemic treatment of micrometastases. Cancer 35: 15-24
17. Sellwood RA, Kuper SW, Burn JI, Wallace EN (1965) Circulating cancer cells: the influence of surgical operations. Br J Surg 52: 69-72
18. Swinton NW, Legg MA, Lewis FG (1964) Metastasis of cancer of the rectum and sigmoid flexure. Dis Colon Rectum 7: 273-277
19. Taylor I, Rowling JT, West C (1979) Adjuvant cytotoxic liver perfusion for colorectal cancer. Br J Surg 66: 833-837
20. Taylor I, Mullee MA, Machin D (1984) Adjuvant therapy of colorectal cancer with portal vein cytotoxic perfusion. In: Jones S, Salmon S (eds) Adjuvant therapy of cancer IV, Grune and Stratton, New York, p 481
21. Turnbull RB (1970) Cancer of the colon: 5-10 year survival rates following resection utilizing the isolation technique. Ann R Coll Surg Engl 46: 243-250
22. Wanebo H (1984) A staging system for liver metastases from colorectal cancer. Proc ASCO 3: 143, C-560
23. Wiggers T, Arends JW, Jeekel J, et al. (1983) The no-touch isolation technique in colon cancer. A prospective controlled trial. J Exp Clin Cancer Res 2: 37

Diagnosis and Staging

The Role of the Pathologist in the Clinical Management of Malignant Liver Tumors

P. P. Anthony

Postgraduate Medical School, University of Exeter, Devon, Great Britain

Introduction

A multiplicity of different tumours can arise in the liver, each with its own distinctive pathology but many of these are rarities and useful information about them is scant. In tropical Africa and Southeast Asia, liver cell (hepatocellular) carcinoma is one of the commonest of all malignancies but this tumour is rare in Western countries and is seldom amenable to surgery. Bile duct carcinoma (cholangiocarcinoma) is next in importance. It occurs more or less equally throughout the world except in Southeast Asia, where a high incidence is seen in those infested with liver flukes. All other primary tumours are rare though some, like liver cell adenoma, hemangiosarcoma and tumours occurring in children, are of considerable interest. In Western countries, secondary tumours, particularly those from primary carcinomas of the gastrointestinal tract, breast and lung, are by far the commonest and their presence is no longer regarded as hopeless for the patient.

The etiology, manifestations and morphological appearances of liver tumours have been described in detail over the years [2, 3, 5, 8, 16, 19, 20] and, in this paper, only those pathological aspects are discussed that are especially relevant to clinical management.

To further this aim, a series of questions have been put and answers attempted, within the necessary limitations of our current knowledge. Benign tumours, tumour-like lesions and metastatic tumours are considered alongside primary malignant tumours.

How Much Reliance Can Be Placed on Diagnosis by Needle Biopsy or Aspiration Cytology?

Table 1 tabulates the reliability score for each individual type of tumour. The question asked is really in two parts. First, which tumours are likely to yield an adequate sample for diagnosis and by what means? Second, what are the likely limits of accuracy by a reasonably experienced pathologist? In the scoring, the two have been combined for the sake of simplicity and the evaluation rests partly on established knowledge and partly on what may reasonably be expected to be found if the attempt is made. Many are rare tumours that have been diagnosed only after resection or at autopsy.

As far as *benign tumours* are concerned [12] much help is not likely from the pathologist prior to surgery. *Liver cell adenoma* [18] forms a soft vascular mass from which only fragments are obtained by needle biopsy and these consist of liver tissue little different from normal. Only the total absence of portal tracts and bile ducts gives any clue to the diagno-

Table 1. The reliability of biopsy compared with cytology in the main types of tumour in the liver

Type of tumour	Reliability of diagnosis by	
	Biopsy	Cytology
Benign		
Liver cell adenoma	+	−
Bile duct cystadenoma	−	+
Bile duct papillomatosis	+++	++
Hemangioma	−	−
Granular cell tumour	+++	−
Malignant		
Liver cell carcinoma	+++	+
Bile duct carcinoma	++	++
Bile duct cystadenocarcinoma	−	+
Hepatoblastoma	+++	+
Primary carcinoid tumour	++	−
Hemangiosarcoma	+++	+
Other sarcomas	++	+
Primary lymphoma	+++	+
Tumour-like lesions		
Focal nodular hyperplasia	++	−
Mesenchymal hamartoma	++	−
Peliosis	++	−
Cysts	−	+

For explanations see text

sis. Aspiration cytology yields virtually normal liver cells. *Bile duct cystadenoma* [13] can only be aspirated: a mucoid fluid is obtained which may contain papillary epithelial clumps. *Bile duct papillomatosis* [15] results in the passage of tumour fragments and blood clots down the common bile duct: these should be taken for both histology and cytology and the lumen irrigated to obtain further material. All types of *hemangioma* [10], with the possible exception of infantile hemangio-endothelioma, will yield only blood. Benign connective tissue tumours are small and clinically irrelevant and are found by chance, except *granular cell tumour* of the biliary tract [1]. This tends to project into the lumen and can be biopsied at endoscopy. The histological appearances are unmistakeable.

Liver cell (hepatocellular) carcinoma [2, 3, 5, 19] almost invariably presents late, i.e. it is large when the patient is first seen. This is particularly so in the tropics. In Western countries, sudden and unexpected deterioration in the condition of a cirrhotic patient with pain, weight loss and ascites points to the development of the tumour. Biopsy of a palpable mass is nearly always successful and even a small amount of tissue yields sufficient material for diagnosis. Characteristically, trabecular or plate-like fragments are seen which may be covered, on the outside, by an endothelial lining (Fig. 1). The various histological (trabecular, pseudoglandular, compact) and cytological (hepatic, clear cell, pleomorphic) subtypes are important for histological diagnosis and differentation from other, particularly secondary, tumours but are of no interest for clinical management: the course is the same. However, "good prognosis" types do exist and are discussed below. Conventional special stains, tissue localisation of alpha-fetoprotein, carcinoembryonic antigen,

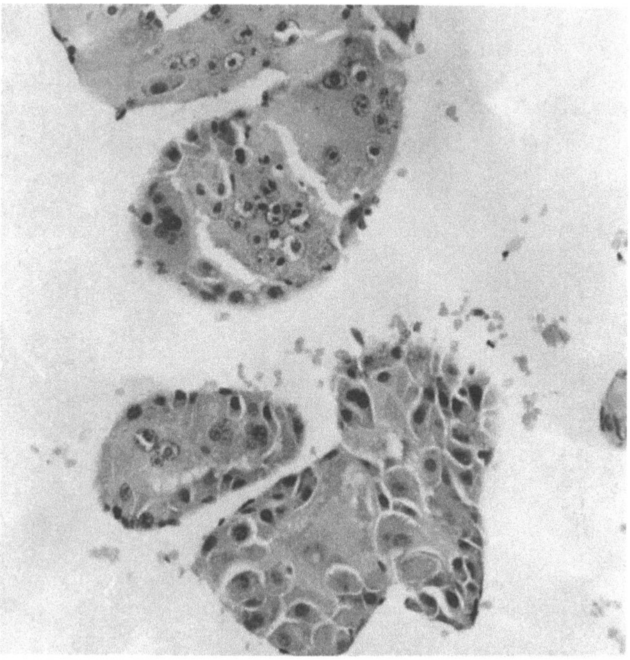

Fig. 1. Characteristic "roll-off" phenomenon seen in small fragments of liver cell carcinoma obtained by needle biopsy. Thick neoplastic liver cell cords show multinucleation and pleomorphism. A flat endothelial lining is barely visible on the surface of the fragments. H&E, ×200

alpha-1-antitrypsin, chorionic gonadotrophin, etc. and electron microscopy may all have to be employed but the diagnosis is simple in the majority. On rare occasions, tumour tissue is obtained for diagnosis from the portal or major hepatic veins or from the lumen of the common bile duct which may all be involved. Aspiration cytology is unreliable for two reasons: one, liver cell carcinoma is often cytologically well differentiated (Fig. 2); two, non-neoplastic, cirrhotic or dysplastic liver cells may appear highly abnormal. Claims have been made to the contrary [21] but features alleged to be pathognomonic, like intracytoplasmic bile, are too infrequently seen or do not necessarily indicate malignancy. As the tumour is rare in Western countries it is wise to refer doubtful or unfamiliar material to an expert.

Bile duct carcinoma [2, 3, 8, 19] is readily recognisable either in a needle biopsy or in a cytological aspirate as an adenocarcinoma. It is quite impossible, however, to be certain that this is a primary as metastatic adenocarcinomas, from pancreas, stomach and colon in particular, look the same. A firm histological diagnosis of a primary adenocarcinoma of intrahepatic bile duct origin can only be made if in situ carcinomatous change is seen in nearby bile ducts (Fig. 3) and this is rare. Neither tumour markers nor electron microscopy are of any further help other than in differentiation from a liver cell carcinoma in cases where a glandular pattern is not obvious. Any amount of proven mucus secretion rules out liver cell carcinoma, however. A small minority of bile duct carcinomas arise near the hilum of the liver giving rise to a characteristic clinical syndrome mimicking primary biliary cirrhosis. A preoperative diagnosis cannot be made and even the interpretation of a biopsy obtained at laparatomy can be quite difficult. *Bile duct cystadenocarcinoma* [13] is not

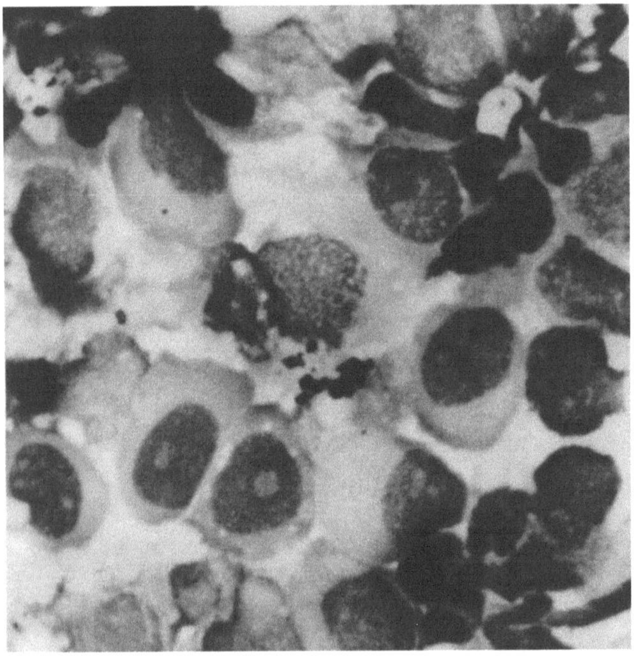

Fig. 2. Fine needle aspirate from a well-differentiated liver cell carcinoma. There is a tendency to a cord-like or pericanalicular arrangement and a large bile droplet is present *(top left)*. Air-dried Romanowsky smear, ×1200

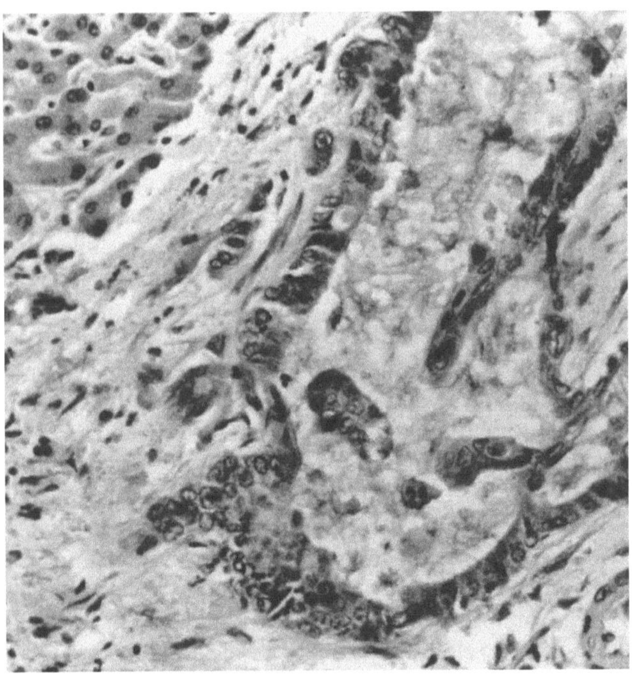

Fig. 3. In situ carcinomatous change in a large bile duct opposite the normal liver *(top left)* bordering on the portal tract. H & E, ×200

likely to yield useful histological material but aspirated fluid almost certainly will contain malignant papillary clumps.

Hepatoblastoma [11] is histologically recognisable as a tumour composed of liver cells in various stages of differentiation and a mesenchymal, usually osteoid, component is frequently present. Aspiration cytology is not likely to be useful. In any event, the presence of a rapidly growing mass in a young child whose blood contains a vastly elevated level of alpha-fetoprotein is a situation which requires no further help from the pathologist.

Carcinoid tumour in the liver is usually a metastasis and may be associated with the characteristic syndrome. Primary carcinoid in the liver is rare and curiously silent: hypoglycaemia due to an unidentified product and secretion of pancreatic polypeptide and of somatostatin are the only known endocrine manifestations. A needle biopsy should provide a diagnosis if the possibility is borne in mind (Fig. 4). They may also arise from major bile ducts and present with obstructive jaundice.

Haemangiosarcoma is readily diagnosable in a needle biopsy and other sarcomas, all rare [10], reasonably so. Lymphomatous involvement of the liver is usually secondary.

Tumour-like lesions, listed in Table 1 [2, 3] are not difficult to diagnose in biopsy material, in the appropriate clinical setting, including radiology. Aspiration cytology is unlikely to be of any use.

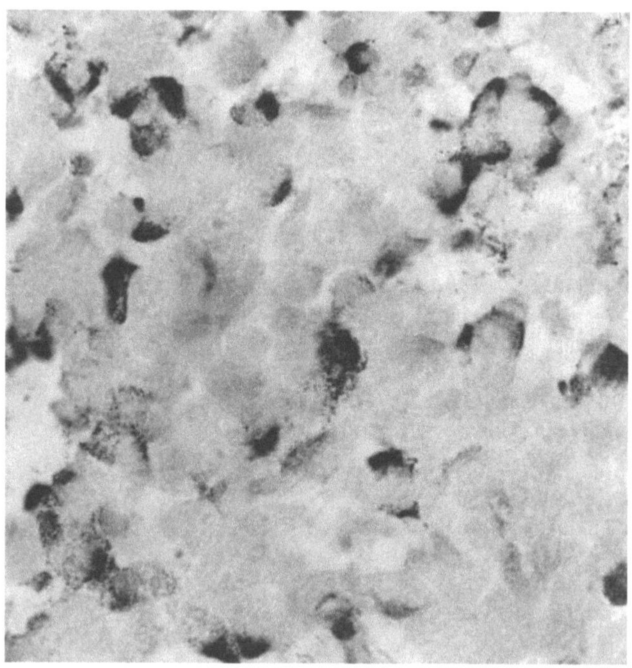

Fig. 4. Primary carcinoid tumour of liver, initially regarded as liver cell carcinoma, from a 36-year-old woman; no attempt was made at resection and the patient remained alive for 2 years when the biopsy was reviewed. Cohesive, relatively uniform cells contain neurosecretory granules. Only somatostatin could be demonstrated by immunohistology. Grimelius' method, $\times 800$

Can the Source of a Metastatic Tumour Be Identified from Its Morphology?

The problem of identifiying the primary source of a metastasis in the liver is a difficult one. In general, the tumour may show glandular or squamous differentiation or be of a special type with a unique morphology. The commonest are *adenocarcinomas* and no more than a tentative suggestion from a list of probabilities is usually possible. Carcinomas of the gastrointestinal tract, breast and lung account for the majority. *Squamous cell carcinomas* metastasize to the liver much less commonly, lung excepted. Little further help can be expected from immunohistology for tumour markers or from electron microscopy. Aspiration cytology is often successful and provides information that is as much or only little less than that obtained from a needle biopsy. *Special types of tumour* in which morphology and special techniques indicate the likely primary source and/or a useful line of therapy include *oat cell carcinoma of lung, hypernephroma, melanoma, carcinoid and islet cell tumours, carcinomas of the prostate and of the thyroid, malignant teratoma* and *lymphoma*. Metastatic sarcomas in the liver are readily identifiable but are rare and seldom amenable to treatment.

Which Primary Tumours Are Likely to Be Solitary or Multiple?

Table 2 attempts a tabulation of the likelihood of a tumour to be solitary or multiple and is, by necessity, an oversimplification. *Always* means nearly always, i. e. there are few exceptions on record. *Usually* and *rarely* vary in strength of meaning with the tumour in

Table 2. The likelihood of individual types of liver tumour to be solitary or multiple

Type of tumour	Solitary	Multiple
Benign		
Liver cell adenoma	Usually	Rarely
Bile duct cystadenoma	Always	-
Bile duct papillomatosis	-	Always
Hemangioma	Usually	Rarely
Granular cell tumour	Always	-
Malignant		
Liver cell carcinoma	Rarely	Usually
Bile duct carcinoma	Rarely	Usually
Bile duct cystadenocarcinoma	Always	-
Hepatoblastoma	Usually	Rarely
Primary carcinoid tumour	Usually	Rarely
Hemangiosarcoma	Rarely	Usually
Other sarcomas	Usually	Rarely
Primary lymphoma	Usually	Rarely
Tumour-like lesions		
Focal nodular hyperplasia	Usually	Rarely
Mesenchymal hamartoma	Always	-
Peliosis	-	Always
Cysts	Rarely	Usually

For explanations see text

question from 70%-90% to 30%-10%. Most common malignant tumours, notably liver cell and bile duct carcinomas and hemangiosarcoma, involve both lobes of the liver though the main mass is located in only one, which is usually the right lobe. This multiplicity may not be evident at the time of surgery but recurrence soon follows. The larger the tumour, the greater is the likelihood of "satellite" deposits. In liver cell carcinoma, for example, tumours over 5 cm in size are probably never curable. An exception is fibrolamellar carcinoma, which is often solitary, large and found as often, or perhaps even more commonly, in the left lobe. Some tumours and tumour-like lesions, notably hemangioma, liver cell adenoma or carcinoma, leiomyosarcoma, focal nodular hyperplasia and hamartoma, may become pedunculated but this is excessively rare. It has been suggested that, in some instances at least, the growth may have originated in an accessory lobe.

Are There Subtypes of Liver Tumours with a Better Prognosis?

The clear cell variant of liver cell carcinoma has been alleged to carry a better than average prognosis but survival is prolonged by a few weeks only [14]. Three special types of liver cell carcinoma exist, however, of which two are particularly important.

Fibrolamellar carcinoma [4, 7] was first definitively described by Peters [19]. It is rare: some 54 cases were on record by early 1984 and a few more reports are in the press. It affects adolescents and young adults of either sex; it appears, in fact, to be slightly commoner in females. The tumour is usually large, solitary and found rather more commonly in the left lobe of the liver. Alpha-fetoprotein in the blood is normal or slightly raised but a vitamin B_{12}-binding protein and neurotensin are commonly present [6]. The histological experiences are highly characteristic (Fig. 5). Electron microscopy shows numerous mitochondria, cytoplasmic inclusions and intracellular lumina; copper-binding protein and alpha-1-antitrypsin have also been demonstrated. Growth is slow and most cases are amenable to surgery. Berman et al. [4] recorded 2 and 5-year survival rates of 82% and 63% respectively.

Minute or encapsulated liver cell carcinoma is most frequently seen in Japan, where it represents 10% or so of all liver cell malignancy [17]. The characteristics are a small size (generally 3-5 cm), slow growth, a fibrous capsule (Fig. 6), which is often thick enough to show up as a bloodless rim on angiography, a well-differentiated trabecular structure and cytology and lack of vascular invasion. Most are found in small livers with advanced cirrhosis which may present problems for the surgeon but, being solitary, complete resection is technically possible.

Pedunculated liver cell carcinoma is not yet established as an entity but some 15 cases are on record [9]. Patients tend to be old and relatively free from symptoms though the tumours are quite large. They are highly amenable to resection and patients do well.

The only subtype of bile duct carcinoma that has a distinctly better prognosis is *bile duct cystadenocarcinoma,* which should always be resected if at all possible. *Adeno- and squamous cell carcinomas* arising in pre-existing cysts and congenital malformations may, similarly, be resectable but some of these are multiple. *Well-differentiated bile duct carcinomas* grow slowly and may even become calcified, patients surviving for two to three years. *Hilar adenocarcinomas* generally are slow growing and useful palliation is possible. *Hepatoblastomas* with a well-differentiated epithelial component have been reported to carry a better prognosis. *Primary carcinoid tumours* should always be resected and do well.

Epithelioid hemangioendothelioma is a special subtype of hemangiosarcoma that has only recently been recognized [22]. It occurs in the liver, usually in middle-aged females, and growth is slow: a third or so of patients survive for 5 years or more.

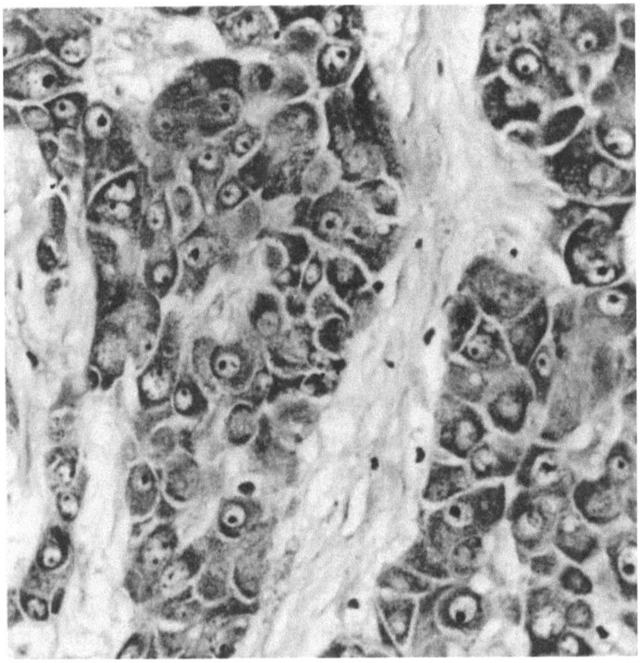

Fig. 5. Fibrolamellar carcinoma: groups and strands of large, polygonal, mitochondrion-rich cells embedded in a lamellar connective tissue stroma. Altmann's method, × 300

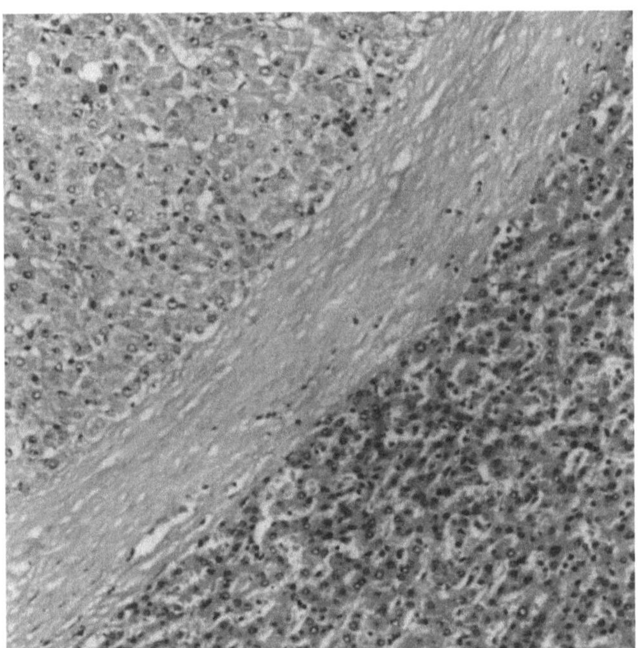

Fig. 6. Minute, encapsulated liver cell carcinoma *(top left)* separated by a thick capsule from the surrounding liver *(bottom right)* H & E, × 80

Summary and Comments

This brief outline of the uses and limitations of histopathological and cytological diagnosis clearly indicates that morphological investigation plays a key role in the management of patients with liver tumours. The best results are obtained by close cooperation between surgeon, radiologist and pathologist and the latter must be prepared to use modern techniques to arrive at the most exact diagnosis. The presence of a malignant tumour in the liver, whether it be primary or secondary, should no longer be regarded as an inevitable death warrant for the patient.

References

1. Aisner SC, Khaneja S, Ramirez O (1982) Multiple granular cell tumours of the gallbladder and biliary tree. Arch Pathol Lab Med 106: 470-471
2. Anthony PP (1981) The pathology of primary cancer of the liver. In: Friedman M, Ogawa M, Kisner D (eds) Diagnosis and treatment of upper gastrointestinal tumours. Excerpta Medica, Amsterdam, p 79
3. Anthony PP (1985) Tumours and tumour-like lesions of the liver and biliary tract. In: MacSween RNM, Anthony PP, Scheuer PJ (eds) Pathology of the liver, 2nd edn. Churchill Livingstone, Edinburgh (in press)
4. Berman MM, Libbey NP, Foster JH (1980) Hepatocellular carcinoma polygonal cell type with fibrous stroma - an atypical variant with a favourable prognosis. Cancer 46: 1448-1455
5. Cameron HM, Linsell DA, Warwick GP (eds) (1976) Liver cell cancer. Elsevier, Amsterdam
6. Collier NA, Weinbren K, Bloom SR, Lee YC, Hodgson HJF, Blumgart LH (1984) Neurotensin secretion by fibrolamellar carcinoma of the liver. Lancet 1: 538-540
7. Craig JR, Peters RL, Edmondson HA, Omata M (1980) Fibrolamellar carcinoma of the liver: a tumour of adolescents and young adults with distinctive clinico-pathologic features. Cancer 46: 372-379
8. Gibson JB, Sobin LH (1978) Histological typing of tumours of the liver, biliary tract and pancreas. International histological classification of tumours No. 20. World Health Organisation, Geneva
9. Horie Y, Katoh S, Yoshida H, Imaska T, Suou T, Hirayama C (1983) Pedunculated hepatocellular carcinoma. A report of three cases and review of literature. Cancer 51: 746-751
10. Ishak KG (1976) Mesenchymal tumours of the liver. In: Okuda K, Peters RL (eds) Hepatocellular carcinoma. Wiley, New York, p 247
11. Ishak KG, Glunz PR (1967) Hepatoblastoma and hepatocarcinoma in infancy and childhood. Report of 47 cases. Cancer 20: 396-422
12. Ishak KG, Rabin L (1975) Benign tumours of the liver. Med Clin North Am 59: 995-1013
13. Ishak KG, Willis GW, Cummins SD, Bullock AA (1977) Biliary cystadenoma and cystadenocarcinoma. Report of 14 cases and review of the literature. Cancer 38: 322-338
14. Lai CL, Wu PC, Lam KC, Todd D (1979) Histologic prognostic indicators in hepatocellular carcinoma. Cancer 44: 1677-1683
15. Mercadier M, Bodard M, Fingerhut A, Chigot JP (1984) Papillomatosis of the intrahepatic bile ducts. World J Surg 8: 30-35
16. Munoz N, Linsell A (1982) Epidemiology of primary liver cancer. In: Correa P, Haenszel W (eds) Epidemiology of cancer of the digestive tract. Nijhoff, The Hague, p 161
17. Nakashima T, Okuda K, Kojiro M, Jimi A, Yamaguchi R, Sakamoto K, Ikavi T (1983) Pathology of hepatocellular carcinoma in Japan; 232 consecutive cases autopsied in ten years. Cancer 51: 863-877

18. Nime F, Pickren JW, Vana J, Aronoff BL, Baker HW, Murphy GP (1979) The histology of liver tumours in oral contraceptive users observed during a national survey by the American College of Surgeons Commission on Cancer. Cancer 44: 1481-1489
19. Okuda K, Peters RL (eds) (1976) Hepatocellular carcinoma. Wiley, New York
20. Remmer H, Bolt HM, Bannasch P, Popper H (eds) (1978) Primary liver tumours. Falk Symposium 25. MTP Press, Lancaster
21. Tao LC, Ho CS, McLoughlin MJ, Evans WK, Donat EE (1984) Cytologic diagnosis of hepatocellular carcinoma by fine needle aspiration biopsy. Cancer 53: 547-552
22. Weiss SW, Enzinger FM (1982) Epithelioid haemangioendothelioma. A vascular tumour often mistaken for a carcinoma. Cancer 50: 970-981

Significance and Limitations for Diagnostics and Follow-up

P. Gerhardt, M. Just, and K. Weidenhammer

Abteilung Röntgendiagnostik, Chirurgisches Zentrum der Universität Heidelberg,
Im Neuenheimer Feld 110, 6900 Heidelberg, FRG

Diagnostic imaging is now of a standard which permits it to have a substantial influence on the selection of therapy in many diseases. The spectrum of these diagnostic modalities comprises scintigraphy, angiography, sonography, CT scan, and now NMR, and the advantages and disadvantages of these techniques are discussed in this paper. The biological effect of ionizing radiation will not be considered in this evaluation, but only the diagnostic benefit and practicability of the method.

The identification of any focal lesion with the imaging methods in question depends on spatial resolution and contrast resolution. These, together with the invasiveness and cost, are the significant parameters for us. As numerous models of various technical types of equipment are in use there is no doubt that comparisons are very difficult; for example, the ultrasound and CT findings recorded by different investigators are not directly comparable. *Radionuclide scanning* is now rarely used for screening or for follow-up of pathologic lesions of the liver. Centrally located masses in the liver are often missed, so that false-negative results are frequent. This is also the case in peripheral lesions smaller than 20 mm in diameter, as the spatial resolution of scintigraphy is inferior to that of other techniques. While some authors still consider a radionuclide scan the diagnostic procedure of choice [15, 22, 29], this may be due to the use of older sonographic or CT instruments.

Angiography has declined in significance, as for screening and follow-up. This method is invasive; and in addition small tumors located at the periphery are rarely identified, so that the sensitivity required is not achieved.

On the other hand, angiography is indispensable for the planning of regional therapy.

Sonography is of major importance for the diagnosis of liver masses. This method combines many advantages, including noninvasiveness, sufficient spatial resolution with the detection of focal lesions of about 5-10 mm in diameter, and immediate availability. Furthermore, the examination can be repeated several times and the costs are relatively low. The substantial disadvantage of sonography is the dependence of the results on the examiner's training, experience, and capacity for self-criticism. No other diagnostic imaging procedure yields such a high number of false results.

CT scan is the most successful method of detecting tumors of the liver, especially when contrast material is used. In sensitivity, specificity, and accuracy it is superior to all other methods. The advantages are the standardization of the examination procedure, the reproducibility of the collected data, and the possibility of creating additional planes by reformatting. The determination of absorption values allows some degree of tissue characterization. The demonstration of the topography and the expansion of the tumor is very

Recent Results in Cancer Research. Vol 100

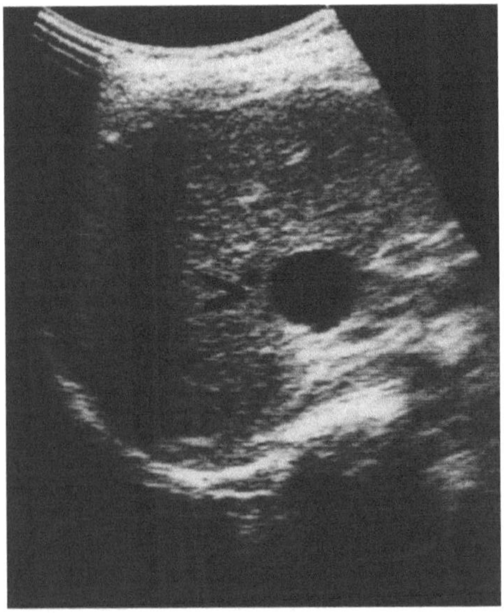

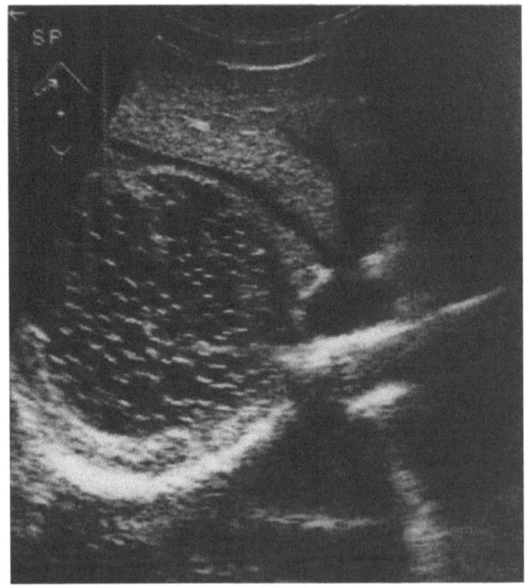

Fig. 1 *(Left).* Cyst in the right liver lobe; echofree, well-defined lesion with a diameter of 20 mm; 3.5 MHz real-time sonography

Fig. 2 *(Right).* Echinicoccus cyst in the right liver lobe, 25 × 120 mm in diameter; 3.5 MHz real-time sonography

valuable in the precise planning of therapy [8, 9]. The main disadvantages of CT scan are the high cost, the susceptibility to artifact production, and the need for an IV contrast agent, in many cases.

Some examples may demonstrate the diagnostic potentials of the imaging methods in question.

With the use of sonography, cysts are seen as echofree ball-shaped areas greater than approximately 5 mm in diameter. The position of the transducer is shown on the screen. The typical sonographic finding with cysts is apparent amplification of echoes behind lesions. This is in contrast to the image found with stones in the gallbladder, for example, where a "sound shadow" is characteristic (Fig. 1). The findings in the example of hydatid disease shown in Fig. 2 correspond to multiple echofree areas confirmed by echogenic walls (Fig. 2).

Solid primary tumors of the liver and liver metastases can be detected if their diameter is greater than approx. 10 mm. Masses with low echogenicity are usually harder to find than those with higher echogenicity, regardless of whether primary or secondary tumors are concerned [26]; that is why there is no correlation between the sonographic appearance of metastases and of primary tumors.

The diameter of the lesion, indicated by the area of abnormal reflex pattern, can be measured precisely, as in the metastasis of a carcinoma of the colon shown in Fig. 3. The diameter in this example is 45 mm. Furthermore, with modern sonographic instruments it is possible to record the grayscale pattern of echo intensity within a certain area, thus generating the histogram function [10]. This gives quite an objective idea of the reflex pattern. The metastasis, illustrated in Fig. 3 proved to have a reflex density of 27, as against 15 in healthy liver tissue. Echogenic metastases are conspicuously frequent with tumors of the gastrointestinal tract.

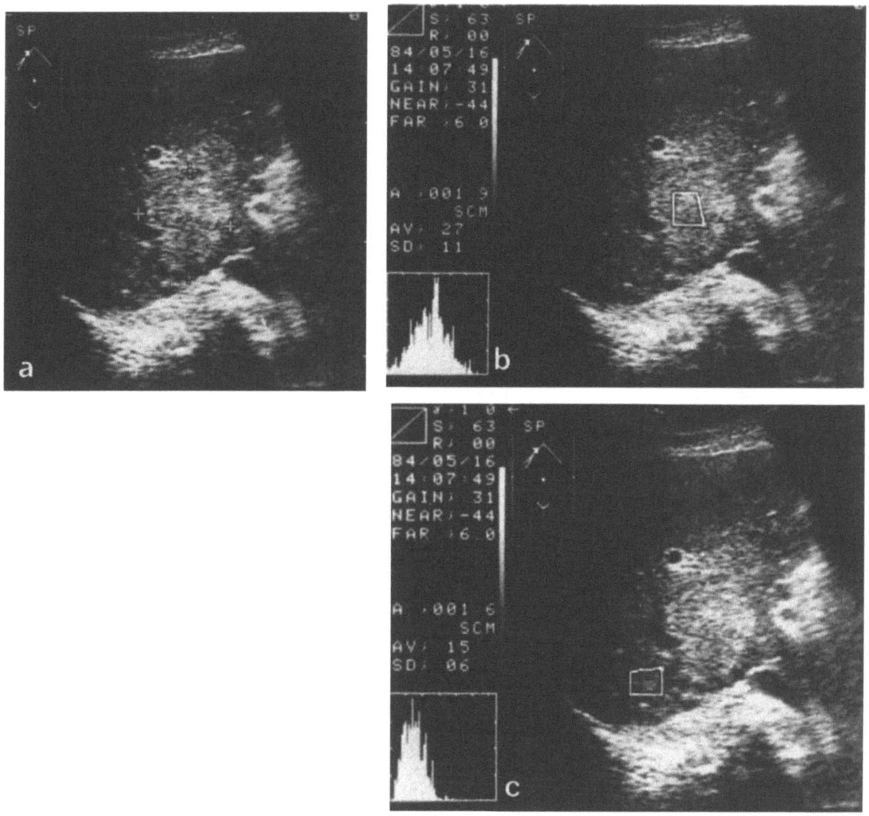

Fig. 3 a–c. Liver metastases of a colon carcinoma; 3.5 MHz real-time sonography. **a** Diameter of the metastasis is 45 mm in two planes. **b** Histogram of the metastasis; medium echo density of 27. **c** Histogram of normal liver tissue; medium echo density of 15

In the case of this liver metastasis from a carcinoma of the sigmoid colon there was increased echointensity with an average of 31, against which the normal tissue had only 21 (Fig. 4).

Another criterion for the existence of metastases, which in our experience are especially frequent in the presence of primary tumors of the gastrointestinal tract, is a circle of reduced echogenicity surrounding the lesion. This also holds if the echointensity of metastases is only slightly different from that of healthy liver tissue (Fig. 5).

As illustrated in Figs. 5 and 6, metastases are identified by the presence of echofree margins. In one example (Fig. 5) the echointensity amounts to 16, compared with 13 in healthy liver tissue, while in the other (Fig. 6) it is 19 both in the metastases and in the normal liver tissue. Although according to the literature the pattern of echoes does not depend on the degree of blood supply, our experience has shown that most echogenic metastases are better supplied with blood than masses with low echodensity. This observation has derived from comparison of the sonograms of the lesions in question with the corresponding angiograms.

In the field of oncology the CT scan has become accepted as the most important of the imaging procedures.

In addition to sonography, it is mandatory before many therapeutic procedures. Wit-

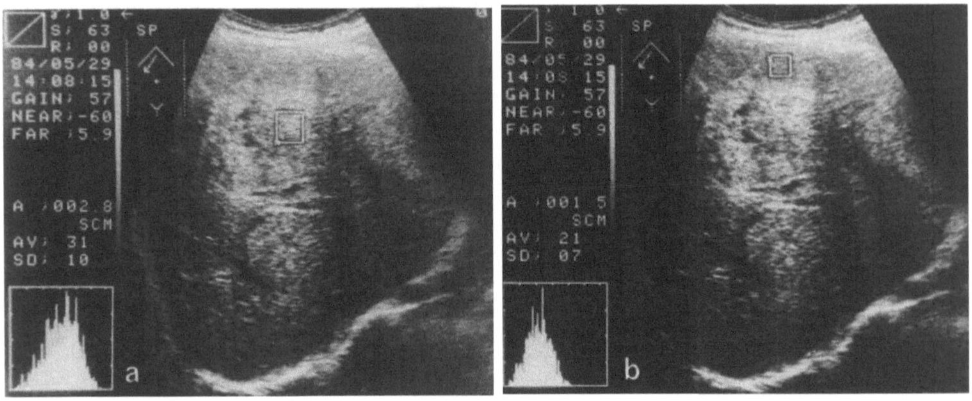

Fig. 4 a, b. Metastasis in the liver of a carcinoma of the sigmoid colon: mean echo density of the metastasis (**a**) is 31 while that of normal liver tissue (**b**)is 21. 3.5-MHz real-time sonography

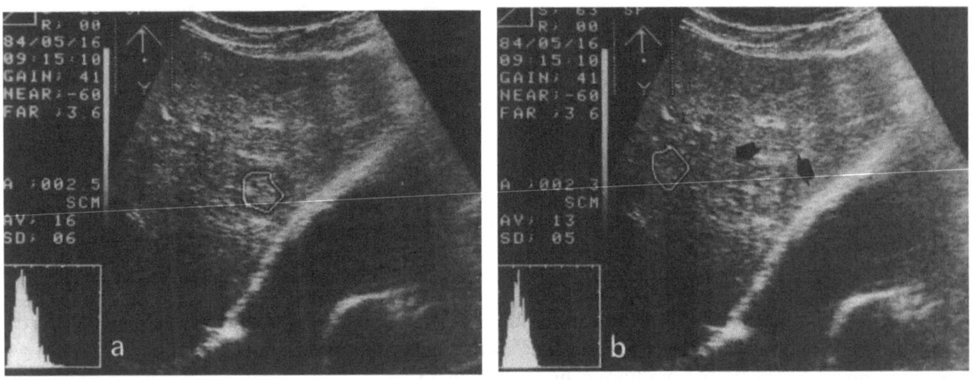

Fig. 5. a, b. Metastasis in the liver of a carcinoma of the colon. The metastasis has a margin of low echogenicity. The echo density of the metastasis (**a**) amounts to 16, as against 13 in the normal liver parenchyma. 3.5-MHz real-time sonography

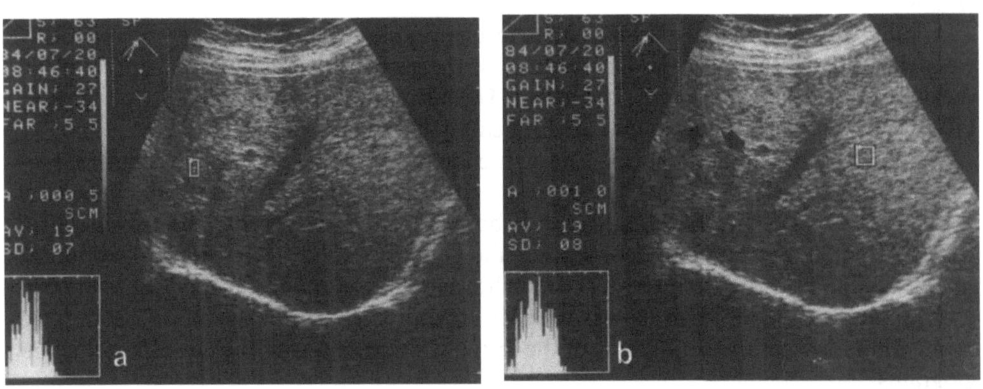

Fig. 6. Metastasis in the liver of a carcinoma of the colon. Margin of low echogenicity around the metastasis has an identical echo density (19) to the normal liver tissue. 3.5-MHz real-time sonography

tenberg et al. [30] have examined the influence of CT scan on therapy planning, (Tables 1 and 2). In 51% of 623 patients they found the clinical diagnosis confirmed, whereas in 35% there was some uncertainty and in 14% the treatment had to be modified. In 56 of 290 patients a planned operation was not performed because the diagnosis was revised. On the other hand, in 8 of 331 patients an operation was performed that had not been planned before.

With more advanced CT instruments it is possible to detect lesions as small as 5 mm in diameter, especially if IV contrast medium is used.

Figure 7 shows two metastases of a carcinoid of the small bowel, demonstrating that a very small difference in absorbtion values can cause a false-negative finding. In the corresponding sonogram, the metastasis in the right liver lobe can be clearly demonstrated by an echofree margin as a lesion with a diameter of 28–40 mm. The echointensity of 15 is the same in the metastasis as in the normal liver tissue. The average echodensity in the portal vein is 4 (Fig. 8).

Since both small hypodense masses and larger isodense masses in the liver can be missed by regular CT scanning angio-CT scanning was established for better visualization of these lesions. In this examination scanning of the liver is performed in rapid sequences and at various levels after IV administration of a bolus of contrast material [7, 12, 17]. In Figs. 9 and 10, showing two metastases of a carcinoma of the colon in the right lobe of the liver, good demarcation of the hypodense masses is easily seen against the normal liver tissue, being enhanced by contrast material. In the angiogram both metastases are seen to be localized in an area of hypervascularization, with enhanced contrast in the parenchymal phase.

For the detection and follow-up of hepatocellular carcinoma, the usefulness of sonography, dynamic CT scan, and angiography is comparable [13, 16, 23]. In the example of a hepatocellular carcinoma shown in Figs. 11 and 12 the clearly defined area of the lesion in the right lobe with density values of 34 Hounsfield units (HU) is demonstrated. Sonogra-

Table 1. Influence of CT result during diagnostic procedure ($n = 623$). (After Wittenberg et al. [30])

Adverse effect or no influence	35%
Increased physican confidence	51%
Contributed to a change in therapy	14%

Table 2. Influence of CT on therapy planning. (Wittenberg et al. [30])

Surgery use	No. of patients (%)
Surgery planned	290
Appropriately avoided	56 (19)
Inappropriately avoided	0
Surgery not planned	331
Appropriately prompted	8 (2)
Inappropriately prompted	4 (1)
Total	621

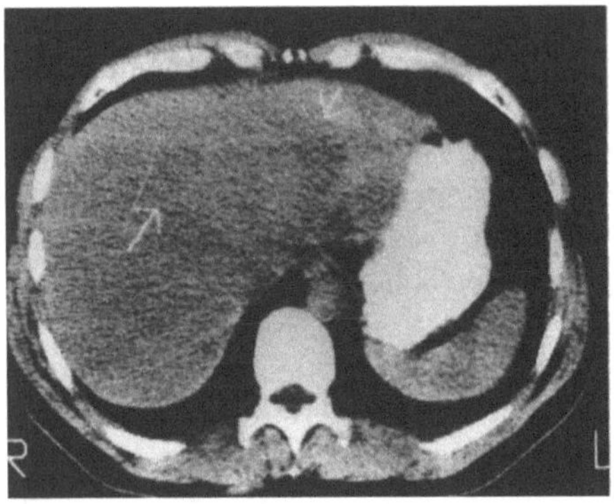

Fig. 7. Computer tomography without contrast material. Metastases of a carcinoid of the small bowel are found in the right and left liver lobes. There is only a small difference from normal liver tissue in the absorption values

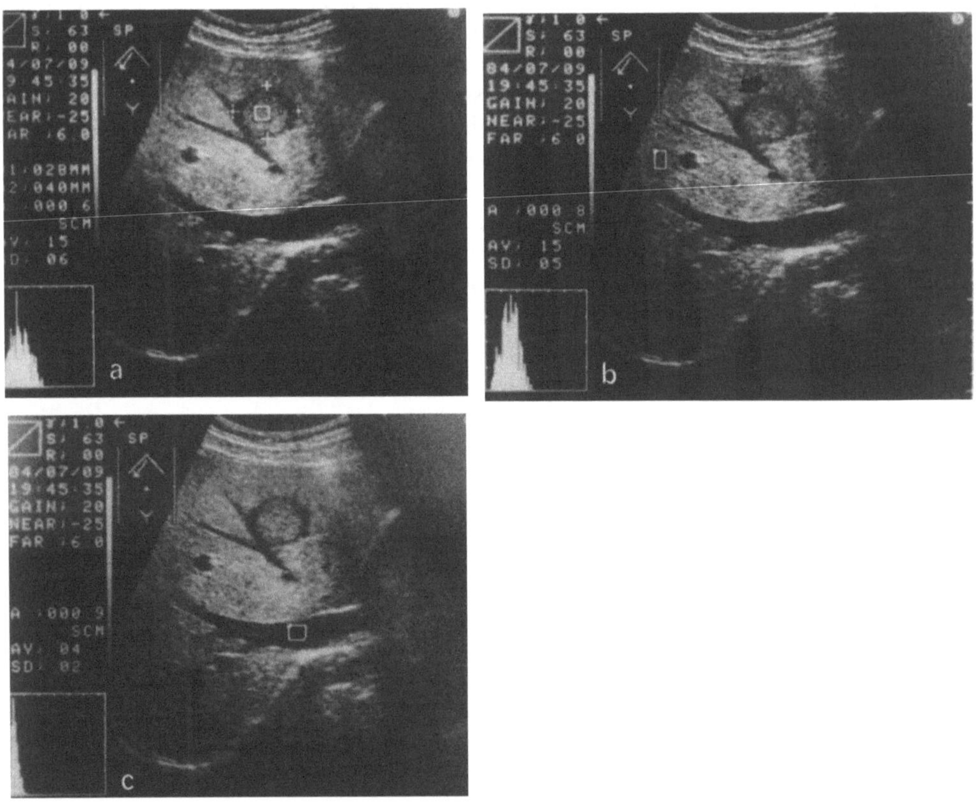

Fig. 8 a–c. Metastasis of a carcinoid of the small bowel (same case as Fig. 7) with diameters 28 × 40 mm and medium echo density of 15 (**a**). Normal liver tissue also has a mean echo density of 15 (**b**), while the portal vein has a medium echo density of 4 (**c**). The metastasis is surrounded by a markedly low density margin. 3.5-MHz real-time sonography

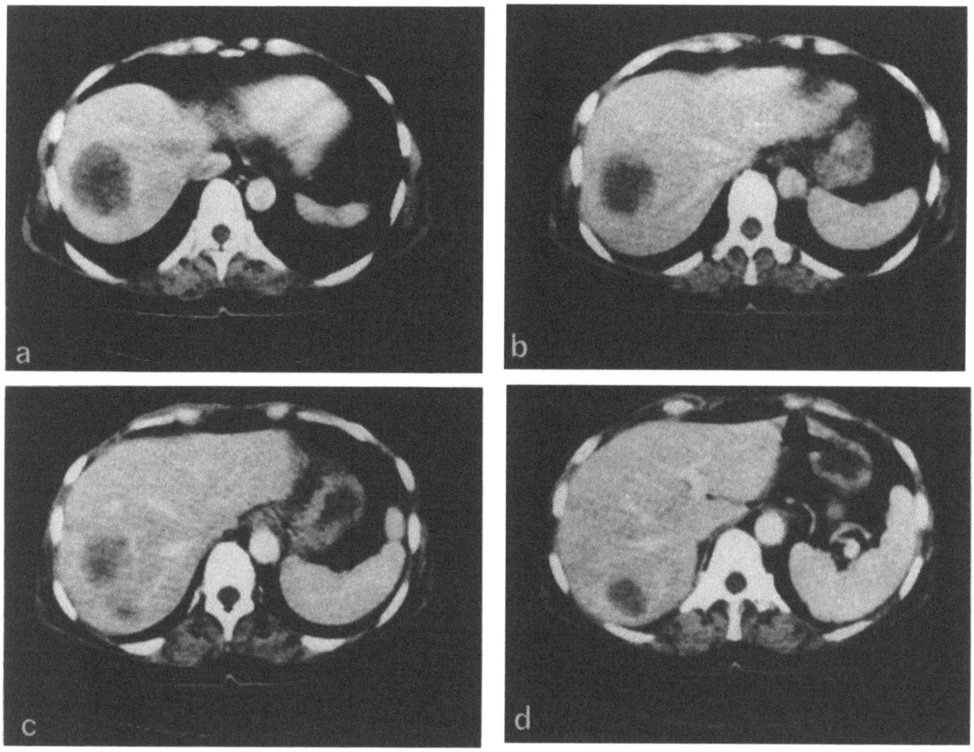

Fig. 9 a–d. Angio-CT showing two metastases in the right liver lobe. The hypodense lesions are well delimited after iv. injection of a bolus of contrast medium (**a–d** consecutive slices from cranial to caudal)

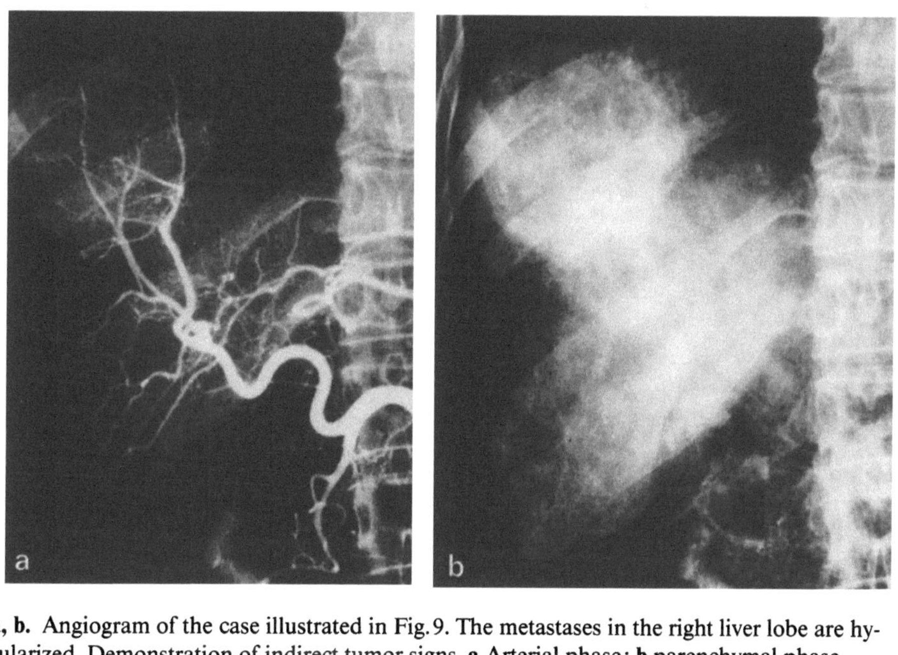

Fig. 10 a, b. Angiogram of the case illustrated in Fig. 9. The metastases in the right liver lobe are hypervascularized. Demonstration of indirect tumor signs. **a** Arterial phase; **b** parenchymal phase phically, the tumor is seen to be markedly echogenic with an echointensity of 21, as against 14 in the normal liver tissue; infiltration of the liver veins must also be suspected.

On the angiogram, the tumor is identified as an area of hypervascularization without detectable AV shunts.

In the CT scan the density values for an abscess of the liver can be similar to that for a liver tumor, as in the case shown in Fig. 13, with 25 HU. Sonography makes it relatively easy to differentiate an abscess from a tumor, as abscesses have significantly lower echointensity. In the case illustrated in Fig. 14 the mean echodensity is 6, as against 14 in the normal tissue.

The advantage of an angio-CT scan in the case of inconclusive findings is demonstrated in Fig. 15. In a patient with a history of breast cancer, on ultrasound examination an echogenic mass was detected in the liver with average echodensity values of 27, as against 18 in normal liver tissue.

The suspicion that a metastasis was present could not be confirmed by dynamic CT scan. The unrecognized mass seen on the regular scan and immediately after the injection of the bolus became almost isodense 9 min after administration of the contrast medium. This finding is typical of a hemangioma (Fig. 16).

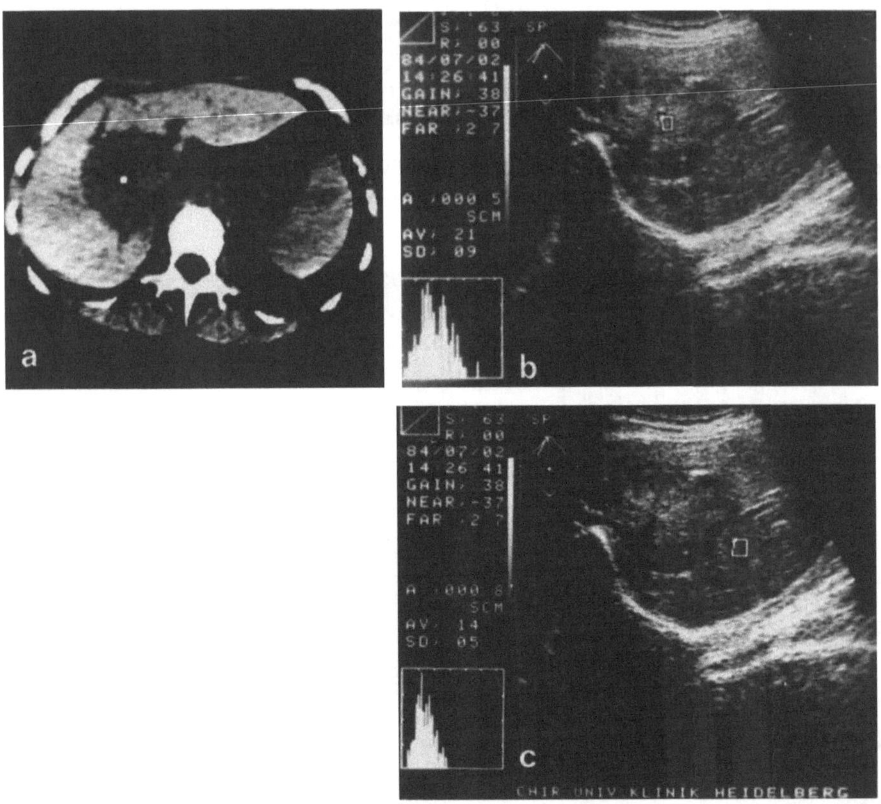

Fig. 11 a–c. Primary hepatocellular carcinoma. The CT image shows a well-defined hypodense lesion in the right liver lobe (**a**). Sonography reveals an echogenic lesion with a relatively low echogenic margin. The mean echo density of the tumor is 21, as compared to 14 in normal liver tissue (**b, c**). 3.5-MHz real-time sonography

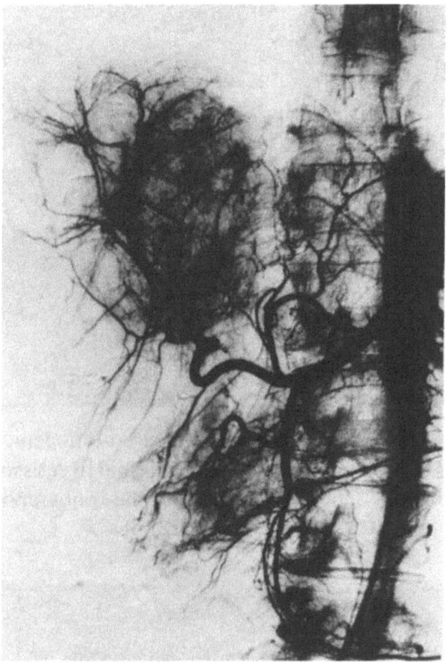

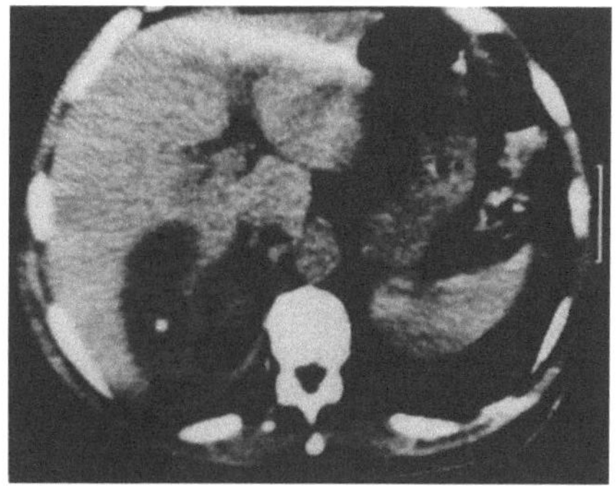

Fig. 12 *(Left).* Celiacography in the patient shown in Fig. 11. Demonstration of the hypervascularized primary hepatocellular carcinoma

Fig. 13 *(Right).* CT of a retroperitoneal abscess with involvement of the right liver lobe. Well-delineated hypodense area with absorption values of 15 HU

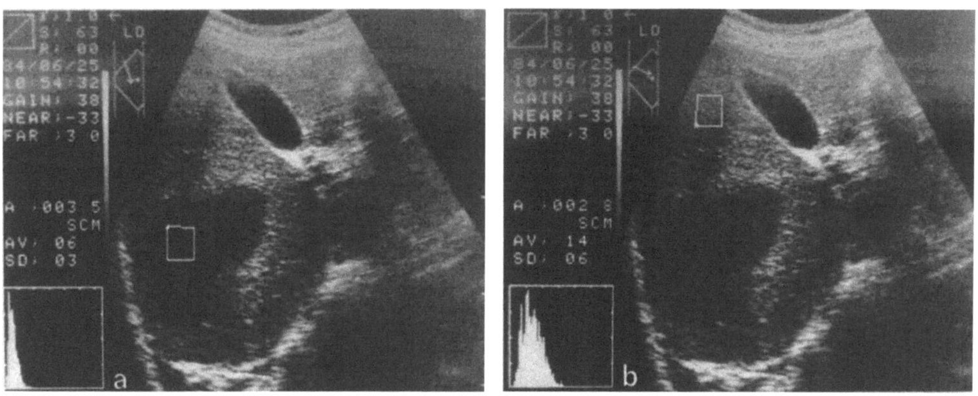

Fig. 14 a, b. Same case as Fig. 13. Sonogram of the right liver lobe. Area with almost no echogenicity; echo density is 6, as against 14 in normal liver tissue (means) 3.5-MHz real-time sonography

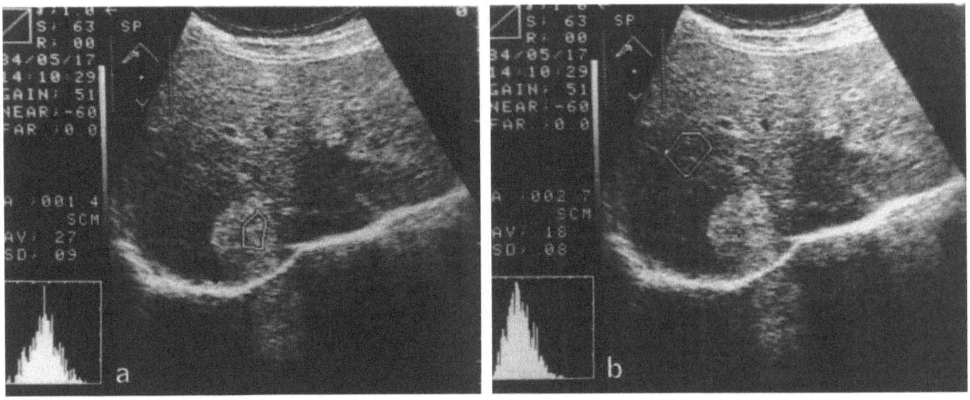

Fig. 15 a, b. Sonogram of the right liver lobe, revealing a lesion with markedly increased echogenicity near the diaphragm. The mean echo density amounts to 27, compared with 18 in normal liver tissue (**a**, **b**). Suspicion of metastasis with known carcinoma of the breast. 3.5-MHz real-time sonography

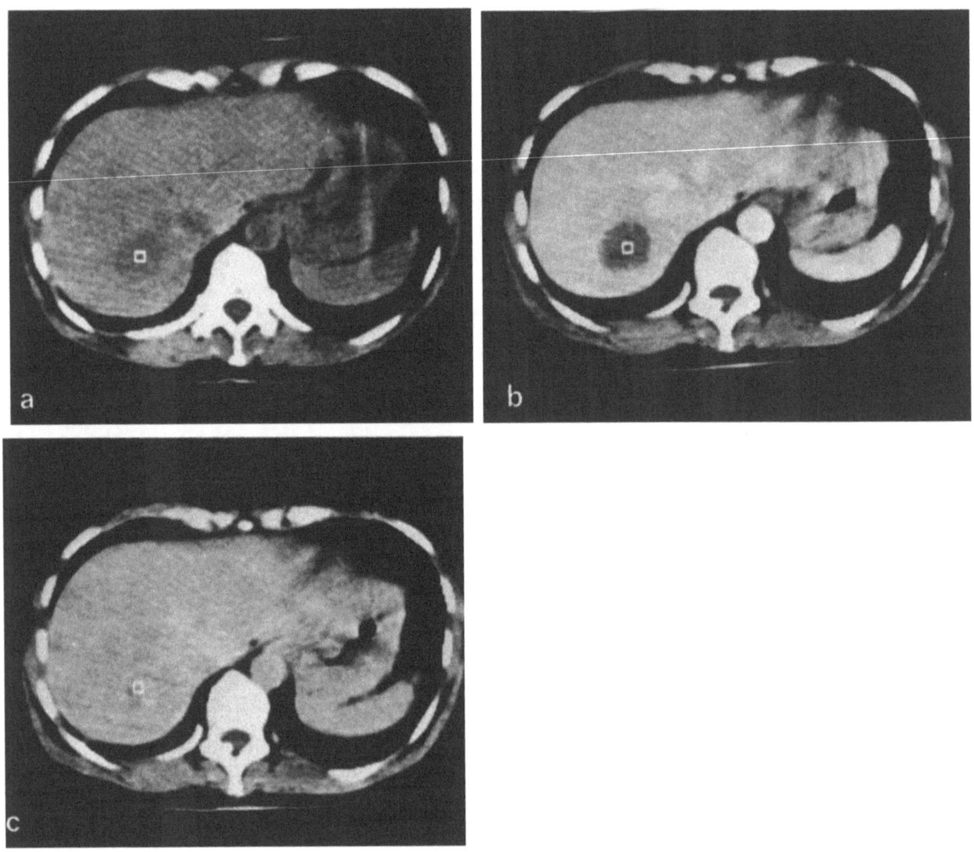

Fig. 16 a–c. Same case as Fig. 15. Dynamic CT with iv. bolus injection of contrast medium. **a** Before contrast mediums; **b** after injection, enhancement of portal vein system, clear demarcation of pathologic area; **c** at 9 min after injection of contrast medium, no difference in absorption values of the lesion and normal liver tissue. Typical findings for hemangioma

Table 3. Literature review of sensitivity, specificity, and accuracy of scintigraphy for the evaluation of liver lesions

n	Sensitivity	(%)	Specificity (%)	Accuracy (%)	Publication
424		83	75	77	Lunia et al. [14]
94		94	67	90+82	Snow et al. [22]
80		79	81	80	Smith et al. [21]
305		76.6	92.6	76	Arnaud et al. [1]
84		-	-	79	Knopf et al. [11]
21		89	100	-	Engel et al. [5]
Hemangioma, 99^{m} Tc-red blood cell imaging					
33	Lesions < 3 cm∅			12.1	Sheu et al. [20]

Table 4. Literature review of sensitivity, specificity, and accuracy of sonography for the evaluation of liver lesions

n	Sensitivity	(%)	Specificity (%)	Accuracy (%)	Publication
120		-	-	92	Taylor and Carpenter [25]
100		83	97	93	Sullivan et al. [24]
94		75	50	81+85	Snow et al. [22]
78		-	70	-	Martinez et al. [15]
356		90.6	97.6	94.4	Beyer et al. [3]
80		61	94	80	Smith et al. [21]
305		93.6	97.7	97	Arnaud et al. [1]
251	Octoson	92.6	-	92.8	Fiegler et al. [6]
	Realt-time	82.6	-	86.8	
33	Lesions < 3 cm∅		-	93.9	Sheu et al. [20]
30	Hepatoma	96	100	-	LaBerge et al. [13]
163		92	80	85	Vatter et al. [27]

Table 5. Literature review of sensitivity, specificity, and accuracy of CT for the evaluation of liver lesions

n	Sensitivity	(%)	Specificity (%)	Accuracy (%)	Publication
94		96	86	95+91	Snow et al. [22]
161		85,5	97,5	94,4	Beyer et al. [3]
80		76	89	84	Smith et al. [21]
84		-	-	98	Knopf et al. [11]
81		88	88	-	Berland et al. [2]
97		89	94	-	Danielson et al. [4]
33	Lesions < 3 cm∅		-	84,3	Sheu et al. [20]
30	Hepatoma	96	100	-	LaBerge et al. [13]
109		88	76	89	Vatter et al. [27]
62	Angio-CT	-	-	90	Rossi et al. [19]
64	Angio-CT	96	-	97	Kober et al. [12]
251	Angio-CT	95,7	-	96	Fiegler et al. [6]

A review of the literature on imaging procedures in liver tumors reveals that the radionuclide scan has demonstrated sensitivity in 76%-94% of cases, specificity of 67%-92% for malignant tumors, and accuracy of 76%-82% (Table 3).

Obviously, these results are surpassed by those obtained with ultrasound examination and CT scanning (Table 4 and 5), for both of which comparable figures are reported. The best results, however are achieved with dynamic CT scan. Therefore, all inconclusive findings ought to be controlled by this technique, especially if a malignant tumor cannot be ruled out. Because of the limited availability of CT scanning at present, ultrasound is usually the first diagnostic tool, unless the history or the clinical findings suggest liver disease. If the quality of the examination is good the diagnostic reliability is high. Therefore, in clinical practice, ultrasonography is the first method applied in the sequence of imaging procedures, although in terms of accuracy dynamic CT scan seems to be the most valuable. With the introduction of a new contrast medium, ethiodized oil emulsion (EOE-13), an aqueous solution of an iodized oil, CT scanning will probably become even more accurate for the evaluation of liver masses [28].

However, this progress may soon be obsolete, as similar results have already been accomplished with NMR [18]. Thus, it is our desire and hope that improved diagnostic imaging may also improve the outcome of primary and metastatic liver tumors.

References

1. Arnaud JP, Daly R, Adloff M (1982) Comparison of sonography and scintigraphy in the detection of liver metastases in patients with colorectal carcinoma. J Radiol 63: 96-100
2. Berland LL, Lawson TL, Foley WD, Melrose BL, Chintapalli KN, Taylor AJ (1982) Comparison of pre- and postcontrast CT in hepatic masses. AJR 138: 853-858
3. Beyer D, Friedmann G, Mödder U (1982) Leberdiagnostik mit bildgebenden Verfahren. Internist 23: 66-74
4. Danielson K, Sheewy P, Stephens D, Hattery R, LaRusso N (1983) Computed tomography and peritoneoscopy for dectection of liver metastasies: Review of the Mayo Clinic experience. J Computer Assist Tomogr 7: 230-234
5. Engel MA, Marks DS, Sandler MA, Shetty P (1983) Differentiation of focal intrahepatic lesions with ^{99m}Tc-red blood cell imaging. Radiology 146: 777-782
6. Fiegler W, Schütz H, Claussen C, Schörner W, Felix R (1984) Herdförmige Lebererkrankungen - Vergleichsstudie Computertomographie, konventioneller Ultraschall, automatisierter Multisektorscanner (Octoson). Fortschr Röntgenstr 141: 71-74
7. Freeny PC, Marks WM (1983) Computed Tomographic Arteriography of the liver. Radiology 148: 193-197
8. Gerhardt P (1983) Indikation und Leistungsfähigkeit der Computertomographie in der chirurgischen Diagnostik. Dtsch Ärztebl 80: 1-12
9. Gerhardt P, Terwey B (1982) Computertomographie und Sonographie zur Metastasenerkennung. Verh Dtsch Krebs Ges 3: 359-372
10. Green B, Bree RL, Goldstein HM, Stanley C (1977) Greyscale ultrasound evaluation of hepatic neoplasms: patterns and correlations. Radiology 124: 203-208
11. Knopf DR, Torres WE, Fayman WJ, Pjsones PJ (1982) Liver lesions: Comparative accuracy of scintigraphy and computed tomography. AJR 138: 623-627
12. Kober B, Gamroth A, Kimmig B, Weber M, Hermann HJ, zum Winkel K (1984) Angio-CT in der Diagnostik von Lebermetastasen colorektaler Tumoren. Röntgenpraxis 37: 330-333
13. LaBerge JM, Laing FC, Federle MP, Jeffrey RB, Lim RC (1984) Hepatocellular carcinoma: Assessment of resectability by computed tomography and ultrasound. Radiology 152: 485-490
14. Lunia S, Parthasarathy K, Bakshis, Bender M (1974) An evaluation of the Tc-^{99m} sulfur colloid

liver scintiscans and their usefulness in metastatic work-up: a review of 1424 studies. J Nucl Med 16: 62-65
15. Martinez CL, Navarro IA, Mengual P, Arbues J, Baringo T, Sosono F (1981) Scintigraphy and echotomography in the diagnosis of hepatic masses. Rev Esp Enferm Apar Dig 60: 579-588
16. Mathieu D, Grenier P, Lardè D, Vasile N (1984) Portal vein involvement in hepatocellular carcinoma: Dynamic CT features. Radiology 152: 127-132
17. Matsui O, Kadoya M, Suziki M, Inoue K, Itoh H, Ida M, Takashima T (1983) Work in progress: Dynamic sequential computed tomography during arterial portography in the detection of hepatic neoplasms. Radiology 146: 721-727
18. Moss AA, Goldberg HI, Stark DB, Davis PL, Margulis AR, Kaufmann L, Crooks LE (1984) Hepatic tumors: Magnetic resonance and CT appearance. Radiology 150: 141-147
19. Rossi P, Rovighi L, Tipaldi L, Bompiani C, Simonetti G (1981) High-contrast enhancement of the liver in CT by repeated doses of contrast medium. Eur J Radiol 1: 126-131
20. Sheu J, Sung J, Chen D, Yu J-Y, Wang T-H, Su C-T, Tsang Y-M (1984) Ultrasonography of small hepatic tumors using high-resolution linear-array real-time instruments. Radiology 150: 797-802
21. Smith TJ, Kemeny MM, Sugarbaker PH, Jons AE, Vermess M, Shawker TA, Edwards BK (1982) Prospective study of hepatic imaging in the detection of metastatic disease. Ann Surg 195: 486-491
22. Snow JH, Goldstein HM, Wallace S (1979) Comparison of scintigraphy, sonography and computer tomography in the evaluation of hepatic neoplasms. AJR 132: 915-918
23. Subramanyam BR, Balthazar EJ, Hilton S, Lefleur RS, Horii SC, Raghavendra BN (1984) Hepatocellular carcinoma with venous invasion: sonographic-angiographic correlation. Radiology 150: 793-796
24. Sullivan DC, Taylor KJW, Gottschalk A (1978) The use of ultrasound to enhance the diagnostic utility of the equivocal liver scintigraph. Radiology 128: 727-732
25. Taylor KJW, Carpenter DA (1975) Comparison of radioisotope and ultrasound examination in the investigation of hepatobiliary disease. In: White DN (ed) Ultrasound in medicine, vol 1. Plenum, New York, pp 159-167
26. Triller J, Fuchs WA (1980) Abdominale Sonographie. Thieme, Stuttgart, pp 37-38
27. Vatter J, Brecht G, Franken T, Harder T (1984) Die Wertigkeit der Ultraschalluntersuchungen beim Screening von Lebermetastasen und von einer Leberbeteiligung bei malignen Systemerkrankungen. Fortschr Roentgenstr 140: 162-167
28. Vermess M, Lau HM, Adams MD, Hopkins RM, Hoey GB, Grimes G, Chatterji DC, Girton M, Doppman JL (1982) Biodistribution study of ethiodized oil emulsion 13 for computed tomography of the liver and spleen. J Comput Assist Tomogr 6: 1115-1119
29. Wallace S, Chuang VP (1982) The radiological diagnosis and management of hepatic metastases. Radiology 22: 56-64
30. Wittenberg J, Fineberg HV, Ferucci JF Jr, Simeone JF, Müller PR, van Sonnenberg E, Kirkpatrick RH (1980) Clinical efficiency of computed body tomography. AJR 134: 1111-1120

Pathological Changes in the Liver and Computed Tomography

K. Weinbren and L. H. Blumgart

Royal Postgraduate Medical School, Hammersmith Hospital, DuCane Road,
London W12 OHS, Great Britain

The constant form and position of the liver in the upper abdomen and its predictable relative size are properties which have been regarded as favourable for investigation of pathological changes by the use of imaging procedures. As more experience with these procedures has been gained over the past few years, confidence has grown and plans for therapy have become more and more influenced by interpretation of the images generated by the new techniques. The problem of validating such interpretations is difficult in many situations for a variety of reasons, not least of which is that with successful therapy the lesions may regress and morphological confirmation may never be available. Validation has therefore become a matter of concordance by other equally unvalidated imaging procedures [1] or agreement with clinical assessment of the patient's state of progress [2]. If, for example, a small doubtful lesion is replaced after an interval of time by a larger and undoubted cancer, then the first image is thus confirmed.

Other attempts at validation have involved a comparison of structural changes in organs found at autopsy examination [3] with the images generated by computed tomography of such an organ. There are inherent difficulties in all of these approaches, as, in the case of comparators, other procedures are often known to yield false-negative or false-positive [3] findings and, in the case of clinical confirmation, this is subject to error because of the dynamics of ischaemia and reactive, invasive and a host of other processes which involve a tumour in an organ and which clearly vary with time.

The images generated by a scanning procedure applied to an organ removed at autopsy and placed on flat surfaces are likely to be distorted by the change in the form of the organ, by the collapse of vascular spaces and by the absence of blood flow. Sometimes post-mortem autolysis may contribute to the difficulty by gas formation or pooling of blood or other fluids. All these difficulties apply to computed tomography of the liver and it seemed important to try to define the limitations of this imaging procedure by comparing the scans with tissues if they became available shortly after the tomographic studies were done. Liver specimens were included in this series if the computed tomography was performed within the previous 10 days and consisted of resected parts of liver or autopsy specimens. The in vivo form of the liver was retained or restored by using perfusion equipment which recirculated a mixture of equal parts of 10% formalin and 2.5% glutaraldehyde into portal or hepatic vessels at a maximum pressure of 20 cm water (Fig. 1).

Next, an attempt was made to match the planes generated by the CT scan with comparable slices taken from the fixed specimen. To this end a polypropylene frame was constructed which accommodated the resected specimen and which permitted sectioning at

Recent Results in Cancer Research. Vol 100

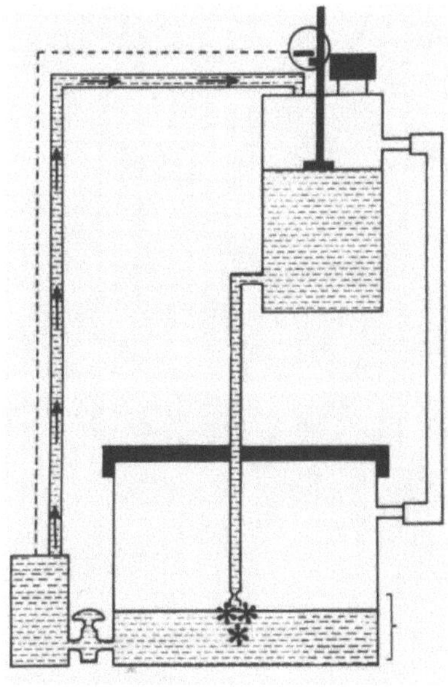

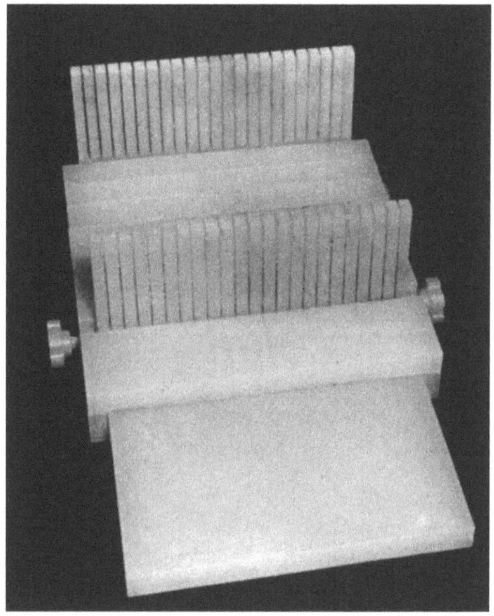

▲ **Fig. 1** *(Upper left).* Diagram of perfusion-fixation equipment

Fig. 2 *(Upper right).* Polypropylene frame for orientating fixed specimen

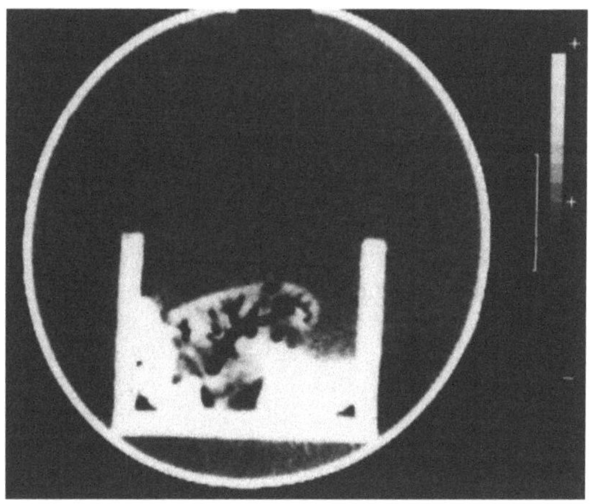

Fig. 3. Computed tomography scan of specimen in frame

the 8-mm intervals currently used in scanning (Fig. 2). At first, the specimen was placed in the frame and orientated so that its position coincided with that in vivo and then sectioned, but after the first few this step was not used and slices and generated images were moderately comparable (Fig. 3). The procedure was then to observe morphological changes and check whether the relevant lesions were visible on the generated scan (Fig. 4). In a sense, the exercise was rather less a validation of diagnostic efforts than an attempt to construct parameters within which the scans might be evaluated. This work is ongoing and the identification of anatomical changes in this way is useful for other imaging procedures. The present report refers to 45 CT scans and surgically resected liver lobes or whole livers removed at autopsy within 10 days and perfused, fixed and sliced as described.

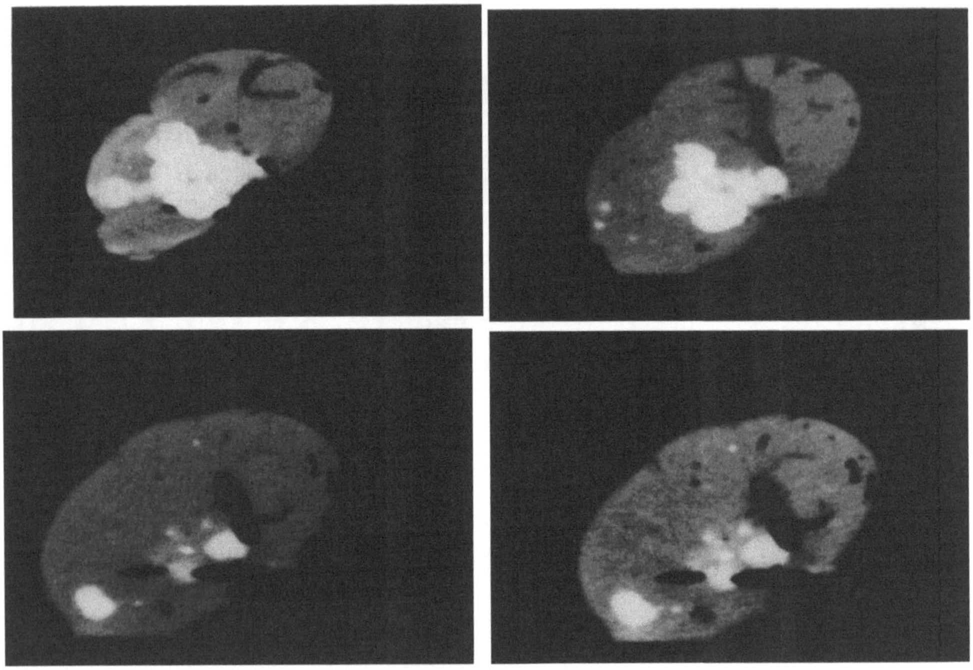

Fig. 4. Orientation using characteristics (calcified foci) of specimen

In essence, the results indicate that correlation between lesions and contrast images depend on form, dimensions, site, extent of necrosis, organisational changes within specific lesions and relationship to extrahepatic tissues. Most of the correlations which might have been anticipated were in fact observed, but there were certain aspects which seem to be worth remarking on.

Form

An alteration of contour was easily displayed (Figs. 5-7).

Dimensions and Site

The dimensions of the solid tumours which were encountered on tissue slices were recorded and the relevant image scans checked for the presence of such lesions. Of discrete tumour deposits which were observed on tissue slices, ranging from 0.2 to 10 cm diameter, those under 0.8 cm were not detectable on the CT scan film and approximately 50% of those of 1-1.5 cm diameter were seen. Of tumours 2 cm or greater almost all in peripheral liver tissue were identified, but tumours at the hilum, usually cholangiocarcinoma, were not discerned on the scan film. There was nothing to suggest a peculiar attenuation of cholangiocarcinoma as opposed to hepatocellular or metastatic tumours and thus it was concluded that the site was probably inaccessible, particularly in view of the major vascular and ductal structures in this region.

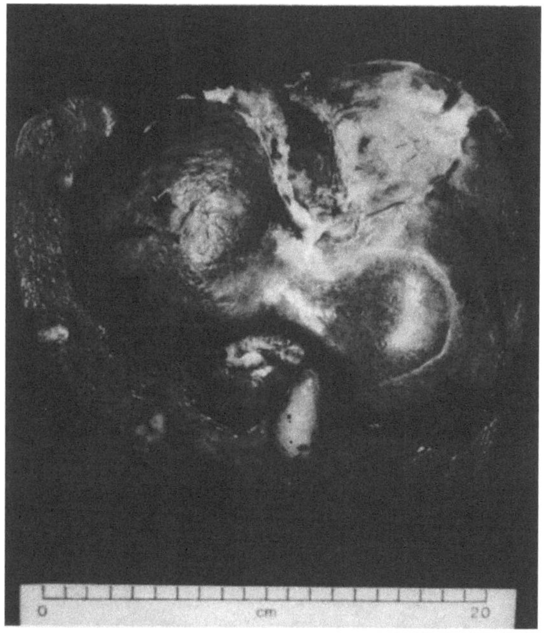

Figs. 5-7. Alteration of form caused by enlarged caudate lobe in hepatic venous ostial occlusion. (Fig. 7 see p. 62)

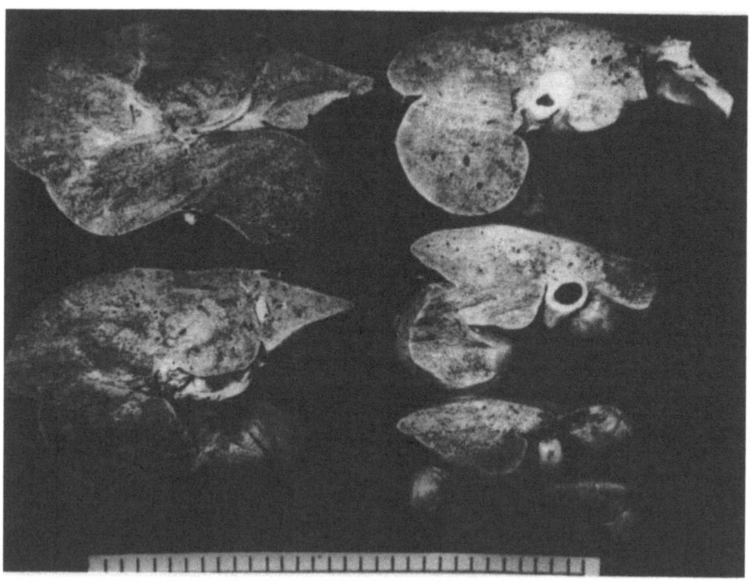

Fig. 6 Legend see Fig. 5

Tumour Necrosis

The degree of attenuation recorded in Hounsfield units in images of necrotic tumour differed from that observed in apparently viable tumour, both of which were less dense than that of otherwise normal liver (Figs. 8, 9). Such necrosis was distinguishable from benign cysts by virtue of the appearance of the wall of the cystic structure and was distinguishable

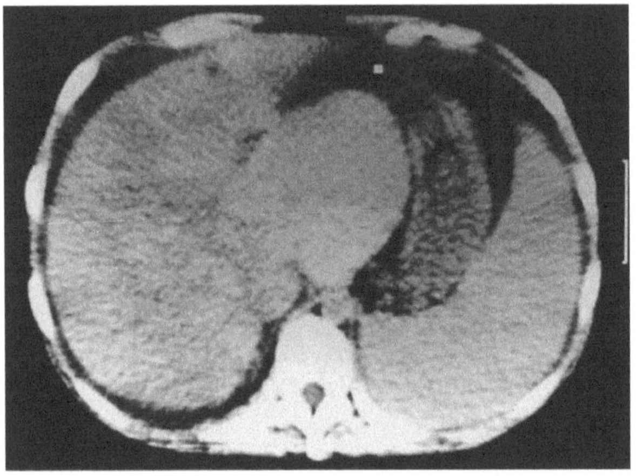

Fig. 7

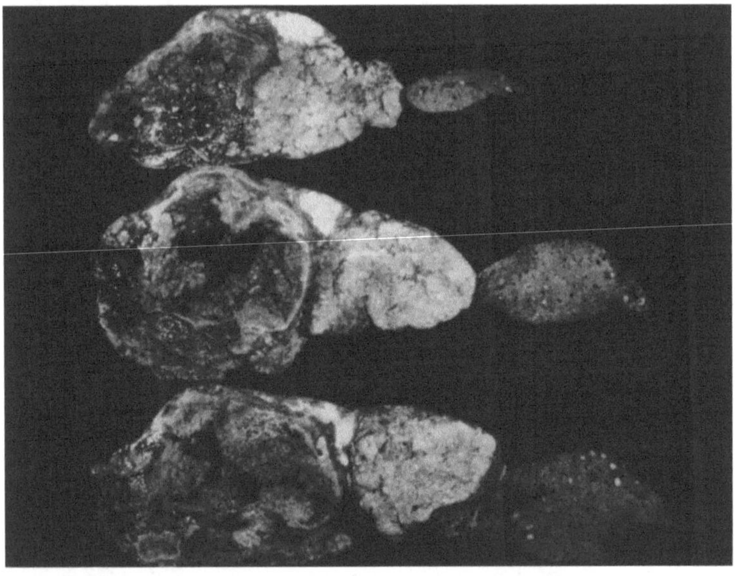

▲ Fig. 8

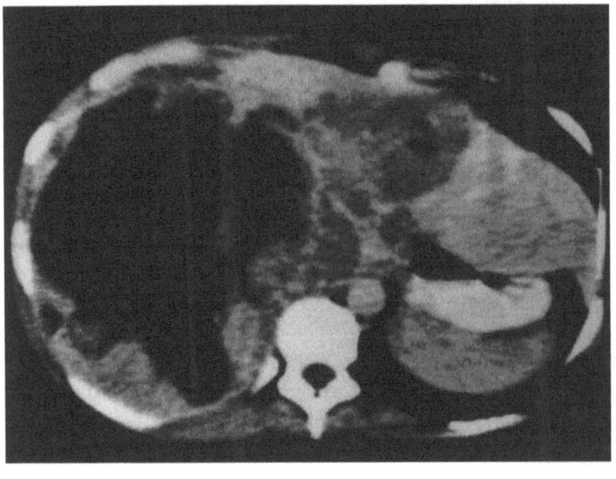

◄ Fig. 9

Figs. 8, 9. Tumour necrosis in specimen and scan

also from dilated ducts by virtue of the shape of distended ducts, usually associated with obstruction. Contrast enhancement has been of value in this respect. Tumour necrosis may be responsible also for changes observed where diaphragm sometimes overlies tumour in the right lobe. In several instances the diaphragm was adherent to the tumour and the decision was taken to resect a small portion with the underlying resected liver. The

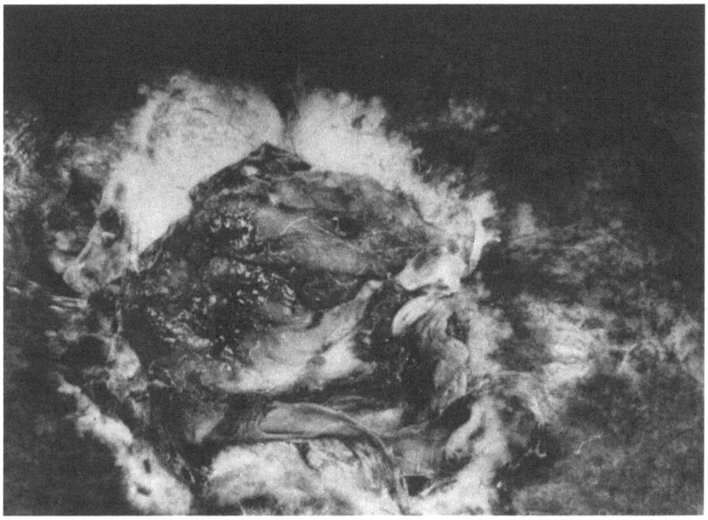

▲ **Fig. 10.** Liver resection with adherent diaphragm

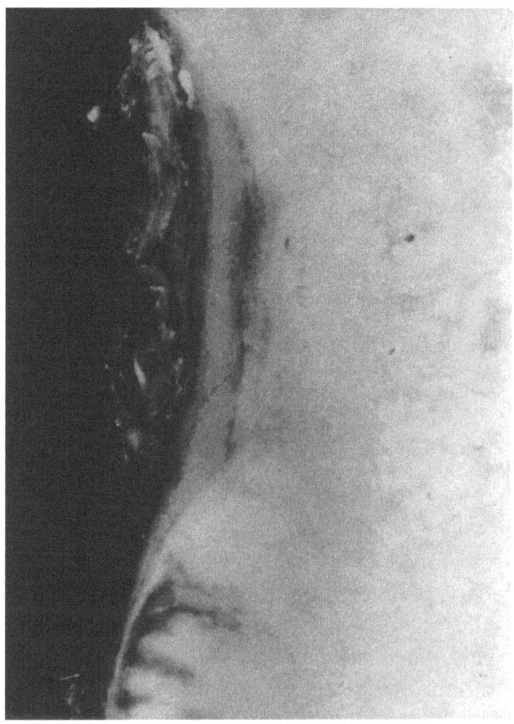

Fig. 11. Slice though diaphragm and underlying liver

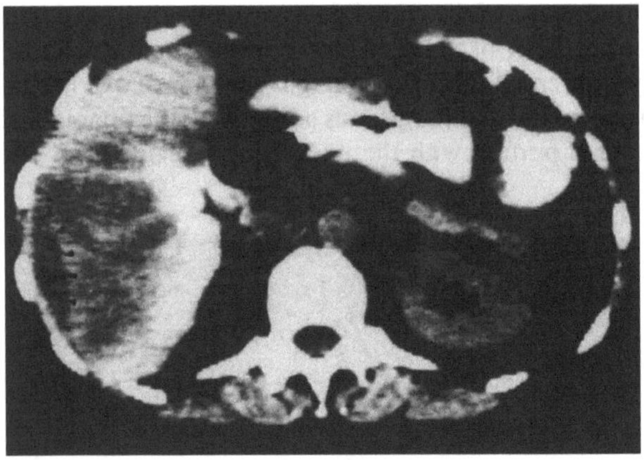

Fig. 12. Computed tomography scan through diaphragm and attached liver

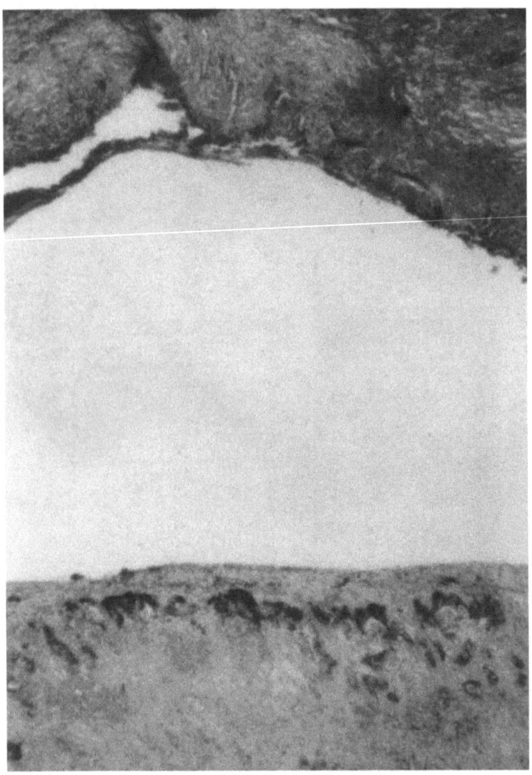

Fig. 13. Section through diaphragm and liver showing granulation tissue

scan image of this region was characteristic, a hypodense region forming a bipointed oval shape reminiscent of a eucalyptus leaf (Figs. 10–13). At first this was construed as a focus of tumour invasion of the diaphragm, but after examination of the resection in several patients, it became clear that the diaphragm was adherent to the umbilicated concavity of the tumour metastasis, the adhesion usually representing an organising process and not due to invasion by malignant tumour (Fig. 13). So far this image has indicated inflammation,

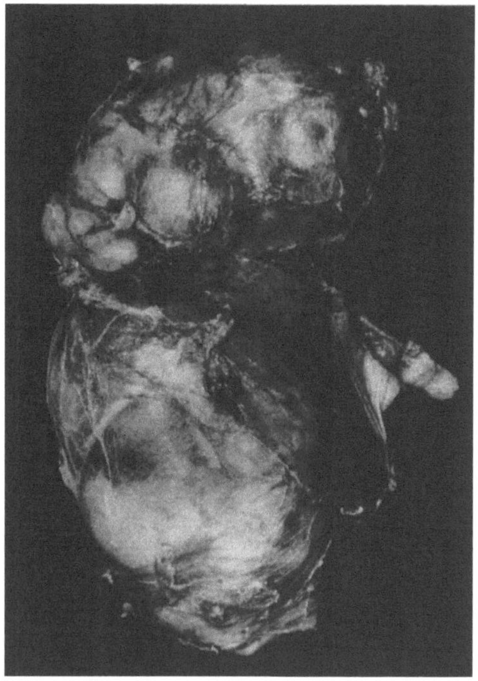

Fig. 14. Leiomyoma of inferior vena cava (resected)

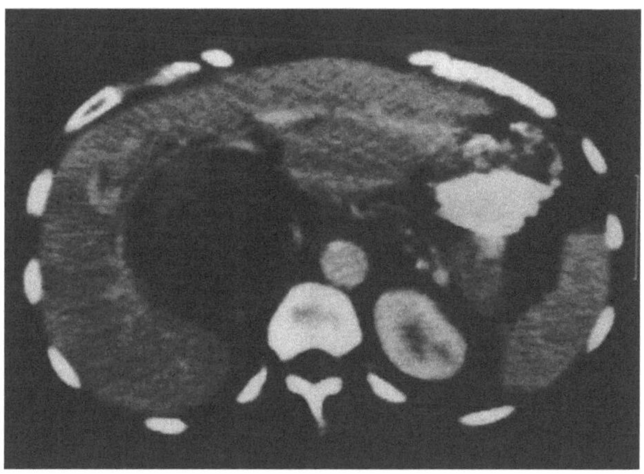

Fig. 15. Computed tomography scan from the same patient as in Fig. 14

but our experience is still limited. In each instance, the tumour was umbilicated and its deeper part was necrotic. On reflection, this perhaps is what ought to have been anticipated, as it is commonplace for tumours to undergo ischaemic necrosis and for necrosis to stimulate an overlying surface inflammatory reaction which after the exsudative phase is organised with formation of fibrous tissue. The outlined sequence is postulated only, but the observations are confirmed in several instances that diaphragmatic adherence does not necessarily indicate tumour invasion. If other cases are similar then it will be encouraging that this sign on the scan may not contraindicate resection therapy on the basis of spread outside the liver.

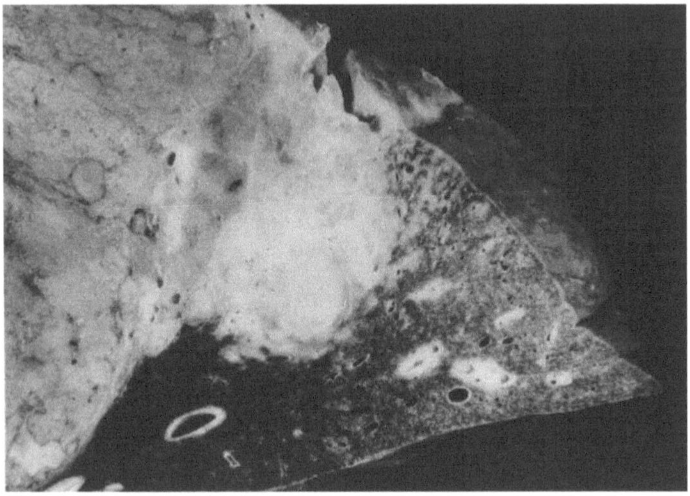

Fig. 16. Focal fibrosis in fibrolamellar carcinoma

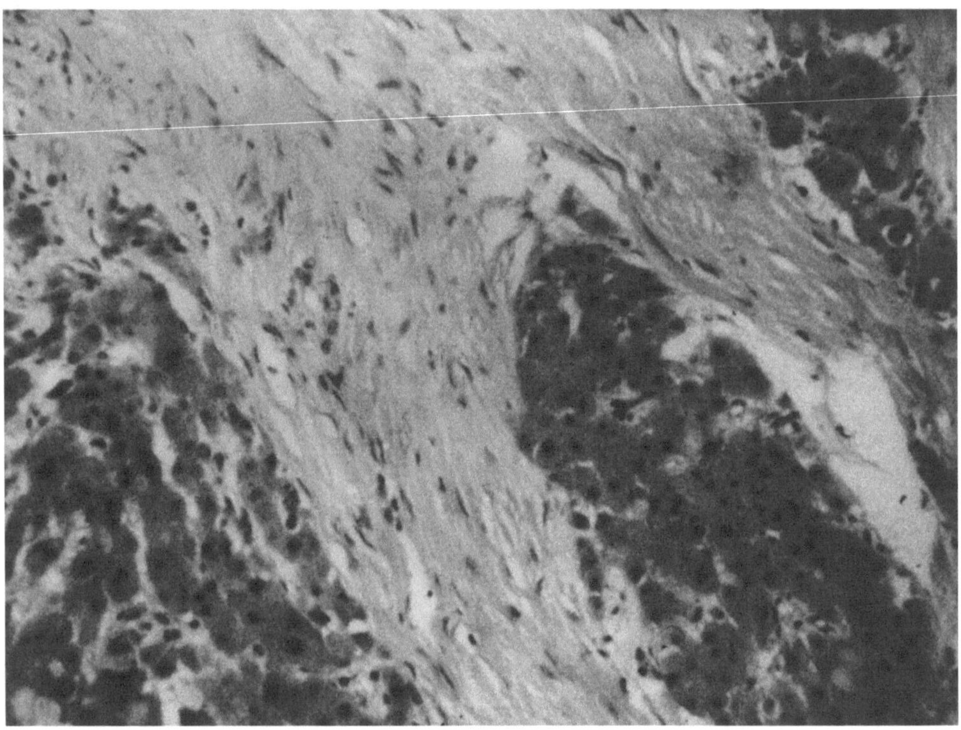

Fig. 17. Section of fibrous region. H & E, × 120

Extrahepatic tumours

Some difficulty has been encountered in extrahepatic tumour masses. Of five such masses, three arising from the posterior abdominal wall, one from the right kidney and one from the inferior vena cava were all recognisable at one or other end of the scan series where liver and tumour were separable. Even isodense images are separable by form, but tumours have usually been hypodense (Figs. 14, 15).

Non-cirrhotic Intrahepatic Primary Tumours

We have not examined primary tumours associated with cirrhosis by this procedure, but have seen two adenomas and ten hepatocellular carcinomas.

The variability of the relationship between tumour cells and fibrous tissue is often not defined by the imaging procedure, but has been highlighted by the dissection procedure adopted in this investigation. In some forms of hepatocellular carcinoma the presence of fibrous tissue is recognised as being an important component by histopathologists [5, 6]. In essence, the combination of large polygonal well-differentiated carcinoma cells and mature fibrous tissue which separates the tumour cells into small islands is regarded as essential for the diagnosis of fibrolamellar hepatocellular carcinoma, and the absence of the fibrous tissue in biopsy material may cause diagnostic difficulty. The use of serial slices has permitted the recognition of the focal nature of the fibrous tissue so that biopsy diagnosis may now be perhaps acceptable on the basis of only the cells (Figs. 16-17).

Acknowledgement: We thank the Department of Radiology for permitting us the use of CT scan films.

References

1. Knopf DR, Torres WE, Fajman WJ, Sones PJ Jr (1982) Liver lesions: comparative accuracy of scintigraphy and computed tomography. AJR 138: 623-627
2. Doppman JL, Dwyer A, Vermess M, Girton M, Sugarbaker P, Miller D, Cornblath M (1984) Segmental hyperlucent defects in the liver. J Comput Assist Tomogr 8: 50-57
3. Scherer U, Santos M, Lisner J (1979) CT studies of the liver in vitro: a report on 82 cases with pathological correlation. J Comput Assist Tomogr 3: 589-595
4. Hosoki T, Toyonaga Y, Araki Y, Mori S (1984) Dynamic computed tomography of isodense hepatocellular carcinoma. J Comput Assist Tomogr 8: 262-268
5. Craig JR, Peters RL, Edmundson HA, Omata M (1980) Fibrolamellar carcinoma of the liver. Cancer 46: 372-379
6. Berman MM, Libby NP, Foster JH (1980) Hepatocellular carcinoma. Polygonal cell type with fibrous stroma - an atypical variant with a favourable prognosis. Cancer 46: 1448-1455

Tumour Markers in the Diagnosis and Management of Patients with Hepatocellular Carcinoma

P. J. Johnson

Liver Unit, King's College Hospital, London SE5 8RS, Great Britain

It is important to recognise from the outset that the criteria on which the value of a tumour marker is based are quite different in respect of diagnosis and management. In this context we mean by management monitoring of response to therapy. With regards diagnosis we are concerned about the specificity and sensitivity of the marker whereas in monitoring therapy the diagnosis has been established and the main requirement of a tumour marker is only that it should be quantitatively related to the viable tumour cell mass. The second concept which is often overlooked is that the value of a marker must be assessed in the appropriate clinical setting. Thus, in the case of hepatocellular carcinoma (HCC), if our putative marker is positive in acute viral hepatitis as well as in HCC, it is of little consequence as there is no difficulty in clinical practice in distinguishing between these two conditions. On the other hand if our marker was also positive in uncomplicated cirrhosis, a condition which it is important and otherwise difficult to distinguish from HCC, the value of the marker would be severely limited. It must also be remembered that a marker which appears very specific having, say, a false-positive rate of 1:100 may still be of limited value if the condition which it diagnoses is expected to occur in only 1:100 cases tested. This again emphasises the need for the marker to be assessed in the appropriate setting – in this case a prospective clinical trial.

Diagnosis of Hepatocellular Carcinoma

There are two main clinical situations in which a serum marker is required and in which any putative marker must be tested. First, does a particular patient, known to have cirrhosis, have a complicating hepatocellular carcinoma? This question would usually have arisen when the patient developed symptoms such as diuretic-resistant ascites or abdominal pain, but it is becoming increasingly well recognised that HCC may, by tumour marker screening, be diagnosed a presymptomatic stage. With increasing interest being shown in the resection of small tumours even in a cirrhotic liver this assumes considerable importance. The second clinical setting is the patient with scan or clinical evidence of a space-occupying lesion within the liver where the clinician wants to know, is this a primary liver tumour as opposed to a secondary tumour or a benign lesion?

By far the most important marker is serum alpha-fetoprotein (AFP), the basic biology of which has been extensively reviewed [2, 16]. Radioimmunoassays which can detect this protein in normal individuals (1–10 ng/ml) are now widely available. Differences be-

Recent Results in Cancer Research. Vol 100

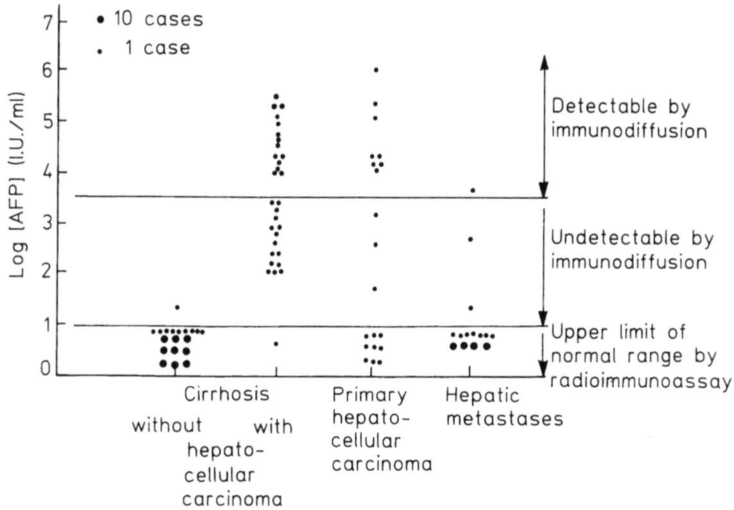

Fig. 1. Value of serum AFP in diagnosing HCC in patients with cirrhosis and distinguishing between primary and secondary hepatic neoplasms

tween patients with and without tumour are thus quantitative not qualitative (Fig. 1). Levels above the normal range are seen in approximately 85% of patients bearing HCC within a cirrhotic liver [13]. In patients with uncomplicated cirrhosis the figure is usually less than 5% but has been reported as being as high as 42% [4]. This is probably due to differences in the composition of the cirrhotic group. In most workers' experience the false-positive results occur mainly in patients with untreated chronic active hepatitis - a condition in which the need for distinction from HCC seldom arises. When this group are excluded the figure is consistently less than 5%. As emphasised earlier, although these figures suggest that AFP would be useful in differential diagnosis, this can only be determined in a prospective clinical study.

In a recent study we measured serum AFP in over 450 patients with biopsy-proven cirrhosis of various etiologies in whom there were no clinical findings or symptoms to suggest the diagnosis of HCC. Patients were followed up until death or for the minimum of 2 years. An elevated level of AFP (> 10 ng/ml) was detected in 63 patients in whom 20 were diagnosed as having HCC, and there were thus 43 false-positive results, which were mainly in patients with chronic active hepatitis. From these data it is possible to determine the sensitivity, specificity and predictive accuracy of the test at various cut-off points. Sensitivity fell from 86% at 10 ng/ml to 62% at 500 ng/ml and specificity rose from 91% at 10 ng/ml to 100% at 500 ng/ml. At the same cut-off points predictive accuracy was 91% and 98% respectively. Thus an AFP level of greater than 500 ng/ml in the setting of cirrhosis was, in our series, diagnostic of HCC development.

Serum AFP levels are elevated in about 50% of HCC patients without cirrhosis and 10% of those with gastrointestinal tumours and metastatic liver disease [9]. However, since, at least in the West, metastatic disease greatly outnumbers cases of HCC, measurement of AFP has little value in practice in distinguishing primary from secondary liver tumour (Fig. 1).

Management

Once the tumour has been diagnosed as hepatocellular carcinoma tumour, markers may be used to monitor response to chemotherapy, resection or transplantation [10]. In the absence of effective therapy serum AFP levels rise exponentially with time, the doubling time being of the order of 40 days (range 6–120 days [5, 15]). With complete surgical removal of the tumour levels fall to the normal range with a half-life of about 4 days, though it should be noted that it does not follow that achieving the normal range necessarily means that all the tumour has been removed. With effective chemotherapy levels also fall. This permits in vivo testing of multiple drugs. Thus the patient may be given a particular chemotherapeutic agent for a short period and the effect of serum AFP observed. If levels fall then chemotherapy should be continued whereas a continued rise indicates that the tumour is resistant and another drug may be tried. This avoids prolonged ineffective and potentially toxic chemotherapy [6] (Fig. 2).

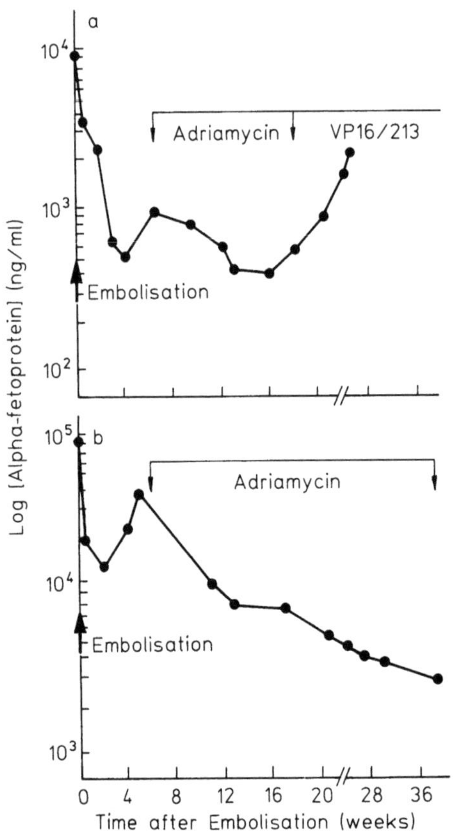

Fig. 2a, b. AFP levels as an indicator for the effectiveness of different therapeutic approaches. **a** Embolisation led to an extensive tumour necrosis shown by falling AFP levels. Continuing therapy with Adriamycin lead to a transient fall in AFP level. After AFP levels rose, therapy with VP 16/213 was initiated, but a further rise in AFP showed the tumour was resistant to this drug. **b** After initial embolisation of the tumour, necrosis occurred, but a rise in AFP levels gave signal of renewed tumour growth. Therapy with Adriamycin led to a continuous fall in AFP levels, indicating tumour regression and effective treatment

Serum levels of AFP may be of prognostic value. A normal AFP level at presentation is associated with a relatively good prognosis. The primary factor predicting better prognosis, however, is probably the absence of cirrhosis, and a normal AFP simply means that the patient is unlikely to have underlying cirrhosis [7]. A rapid AFP doubling time is also a bad prognostic sign [5]. Currently efforts are being made in several units to develop methods of distinguishing between normal and HCC-derived AFP using monoclonal antibodies or on the basis of differential reactivity with various lectins [1]. If successful such approaches could greatly increase the sensitivity and specificity of the test.

Markers Other than AFP

In the specific histological variant of hepatocellular carcinoma, fibrolamellar carcinoma, which affects young people, occurs in a non-cirrhotic liver and is invariably AFP negative, two serum markers have been described. These are vitamin B_{12}-binding protein [14] and neurotensin [1 a], and both may be used to monitor response to therapy. There are HCC-specific isoenzymes of alkaline phosphatase [3] and gamma glutamyl transpeptidase [8] which may make a major impact when quantitative assays become available. Abnormal serum levels of carcinoembryonic antigen and ferritin occur in patients with HCC but are probably not tumour related but simply reflect the underlying chronic liver disease [11, 12].

References

1. Aoyagi Y, Honma A, Suzuki Y, Isemura M, Ichida T, Sasaki H, Ichida F (1984) Measurement of molecular variants of human α-fetoprotein in differential reactivity with lectins and its use in the diagnosis of hepatocellular carcinoma. International Association for Study of the Liver Abstracts, no 184, Berne

1 a. Collier NA, Bloom SR, Hodgson HJF, Weinbren K, Lee YC, Blumgart LH (1984) Neurotensin secretion by fibrolamellar carcinoma of the liver. Lancet I: 538

2. Gitlin D (1975) Normal biology of α-fetoprotein. Ann NY Acad Sci 259: 7-16

3. Higashino K, Ohtani R, Kudo S, Hashinotsume M, Hada T, Kang K-Y, Ohkotchi T, Takahashi Y, Yamamura Y (1975) Hepatocellular carcinoma and a variant alkaline phosphatase. Ann Intern Med 83: 74-78

4. Hirai H, Nishi S, Watabe H (1973) Radioimmunoassay of α-fetoprotein. Protides Biol Fluids 20: 579-587

5. Johnson PJ, Williams R (1980) Serum alpha-fetoprotein estimations and doubling time in hepatocellular carcinoma: influence of therapy and possible value in early detection. J Natl Cancer Inst 64: 1329-1332

6. Johnson PJ, Williams R, Thomas H, Sherlock S, Murray-Lyon IM (1978) Induction of remission in hepatocellular carcinoma with doxorubicin. Lancet 1: 1006-1009

7. Johnson PJ, Melia WM, Palmer MK, Portmann B, Williams R (1981) Relationship between serum alpha-fetoprotein cirrhosis and survival in hepatocellular carcinoma. Br J Cancer 44: 502-505

8. Kojima J, Kanatani M, Makamura M (1980) Electrophoretic fractionation of serum GGTP in human hepatic cancer. Clin Chim Acta 106: 165-170

9. McIntire KR, Waldmann TA, Moertel CG, Go VLM (1975) Serum α-fetoprotein in patients with neoplasms of the gastrointestinal tract. Cancer Res 35: 991-996

10. McIntire KR, Vogel CL, Primack A, Waldmann TA, Kyalwazi SK (1976) Effect of surgical and chemotherapeutic treatment on alpha-fetoprotein levels in patients with hepatocellular carcinoma. Cancer 37: 677-683

11. Melia WM, Johnson PJ, Carter S, Munro-Neville A, Williams R (1981) Plasma carcinoembryonic antigen in the diagnosis and management of patients with hepatocellular carcinoma. Cancer 48: 1004-1008
12. Melia WM, Bullock S, Johnson PJ, Williams R (1983) Serum ferritin in hepatocellular carcinoma. Cancer 51: 2112-2115
13. Melia WM, Wilkinson ML, Portmann BL, Johnson PJ, Williams R (1984) Hepatocellular carcinoma in the non-cirrhotic liver: a comparison with that complicating cirrhosis. Q J Med 53: 391-400
14. Paradinas FJ, Melia WM, Wilkinson ML, Portmann B, Johnson PJ, Murray-Lyon IM, Williams R (1982) High serum B_{12} binding capacity as a marker of the fibrolamellar variant of hepatocellular carcinoma. Br Med J 285: 840-842
15. Purves LR (1973) Primary liver cancer in man as a possible short duration seasonal cancer. S Afr J Med Sci 40: 163-178
16. Sell S, Becker FF (1978) Alpha-fetoprotein. J Natl Cancer Inst 60: 19-26

Cancer Detection by Immunoscintigraphy, Selection, and Clinical Application of Monoclonal Anti-CEA Antibodies and Their F(ab')₂ or Fab Fragments

J.-P. Grob, J.-P. Mach, F. Buchegger, M. Schreyer, F. Mosimann, A. Besson, J. Pettavel, V. von Fliedner, A. Bischof-Delaloye, and B. Delaloye

Ludwig Institute for Cancer Research, Unit of Human Cancer Immunology, 1066 Epalinges/Lausanne, Switzerland

Introduction

The concept of using radiolabeled antibodies capable of localizing the hidden cancer cells [14] has been revitalized by the discovery of the monoclonal antibody (Mab) technology [9]. This discovery has not yet led to the identification of absolutely specific tumor antigens, but has allowed the selection of perfectly homogeneous Mabs which bind with high affinity to tumor-associated markers.

In this review, we shall describe how we selected individual Mabs directed against carcinoembryonic antigen (CEA) [5], which did not cross-react with granulocytes and gave the best tumor localization in the model of nude mice grafted with human colon carcinoma [8, 13]. Using this model, we also demonstrated the superiority of $F(ab')_2$ and particularly Fab fragments from high-affinity Mabs for the localization of relatively small tumor nodules [1]. These Mab fragments were also successfully used in a retrospective clinical study, for the detection of primary and metastatic colorectal carcinomas [4].

The quality of tumor images observed was also due to the optimal energy of the ^{123}I isotope used for labeling the Mab fragments and to the three-dimensional localization of tumor by emission computed tomography (ECT).

In Vitro Screening of Anti-CEA Mab

More than 30 hybridomas producing antibodies binding to CEA were screened, first in vitro by the criteria of high affinity for CEA and low cross-reactivity for granulocytes glycoproteins called NGP [12] or NCA [3]. The affinities measured in 0.15 *M* phosphate-buffered saline for Mabs 192, 35, 202, and 23 were 1.8×10^{10}, 6.5×10^9, 1.9×10^9, and 5.7×10^8 M^{-1}, respectively [8].

When tested by immunoprecipitation with CEA and with semipurified glycoproteins cross-reacting with CEA, the six representative anti-CEA Mabs gave the results summarized schematically in Fig. 1.

Three Mabs, 35, 115, and 73, reacted exclusively with purified CEA; one Mab, 47, reacted with CEA and a glycoprotein of 95 (NCA-95); one Mab reacted with CEA and a glycoprotein of 55 (NCA-55); and one Mab, 202, reacted with CEA and both NCA-95 and NCA-55 [2]. When tested by direct binding on fresh granulocytes or by indirect immunoperoxidase on frozen tissue sections, only Mabs 35, 115, and 73 did not react with

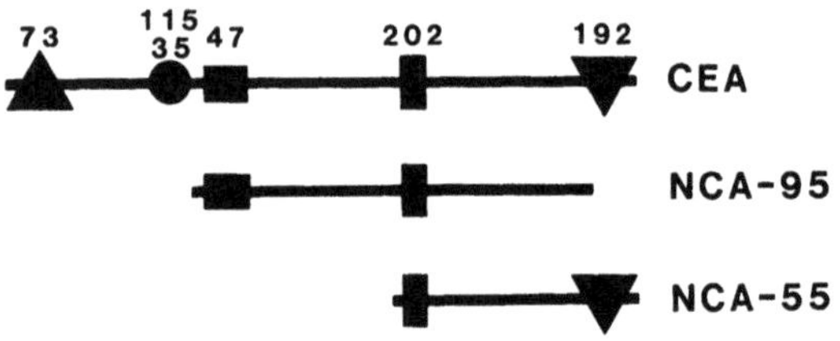

Fig. 1. The five different antigenic determinants recognized by six representative anti-CEA Mabs on the CEA, NCA-95, and NCA-55 molecules. [2]

granulocytes, whereas Mabs 47, 202, and 192 reacted with the surface and the cytoplasm of these cells. Furthermore, Mabs 192 and 202 reacted with bronchiolar and alveolar epithelial cells from normal lung.

These results show that, even when one immunizes with a purified antigen such as CEA, one often obtains Mab cross-reacting with other proteins. That is why the in vitro screening on frozen tissue sections, on fresh cells, and when possible on radiolabeled proteins is essential before using antibodies for immunoscintigraphy or drug targeting.

Mab Selection in Nude Mice Grafted with Human Carcinoma

The model of nude mice heterografted with human tumors has the advantage of testing the capacity of antibodies to reach and bind the antigenic determinants accessible in a living tumor tissue. In that sense it represents the best experimental model for a last selection of Mabs before they can be used in patients. However, one should remember that this experimental model also has precise limitations since in a nude mouse grafted with a human tumor the only human tissue is the tumor and there is no counterpart for the normal human tissues.

For instance, in nude mice grafted with the human colon carcinoma Co-112 [13] we obtained excellent localization with Mabs 192 and 202 [8] but there were limitations in using these Mabs in patients because of their reactivity with granulocytes.

As an example of negative selection, we observed that Mab 73, which was among the most specific Mab in vitro, did not localize well in human colon carcinoma grafted in nude mice. Finally, Mabs 35 and 115 were selected for their excellent specificity in vitro and good tumor localization in vivo.

Tumor Localization of Mab Fragments Tested in Nude Mice

$F(ab')_2$ and Fab fragments from Mabs 35, 115, and 202 were prepared and tested for their capacity to localize, in the human colon carcinoma, Co-112 grafted in nude mice [5]. Groups of four to seven mice were injected simultaneously with ^{131}I-labeled Mab or fragments and with normal IgG or their corresponding fragments labeled with ^{125}I. The mice were dissected 2–5 days later. The results obtained with Mab 35 and expressed as a percentage of the total radioactivity recovered for each isotope per gram tumor and normal tissue are shown in Fig. 2.

It is evident that the ratios of tumor to normal organ antibody concentration increase dramatically with the use of fragments. These ratios were 7 for intact Mab, 25 for $F(ab')_2$, and 85 for Fab. The specificity indices calculated by dividing the tumor to normal organ ratios obtained for antibody by the corresponding ratio obtained for control IgG were 3.4 for intact Mab, 8.2 for $F(ab')_2$, and 19 for Fab [1].

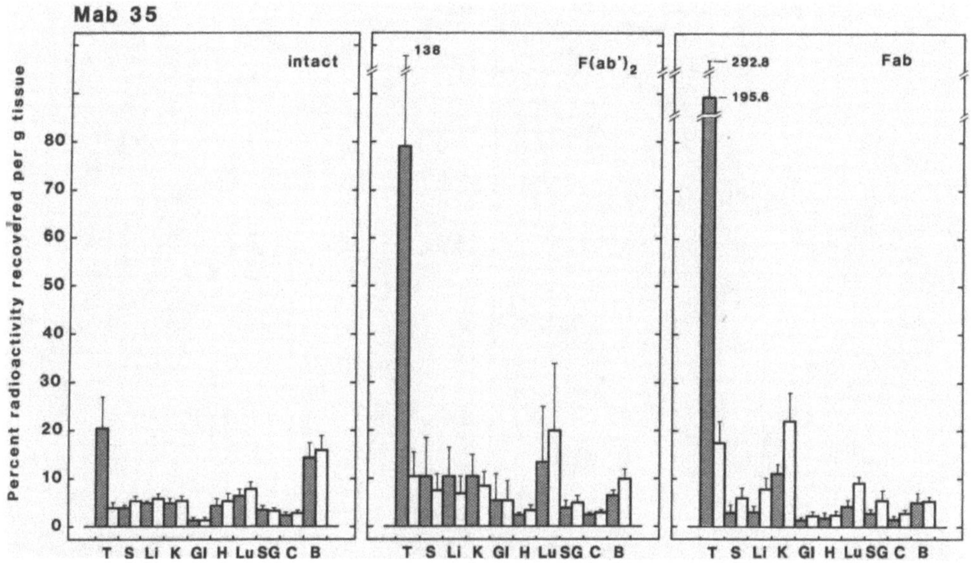

Fig. 2. Distribution of Mab 35 or its fragments *(shaded bars)* and control IgG or fragments *(open bars)* injected simultaneously into nude mice bearing grafts of a human carcinoma. The *vertical lines* represent the standard deviations calculated from groups of four to seven animals per Mab or fragment. *T*, tumor; *S*, spleen; *Li*, liver; *K*, kidneys; *GI*, gastrointestinal tract; *H*, heart; *Lu*, lungs; *SG*, salivary glands; *C*, carcass and head; *B*, blood. [1]

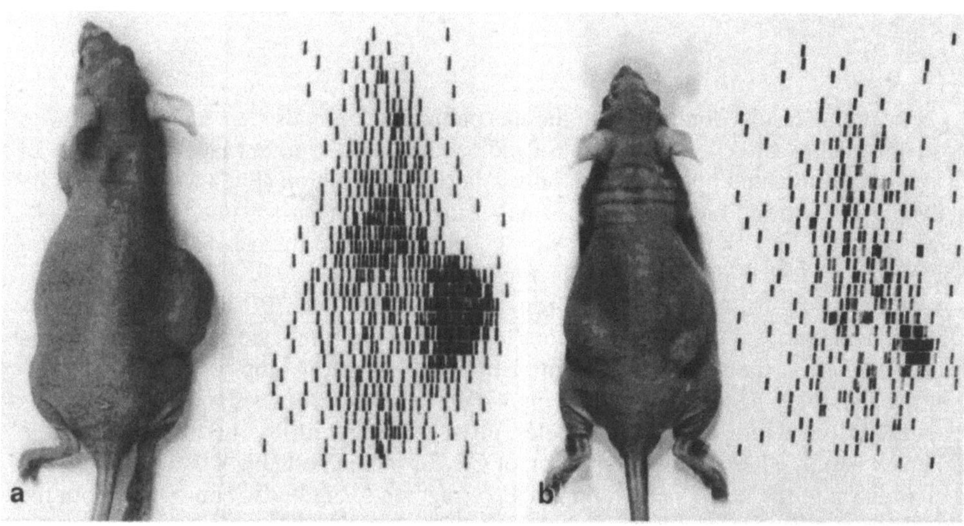

Fig. 3 a, b. Nude mice bearing grafts of the human colon carcinoma Co-112 [13] and corresponding whole body scans. In **a**, the scan was obtained 3 days after injection of intact ^{131}I-labeled Mab 35 and the detected tumor weighed 1.2 g. In **b**, the scan was obtained 2 days after injection of ^{131}I-labeled Fab fragments of Mab 35 and the detected tumor weighed 0.1 g

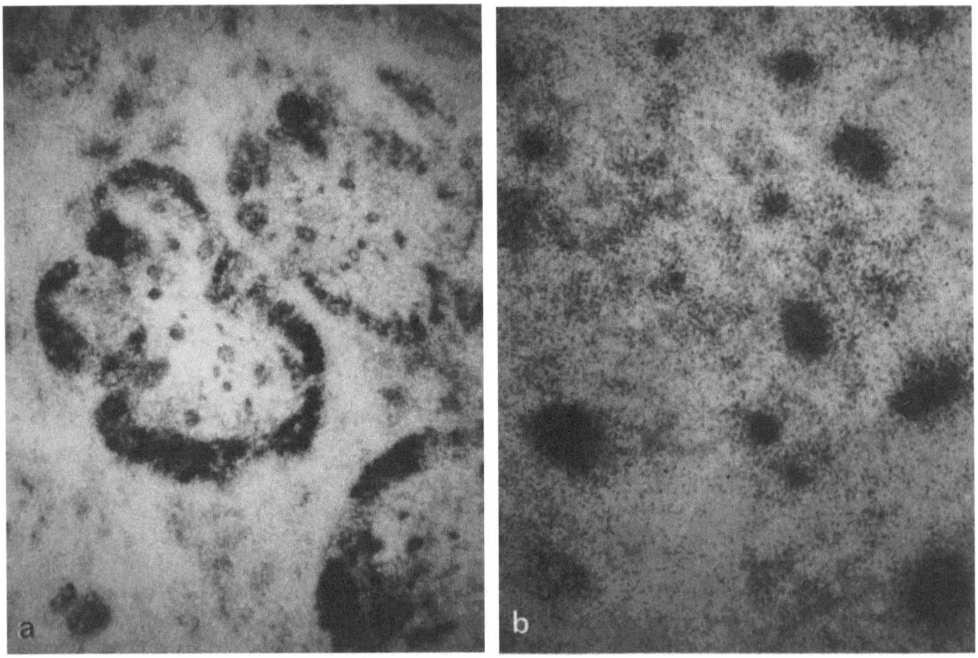

Fig. 4 a, b. Autoradiographs of 8-μm frozen sections from the human colon carcinoma Co-112 grafted in nude mice, obtained 3 days after injection of either intact Mab 35 *(left)* or its Fab fragments *(right)* both labeled with I-125. The *small dots* and *dark areas* correspond to the silver grains due to the radioactivity localized in vivo, whereas the *light staining* corresponds to the immunoperoxidase reaction obtained by incubating the tissue sections with anti-CEA Mab and the avidin-biotin system. **a** × 200, **b** × 400

The scanning results obtained with these experimental animals were in agreement with those obtained by direct measurement of radioactivity. With intact Mab, tumor grafts of 0.5–1 g gave contrasted positive scans only 3 days after injection (Fig. 3 A), whereas fragments of Mab allowed the detection of smaller tumors at an earlier time. The best results were obtained with Fab fragments of Mab 35, which allowed the clear detection of a tumor graft of 0.1 g 48 h after injection [1] (Fig. 3 B).

Autoradiographs of tumor sections from mouse injected with ^{125}I-labeled intact Mabs and fragments showed first that they both localized in the tumor nodules and not in the stromal connective tissue of mouse origin. However, the intact Mabs were localized mostly at the periphery of tumor nodules (Fig. 4 A), whereas the $F(ab')_2$ and Fab fragments penetrated deeper into the tumor nodules, often reacting with the pseudolumen of the malignant glands where the concentration of CEA is the highest (Fig. 4 B).

In addition to the better penetration of Fab fragments, Fig. 4 also shows that both the intact Mab and Fab fragments gave a patchy distribution of radioactivity in malignant tissues, with areas of intense radioactivity and others with almost no radioactivity. These results indicate that if this type of antibodies were to be used for radioimmunotherapy [4] it would be necessary to select an isotope capable of destroying tumor cells within a radius of 100–1000 μm.

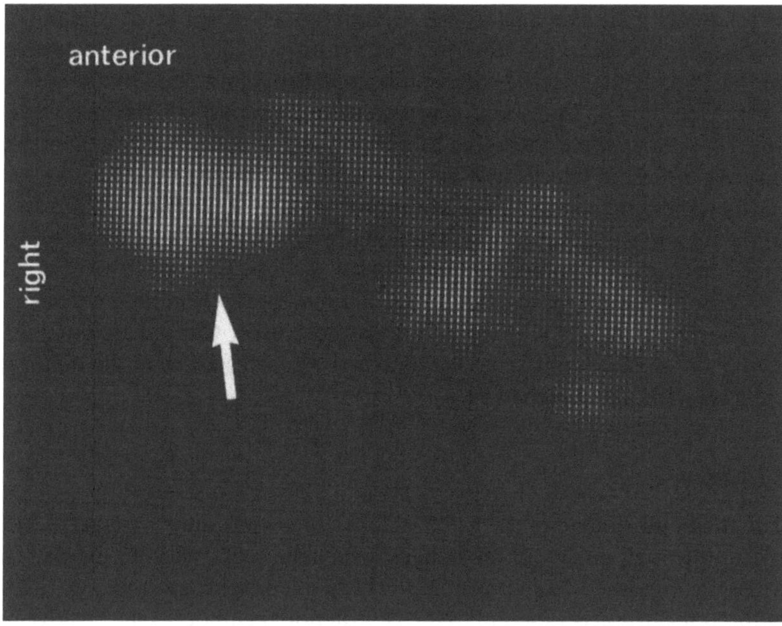

Fig. 5. Emission computed tomography transverse section of the upper part of the pelvis, obtained in a patient with a right colon carcinoma, 48 h after injection of ^{123}I-labeled Fab fragments of Mab 35. The section is shown from below; thus the major area of radioactive uptake *(arrow)* corresponds to the primary colon carcinoma located in the right anterior part of the abdomen. The two symmetrical small radioactive spots correspond to the two iliac vessels detected just below the bifurcation of the aorta

Detection of Carcinoma in Patients Using ^{123}I-Labeled Mab Fragments and ECT

Based on the above experimental results, we tested a series of 23 patients with colorectal carcinoma after injection of $F(ab')_2$ and Fab fragments of Mab 35 labeled with ^{123}I. This isotope, which has a very favorable energy of 159 keV and a relatively short physical period of 13.2 h, proved to be excellent for tomoscintigraphy. ^{123}I was prepared from the ^{127}I(p,5n) ^{123}Xe reaction and provided by the Swiss Federal Institut for Reactor Research at Würenlingen, Switzerland. Using a Siemens dual-head rotating camera, tomographic studies of the pelvis and upper abdomen were performed in all patients at 6 and 24 h after injection and in the majority of patients at 48 h. Other parts of the body such as the thorax and bones were studied only when there was a clinical suspicion of tumor in these areas or when an abnormal radioactive uptake was detected on the whole body scan systematically performed before the tomographic studies. No subtraction techniques were used, but additional scintigraphic studies of the liver with ^{99m}Tc sulfur colloid were regularly performed after the last ^{123}I analysis of the upper abdomen, with the patient remaining in the same position. Sulfur colloid scintigraphy allowed us to identify anatomical landmarks and in some cases to compare filling defects of ^{99m}Tc sulfur colloid with areas of increased ^{123}I antibody uptake.

The overall sensitivity of tumor detection in our series of 23 patients was rather high. In the 13 patients injected with $F(ab')_2$ fragments labeled with ^{123}I, 23 out of 28 tumor sites were detected by ECT. This includes 6/6 primary or recurrent localized carcinomas,

5/8 patients with liver metastases, 0/2 lung metastases (of less than 2 cm diameter and with stable size during a 10-month follow-up) and 12/12 bone metastases (in 2 patients). In the 10 patients injected with Fab fragments, 30 out of 31 tumor sites were detected by ECT, including 6/7 primary or recurrent carcinomas, 6/6 patients with liver metastases, and 18/18 bone metastases (in a single patient). We realize that this very high sensitivity is due in part to the selection of patients with known tumors and to the relatively large size of the tumors detected. The smallest primary tumor detected was a carcinomatous polyp of the rectum weighing 4.5 g and the smallest liver metastases detected were less than 3 cm in diameter as determined by the CT scan.

Figure 5 shows a representative ECT transverse section obtained 48 h after injection of ^{123}I-labeled Fab of Mab 35 in a 76-year-old patient with a carcinoma of the right colon. The major area of radioactive uptake (arrow) corresponds to the tumor, which was surgically resected and weighed 33 g.

Discussion

The major advantage of the use of tomoscintigraphy and ^{123}I-labeled Mab fragment consists in the high quality of the images, which enables tumor accumulation of radioactivity to be distinguished from physiological organ concentration and circulating radioactivity without the artifacts inherent to the subtraction technique. Our positive results in terms of sensitivity should be confirmed in a prospective study in order to prove that this type of immunotomoscintigraphy can compete with the most modern morphological diagnostic methods such as CT scan and nuclear magnetic resonance. Our impression is that for diagnostic purposes Fab fragments of Mab with high affinity for a relatively abundant tumor marker such as CEA represent the best tracer presently available. If one considers the use of Mab for therapy, either by drug targeting or by radiolabeled antibodies, however, the strategy might be different. Fab fragments with their single binding site and their rapid renal excretion may not be optimal and should be replaced by $F(ab')_2$. For drug targeting, a double binding site is probably necessary to provoke internalization. Also for drug targeting, a tumor marker which is more diffusely distributed on the membrane of the malignant cells and not only on their apical side would be more favorable.

Concerning radioimmunotherapy, only three groups have reported results. The group of Order [11] has used semipurified polyclonal antibodies against CEA and ferritin, labeled with therapeutic doses of ^{131}I to treat biliary tract carcinoma and hepatoma, respectively. The moderately optimistic results obtained may be due to the fact that a high percentage of the injected polyclonal antibodies will always accumulate in the liver and therefore may have some usefulness against these two types of liver tumor. Despite great improvement in the dosimetric analysis of the target organ [11] the specificity of the localization in terms of tumor to normal tissue ratios remains difficult to evaluate. Larson et al. [10] have used intact and Fab fragments of Mab directed against the p-97 melanoma-associated antigen in the treatment of this tumor. Despite the repeated injection of relatively high doses (100 mCi) of ^{131}I, the antitumor effect has been very modest. Recently, a research group from the Hammersmith Hospital has reported on the intra-peritoneal, -pleural, or -pericardial injection of Mab anti-milk fat globule antigen [6], labeled with 20 mCi of ^{131}I, in three patients with different types of carcinomas invading these anatomical cavities [7]. The remissions observed, however, are not numerous enough to conclude that they are due to the specificity of the injected radiolabeled antibodies.

In conclusion, the detection of human cancer by radiolabeled antibodies has markedly improved, thanks to Mab selection and fragmentation as well as to the recent advances in nuclear medicine technology. We do not yet know, however, if the tumor uptake of labeled antibodies, which is useful for diagnosis, may justify the administration of larger amounts of radioactivity bound to Mab for therapy.

References

1. Buchegger F, Haskell CM, Schreyer M, Scazziga BR, Randin S, Carrel S, Mach J-P (1983) Radiolabeled fragments of monoclonal anti-CEA antibodies for localization of human colon carcinoma grafted into nude mice. J Exp Med 158: 413-427
2. Buchegger F, Schreyer M, Carrel S, Mach J-P (1984) Monoclonal antibody identify a CEA cross-reacting antigen of 95 KD (NCA-95) distinct in antigenicity and tissue distribution from the previously described NCA of 55 KD. Int J Cancer 33: 643-649
3. Burtin P, Quan PC, Sabine MC (1975) Nonspecific cross-reacting antigen as a marker for human polymorphs, macrophages and monocytes. Nature 255: 714
4. Delaloye B, Bischof-Delaloye A, Buchegger F, von Fliedner V, Grob FR, Volant J-C, Pettavel J, Mach J-P (1986) Detection of Colorectal Carcinom by Emission-computerized Tomography after injection of ^{123}I-labeled Fab or $F(ab')_2$ Fragments from Monoclonal Anti-Carcinoembryonic Antigen Antibodies. J Clin Invest Vol. 77, January 1986 (in press)
5. Gold P, Freedman SO (1965) Demonstration of tumor-specific antigens in human colonic carcinomata by immunological tolerance and absorption techniques. J Exp Med 121: 439
6. Granowska M, Shepherd J, Britton KE, Ward B, Mather S, Taylor-Papadimitriou J, Epenetos AA, Carroll MJ, Nimmon CC, Hawkins LA, Slevin M, Flatman W, Horne T, Burchell J, Durbin H, Bodmer W (1984) Ovarian cancer: diagnosis using ^{123}I monoclonal antibody in comparison with surgical findings. Nuclear Med Commun 5: 485-499
7. Hammersmith Oncology Group and Imperial Cancer Research Fund (1983) Antibody-guided irradiation of malignant lesions: three cases illustrating a new method of treatment. Lancet I: 1441-1443
8. Haskell CM, Buchegger F, Schreyer M, Carrel S, Mach J-P (1983) Monoclonal antibodies to carcinoembryonic antigen: ionic strength as a factor in the selection of antibodies for immunoscintigraphy. Cancer Res 43: 3857-3864
9. Köhler G, Milstein C (1975) Continous cultures of fused cells secreting antibody of predefined specificity. Nature 256: 455-457
10. Larson SM, Carrasquillo JA, Krohn KA, Brown JP, McGuffin RW, Ferens JM, Graham MM, Hill LD, Beaumier PL, Hellström KE, Hellström I (1983) Localization of 131-I-labeled p97-specific Fab fragments in human melanoma as a basis for radiotherapy. J Clin Invest 72: 2101-2114
11. Leichner PK, Klein JL, Siegelman SS, Ettinger DS, Order SE (1983) Dosimetry of I-131 labeled anti-ferritin in hepatoma: specific activities in the tumor and liver. Cancer Treat Rep 67: 647-6518
12. Mach J-P, Pustaszeri G (1972) Carcinoembryonic antigen (CEA): demonstration of partial identity between CEA and a normal glycoprotein. Immunochemistry 9: 1031
13. Mach J-P, Carrel S, Merenda C, Sordat B, Cerottini J-C (1974) In vivo localisation of radiolabeled antibodies to carcinoembryonic antigen in human colon carcinoma grafted into nude mice. Nature 248: 704-706
14. Mach J-P, Buchegger F, Forni M, Ritschard J, Berche C, Lumbroso JD, Schreyer M, Girardet Ch, Accolla RS, Carrel S (1981) Use of radiolabelled monoclonal anti-CEA antibodies for the detection of human carcinomas by external photoscanning and tomoscintigraphy. Immunol Today 2: 239-249

Proposal for Staging Liver Metastases

L. Gennari, R. Doci, F. Bozzetti, and P. Bignami

Istituto Nazionale per lo Studio e la Cura dei Tumori, Via G. Venezian 1, 20133 Milan, Italy

During the past decade there has been an increasing interest in the diagnosis and treatment of liver metastases. The results of treatment reported in the literature are frequently contradictory because different selection criteria of the patients are adopted. As a consequence the comparison of onc therapy with another is difficult or quite impossible. We should try to overcome these difficulties by adopting a common language among oncologists. In other words, we should be forced to use a worldwide accepted classification of liver metastases.

In 1982 we reviewed the main prognostic factors in liver metastases and the published main staging systems in order to propose a new classification [1]. The application of this classification presently concerns metastases from colorectal carcinoma, which seem to be more responsive to treatment than metastases from other sites or histologic types. The classification proposed in 1982 is shown in Table 1. In spite of some criticism regarding the distribution of liver involvement in three groups, i. e., less than 25%, from 25% to 50%, and more than 50%, we still believe the limit of 50% to be accurate. In fact, in our recent analysis of the prognosis of unresected liver metastases from colorectal cancer (Doci et al. in preparation), the survival of patients with the extent of liver involvement grouped according to the criteria previously mentioned (<25%; 25%-50%, >50%) was significantly different (Fig. 1). The observed significant trend loses the prognostic value if the limit between H_2 and H_3 is fixed at 75% of involvement. As regards the time of diagnosis of liver metastases with respect to the primary, survival was not influenced by the fact that metas-

Table 1. Clinical classification of hepatic metastases [1]

H	Synchronous hepatic metastases
rH	Metachronous hepatic metastases
$(r)H_1$	Liver involvement equal to or less than 25%
$(r)H_2$	Liver involvement between 25% and 50%
$(r)H_3$	Liver involvement more than 50%
s	Single metastasis
m	Multiple monolateral metastases
b	Bilateral metastases (both surgical lobes)
i	Infiltration of contiguous structures or organs
F	Impairment of liver function
c	Presence of cirrhosis

Recent Results in Cancer Research. Vol 100

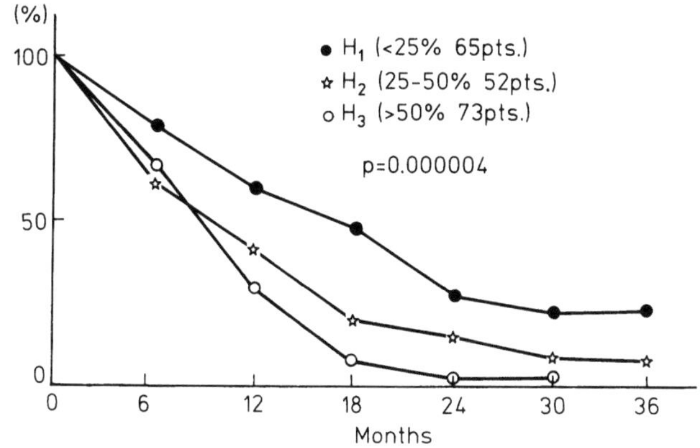

Fig. 1. Actuarial survival of patients with unresected liver metastases from colorectal cancer

tases were synchronous or metachronous; this finding is confirmed by other recent reports. Thus we suggest that the symbol r (recurrence) be excluded from the classification. Moreover, during the 3-year experience we have realized that cirrhosis was a rare finding in patients with liver metastases, so the symbol C can consequently be omitted.

The new simplified classification is presented in Table 2. The proposed classification represents the analytic definition of the main prognostic features of the metastatic disease: the impairment of liver function, the anatomic distribution, and the extent of metastases. Nevertheless, for clinical practice a further simplified system of classification seems necessary. It should maintain the prognostic meaning but also allow planning of the therapeutic approach.

With the aim of achieving these goals, we have combined some groups of the previous classification into a simpler and more comprehensive stage system. This system includes four stages, which are defined in Table 3. The rationale for such a distribution was derived from the analysis of survival, recurrence rate, and distribution of recurrences after hepatic resection or intraarterial chemotherapy of colorectal metastases.

Stage I. When metastatic disease to the liver consists of a single metastasis of limited size, the prognosis is much better: the 5-year survival after surgery ranges from 20% [2] to 42% [3]. In our surgical series the actuarial survival at 3 years of H_{1s} patients is 75% (Fig. 2). In unresected patients the 3-year actuarial survival was 20%. It seems therefore justified to consider, irrespective of treatment results, all patients with single metastasis in the best prognostic stage I. Recurrences were almost equal in local and distant (mainly lung) sites.

Stage II. Patients included in this stage (i.e., H_m, H_b, H_{2s}) had a median postoperative survival ranging from 10 to 14 months and a recurrence rate ranging from 50% to 75% (Table 4). The 2-year actuarial survival of unresected H_{2s}, H_{1m}, and H_{1b} patients was 18%, 20%, and 17% respectively.

Stage III. Patients included in this stage have liver involvement of more than 25% (but with multiple metastases) or more than 50% (independently of the number of lesions). All these patients had a poor prognosis, with a recurrence rate approaching 100% and an almost constant hepatic relapse (Table 5).

Stage IV. The presence of extrahepatic metastases is generally considered a worsening prognostic factor. Even if no consistent data are available about the relationship between

Table 2. Classification of hepatic metastases (1984)

H_1	Liver involvement equal to or less than 25%
H_2	Liver involvement between 25% and 50%
H_3	Liver involvement more than 50%
s	Single metastasis
m	Multiple metastases to one surgical lobe
b	Bilateral metastases
I	Infiltration of adjacent organs or structures
F	Impairment of liver function

Table 3. Proposed staging

Stage		
I	H_{1s}	
II	$H_{1m,b}$	H_{2s}
III	$H_{2m,b}$	$H_{3s,m,b}$
IV	A) "Minimal" intraabdominal extrahepatic disease (detected only at laparotomy)	
	B) Extrahepatic disease	

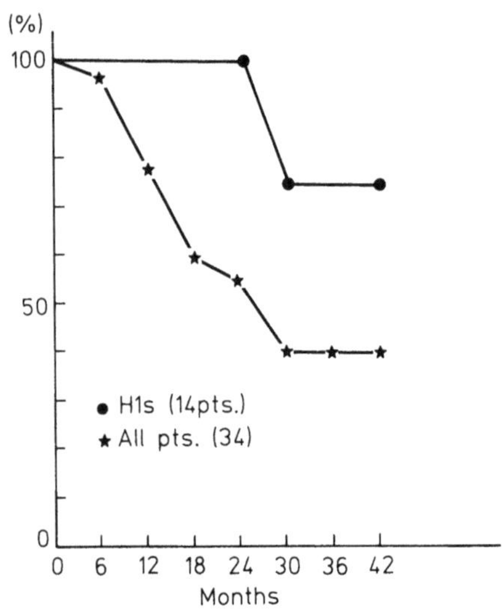

Fig. 2. Actuarial survival of patients with solitary metastasis involving <25% of liver (• H_{1s}) and overall actuarial survival (*) after hepatic resection

the extent of extrahepatic disease and survival, it seems reasonable to distinguish between "minimal" intraabdominal disease discovered only at laparotomy (lymph node metastases, peritoneal implants) and clinically evident growth (peritoneal diffuse carcinosis; lung, bone, soft-tissue metastases). A further analysis is required to confirm the prognostic value of both A and B subgroups.

The prognostic value of the proposed staging system is based on the analysis of our case material, since it is impossible to find confirmation from the other experiences. As previously mentioned, we think that a staging system should also provide some guidelines for

Table 4. Survival and recurrences in stage II patients

	Median survival (months)	% of recurrence		
		Local	Distant	Total
H_{1m}	13.5	75	25	75
H_{1b}	14	50	50	50
H_{2s}	10	-	50	50

Table 5. Survival and recurrences in stage III patients

	Median survival (months)	% of recurrence		
		Local	Distant	Total
H_{2m}	15	40	60	80
H_{2b}	9	100	-	100
H_{3s}	13.5	100	50	100
H_{3m}	8	100	-	100
H_{3b}	23.5	100	-	100

Table 6. Provisional approach to therapy of liver metastases

Stage			Treatment
I	H_{1s}		Resection
II	H_{1m}	H_{2s}	Resection + IHC + (sc?)
	H_{1b}		IHC
III	H_{2m}	$H_{3s,m}$	Resection + IHC + sc
	$H_{2,3b}$		IHC
IV	A		IPC?
	B		sc (new drugs)

IHC, intrahepatic chemotherapy; *sc,* systemic chemotherapy; *IPC,* intraperitoneal chemotherapy

therapy. At present, treatment of hepatic metastases is under intensive investigation and it is obviously impossible to design a therapeutic plan for the different stages. Nevertheless, a hypothetical strategy could be proposed on the basis of the observed site and frequency of recurrences. A provisional multimodal approach is outlined in Table 6. We presently advise only a surgical resection; a recurrence rate of 28% is certainly not low, but the advantages of a postsurgical intrahepatic chemotherapy by portal or arterial route should be balanced against the risks involved in local treatment (surgical risk for positioning of the catheter, complications due to catheter dislodgement, and so on).

In stage II, the surgical resection was followed by either local or distant failure in more than 50% of the cases. Our goal is to improve the disease-free period by giving intrahepatic and perhaps systemic chemotherapy to the resected patients. Patients with bilateral lesions are not suitable for surgery but only for local chemotherapy as a first approach.

Stage III was characterized by the almost total failure of surgery, the value of which is therefore questionable. Nevertheless, resection could have a backup role to facilitate the efficacy of chemotherapy, either local or systemic. In patients with unresectable disease, i.e., in patients with bilateral metastases, we advocate as the first and unique approach a locoregional chemotherapy. Hepatic failure is almost always the cause of death in patients in whom the tumor has extensively invaded the liver. Our goal should be to delay hepatic failure as long as possible.

In stage IV A, i.e., in patients with minimal extrahepatic abdominal disease, intraperitoneal chemotherapy could be performed. Finally, in patients with extraabdominal disease only experimental chemotherapy could be tried.

As regards the criteria of evaluation of responses to treatments, we completely agree with the criteria proposed by Pettavel et al. [4] during the recent meeting in Leiden.

In conclusion, we hope that the present staging system is favorably considered by oncologists and that constructive criticisms and suggestions might lead to a worldwide accepted common language.

References

1. Gennari L, Doci R, Bozzetti F, Veronesi U (1982) Proposal for a clinical classification of liver metastases. Tumori 68: 443-449
2. Foster JH, Berman MM (1977) Solid liver tumours. In: Ebert PA (ed) Major problems in clinical surgery. Saunders, Philadelphia, p 209
3. Wilson SM, Adson MA (1976) Surgical treatment of hepatic metastases from colorectal cancer. Arch Surg 111: 330-334
4. Pettavel T, Leywraz S, Douglas P (1984) The necessity for staging liver metastases and standardizing treatment-response criteria. In: Van de Velde CJH, Sugarbaker PH (eds) Liver metastases. Nijhoff, Dordrecht, p 154

The Staging of Hepatic Metastases Arising from Colorectal Cancer

C. J. H. van de Velde

Department of Surgery, University Hospital, P.O. Box 9600, 2300 RC, Leiden, The Netherlands

Despite over 20 year of intense clinical investigation into the natural history and treatment of hepatic metastases by surgery, chemotherapy, and other treatment modalities, there is no uniform acceptance of any specific treatment. The most important reason for this is obviously that not one treatment has (to date) proved a real breakthrough. All comparisons of treatment results to date have been more or less in vain because the investigators have never referred to standardized criteria for patient selection, magnitude of the metastatic spread, or definition of the responses to the treatment. In fact, the lack of a worldwide accepted classification of liver metastases is responsible for the present difficulty of assessing any treatment in relation to untreated controls. So far no randomized trial including a no-treatment control arm has been reported!

With the advent of many promising new treatment modalities, an increased interest in the surgical (resection) treatment of liver metastases, and a conviction in the value of (multicenter) randomized trials, the need for a uniform staging system becomes more important. It is the purpose of this chapter to review concisely the clinical systems of liver metastasis classification based upon prognostic factors. This will also be related to a proposed International Staging System for Hepatic Metastases. This system was the result of a workshop devoted to this problem [1] and was subsequently simultaneously proposed at the Heidelberg and Houston conferences in September 1984.

A Survey of Staging Systems and Prognostic Factors

The lack of a uniformly accepted staging system has forced authors reporting a specific liver metastases treatment regimen retrospectively to use prognostic variables noted in a historical control group, thus creating institutional staging systems [2]. As long as the results of treatments of patients with two to three small metastases are compared with the results obtained in patients where 80% of the liver volume is replaced by metastatic deposits, assessment of the results will remain extremely difficult to interpret. The overall median survival of patients with untreated liver metastases due to colorectal cancer is in the order of 5 months [3]. The median survival time, however, is not a true indication of survival time as considerable variation exists in the extremes of each group. The lack of uniform reporting of treatment results was noticed by Pettavel as early as 1967 [4], when he proposed the Lausanne classification of liver metastases, which stages them into four stages according to the size of the metastases, liver function, and the presence of hepatomegaly.

Recent Results in Cancer Research. Vol 100

Table 1. Lausanne classification (1984)

Stage I:	PHR less than 25% with stratification F, S, FS
Stage II:	PHR from 25% to 75% with stratification F, S, FS
Stage III:	PHR more than 75% (all patients with FS)

F, abnormal liver function tests; *S*, patient with symptoms

Table 2. Gennari classification (1982)

H	Synchronous hepatic metastases
rH	Metachronous hepatic metastases
(r)H_1	Liver involvement equal to or less than 25%
(r)H_2	Liver involvement between 25% and 50%
(r)H_3	Liver involvement more than 50%
s	Single metastasis
m	Multiple monolateral metastases
b	Bilateral metastases (both surgical lobes)
i	Infiltration of contiguous structures or organs
F	Impairment of liver function
c	Presence of cirrhosis

The Lausanne classification was subsequently revised in 1976 and again in 1983/84 [5]. The final classification is based on the percentage of hepatic replacement by tumor (PHR) and two stratification factors (Table 1).

In 1982, Gennari reviewed six types of classification systems for colorectal metastases to the liver [6]. Taking into account only relevant clinically applicable prognostic factors he proposed a new clinical classification using stages depending on extent of liver involvement (but different, however, from that of Pettavel), and with many subclassifications (Table 2). In 1984 he proposed a revision of his staging system [7].

One main similarity in both staging systems is the inclusion of the degree of hepatic replacement by tumor, a factor mainly appreciated by surgeons. The importance of this staging method has been reported by many authors [5-17]. In most series evaluating prognostic factors by multivariate analysis the PHR emerged as the most significant determinant of survival [8, 9, 14]. The level of significance in the Fortner series [14] (*n*, 117) reached $p = 10^{-6}$, on which basis he divided the patients into three groups: I, PHR $\leqslant$ 50%; II, PHR 55%-80%; and III, PHR > 80%. Bengmark [18] divided his patients into the PHR groups: <20%, 20%-70%; >70%. Finally, Gennari [6] and Petrelli [16] favor a staging in the subsets: $\leqslant$ 25%; 25%-50%; and > 50%. Most authors in this field propose that the stages of PHR should be divided: <25%; 25%-75%; and >75% [1, 5, 9, 11, 12, 15, 17]. Wanebo in his series of 135 patients with unresected liver metastases clearly showed that there was no significant difference between the groups with PHR 26%-50% and 51%-75% in median and mean survival, and advocated the use of the three stages (< 25%; 25%-75%; > 75%) since the differences between these stages were highly significant [15]. Other prognostic factors less frequently used in stratification systems are shown in Table 3. In this table a selection of the 9 main prognostic factors from 15 publications concerning classification systems are reviewed. In evaluating these factors, many subgroups are encountered so that the number of possible separate combinations can easily outnumber the total amount of patients in individual series. Surprisingly, surgery (= resectability),

Table 3. Factors considered in classification systems for liver metastases from colorectal origin

Prognostic factor	Literature references for proposed classification systems													
	Pettavel et al. [5]	Pettavel et al. [5]	Gennari et al. [6]	Almersjö et al. [9]	Dahl et al. [12]	Stehlin et al. [17]	Bengtsson et al. [11]	Wood et al. [19]	El-Domeiri and Mojab [13]	Grage et al. [20]	Fortner et al. [21, 22][a]	Fortner et al. [14][b]	Petrelli et al. [16]	Van de Velde et al. [1]
Hepatic replacement by tumor		*	*	*	*	*	*		*	*		*	*	*
Number of metastases			*					*						
Size of metastases/hepatomegaly	*									*				
Distribution of metastases within the liver			*				*	*	*					
Resectability											*			*
Biochemical impairment of liver function	*	*	*						*	*			*	
Extrahepatic disease									*		*	*	*	*
Performance status													*	
Symptoms		*								*				*

[a] Surgical series (*n*, 65)
[b] Chemotherapy series (*n*, 117)

Table 4. Survival results of hepatic resection for colorectal cancer patients

Literature reference	Number of patients	Survival (%)		
		1 year	3 years	5 years
Adson et al. [23]	141	-	-	25
Attiyeh et al. [24]	25	-	-	40
August et al. [25]	33	94	53	-
Bengmark et al. [26]	39	-	23	-
Fortner et al. [22]	65	89	71	57
Foster [27]	259	-	-	22
Iwatsuki et al. [28]	24	91	73	73
Logan et al. [29]	19	-	-	25
Rajpal et al. [30]	34	85	40	-
Steel et al. [31]	30	90	65	-
Thompson et al. [32]	22	80	38	31
Tsuzuki et al. [33]	14	-	-	40
	705			39

presently the only treatment available for colorectal metastases that has any significant chance of curing the patient, is as yet not included in any overall staging system. Table 4 clearly indicates the value of surgery on the natural history of liver metastases, and thus its use qualifies as a very important factor influencing prognosis. In the proposed International Classification, curatively resected metastases were included as stage 0 disease

Table 5. Proposed International Staging System for hepatic metastases. Selection of liver imaging technique to be made by each institution depending upon their expertise and equipment available

Stage 0:	Curatively resected metastases
Stage I:	P_1 (PHR < 25%), no E, no S
Stage II:	P_2 (PHR 25%–75%), no E, no S
Stage III:	P_3 (PHR > 75%, no E, no S or any P with E and/or S)

E, concurrent extrahepatic disease; *S*, symptoms attributable to liver metastases

(Table 5). This stage obviously is a very broad category which needs further definition. However, the data are not yet available to define this stage better.[1]

An example of the fallibility of small series is that of Adson, who published the largest single institutional series of 141 patients who underwent a liver resection compared with 252 historical controls [23]. Interesting in this series is that an earlier report on surgical treatment (60 patients) indicated that the presence of multiple resectable metastases had an extremely poor effect on prognosis [34]. In his present series (*n*, 141), patients with multiple metastases did just as well as those with solitary metastases. Both in the Adson (surgically treated) series as well as in the Fortner series (chemotherapeutically treated) [14], the presence of extrahepatic disease was a very significant prognostic factor. It was deemed essential to include this important prognostic factor in the hepatic staging system proposed in Table 5. Rather than using performance status, patients are here categorized merely as symptomatic or asymptomatic, similar to the system of Pettavel. It should be noted that this staging system is not a dynamic one. It makes an assessment at a single point in time and has the advantage that it is simple enough for everyday use. For this reason laboratory tests (alkaline phosphatase, bilirubin, carcinoembryonic antigen, lactate dehydrogenase) are not included in the system. These latter, and many other factors are, however, of importance, especially during follow-up.

Apart from acceptance of an indispensable universal staging system for hepatic metastases which can only be revised through analysis of large numbers of patients, standardization of response criteria in reporting treatment results is not the least essential. The two most important end points of any study are quality of life and survival. But at this early stage in our studies, we must first strive to standardize our definitions of progression and regression (analysis of response criteria is thus beyond the scope of this paper).

In conclusion, patients with liver metastasis constitute a (multifactorial) problem in medicine, requiring a cooperative approach to find meaningful answers.

References

1. Van de Velde CJH, Veenhof CHN, Sugarbaker PH (1984) Methodology in the clinical study of hepatic metastases. In: Van de Velde CJH, Sugarbaker PH (eds) Liver metastasis, basic aspects, detection and management. Nijhoff, Boston, pp 358–373

[1] A project has been initiated at the National Cancer Institute, Bethesda, MA, USA in order to define the significant prognostic factors in stage 0 disease by analysis through a central database

2. Balch CM, Urist MM, Soong SJ, McGregor M (1983) A prospective phase II clinical trial of continuous FUDR regional chemotherapy for colorectal metastases to the liver using a totally implantable drug infusion pump. Ann Surg 198: 567-573
3. Jaffe BM, Donegan WL, Watson F, Spratt Jr JS (1968) Factors influencing survival in patients with untreated hepatic metastases. Surg Gynecol Obstet 127: 1-11
4. Pettavel J, Morgenthaler F (1967) Natural history of cancer metastatic to the liver and protracted arterial infusions. 5th International Congress of Chemotherapy, Vienna (abstract)
5. Pettavel J, Leyvraz S, Douglas P (1984) The necessity for staging liver metastases and standardizing treatment response criteria. The case of secondaries of colorectal origin. In: Van de Velde CJH, Sugarbaker PH (eds) Liver metastasis. Basic aspects, detection and management. Nijhoff, Boston, pp 154-168
6. Gennari L, Doci R, Bozzetti F, Veronesi U (1982) Proposal for a clinical classification of liver metastases. Tumori 58: 443-449
7. Gennari L (1984) Proposal for staging liver metastases. (This volume)
8. Cady B, Oberfield RA (1974) Regional infusion chemotherapy of hepatic metastases from carcinoma of the colon. Am J Surg 127: 220-227
9. Almersjö O, Bengmark S, Hafström L (1976) Liver metastases found by follow-up of patients operated on for colorectal cancer. Cancer 37: 1454-1457
10. Bengmark S, Fredlund PE (1978) Temporary dearterialization combined with intra-arterial infusion of oncolytic drug in the treatment of liver tumors. In: Ariel IM (ed) Progress in clinical cancer VII. Grune and Stratton, New York, pp 207-216
11. Bengtsson G, Carlson G, Hafström L, Jonsson PE (1981) Natural history of patients with untreated liver metastases. Am J Surg 141: 586-589
12. Dahl EP, Fredlund PE, Bengmark S (1981) Transient hepatic dearterialization followed by regional intra-arterial 5-fluorouracil infusion as treatment for liver tumors. Ann Surg 193: 82-88
13. El-Domeiri AA, Mojab K (1978) Intermittent occlusion of the hepatic artery and infusion chemotherapy for carcinoma of the liver. Am J Surg 135: 771-775
14. Fortner JG, Silva JS, Cox EB, Golby RB, Gallowitz H, MacLean B (1984) Multivariate analysis of a personal series of 247 patients with liver metastases from colorectal cancer. II. Treatment by intrahepatic chemotherapy. Ann Surg 199: 317-324
15. Wanebo H (1984) A staging system for liver metastases from colorectal cancer. American Society of Clinical Oncology (ASCO) Abstract no C-560
16. Petrelli N, Bonnheim DC, Herrera LO, Mittelman A (1984) A proposed classification system for liver metastasis from colorectal carcinoma. Dis Colon Rectum 27: 249-252
17. Stehlin Jr JS, Hafström L, Greeff PJ (1974) Experience with infusion and resection in cancer of the liver. Surg Gynecol Obstet 138: 855-863
18. Bengmark S, Rosengren K (1974) Angiographic study of the liver after ligation of the hepatic artery in man. Am J Surg 119: 620-624
19. Wood CB, Gillis CR, Blumgart LH (1976) A retrospective study on the natural history of patients with liver metastasis from colorectal cancer. Clin Oncol 2: 285-288
20. Grage TB, Shingleton WW, Jubert AV, Elias E, Aust JB, Poss E (1979) Results of a prospective randomized study of hepatic artery infusion with 5-fluorouracil vs. intravenous 5-fluorouracil in patients with hepatic metastases from colorectal cancer. Front Gastrointest Res 5: 116-129
21. Fortner JG, MacLean BJ, Kim DK, Howland WS, Turnbull AD, Goldiner P, Carlon G, Beattie EJ (1981) The seventies evolution in liver surgery for cancer. Cancer 47: 2162-2166
22. Fortner JG, Silva JG, Golbey RB, Cox EB, MacLean BJ (1984) Multivariate analysis of a personal series of 247 consecutive patients with liver metastases from colorectal cancer. I. Treatment by hepatic resection. Ann Surg 199: 306-316
23. Adson MA, Van Heerden JA, Adson MH, Wagner JS, Ilstrup DM (1984) Resection of hepatic metastases from colorectal cancer. Arch Surg 119: 647-651
24. Attiyeh FA, Wanebo HJ, Stearns MW (1978) Hepatic resection for metastasis from colorectal cancer. Dis Colon Rectum 21: 160
25. August DA, Ottow RT, Sugarbaker PH (1985) Clinical perspective of human colon cancer metastasis. Cancer Metast Rev (in press)

26. Bengmark S, Hafström L, Jeppsson B, Jönsson PE, Rydén S, Sundqvist K (1982) Metastatic disease in the liver from colorectal cancer: an appraisal of liver surgery. World J Surg 6: 61-65
27. Foster JH (1978) Survival after liver resection for secondary tumors. Am J Surg 135: 389
28. Iwatsuki S, Shaw Jr BW, Starzl TE (1983) Experience with 150 liver resections. Ann Surg 197: 247-253
29. Logan SE, Meier SJ, Ramming KP, Morton DL, Longmire Jr WP (1982) Hepatic resection of metastatic colorectal carcinoma. Arch Surg 117: 25-28
30. Rajpal S, Dasmahapatra KS, Ledesma EJ, Mittelman A (1982) Extensive resections of isolated metastasis from carcinoma of the colon and rectum. Surg Gynecol Obstet 155: 813-816
31. Steele Jr G, Osleen RT, Wilson RE, Brooks DC, Mayer RJ, Zamchek N, Ravikumar TS (1984) Patterns of failure after surgical cure of large liver tumors. Am J Surg 147: 554-559
32. Thompson HH, Tompkins RK, Longmire WP Jr (1983) Major hepatic resection. A 25-year experience. Ann Surg 197: 375-388
33. Tsuzuki T, Ogata Y, Iida S, Shimazu M (1984) Hepatic resection in 125 patients. Arch Surg 119: 1025-1032
34. Wilson SM, Adson MA (1976) Surgical treatment of hepatic metastases from colorectal cancer. Arch Surg 111: 330-334

Indications for Treatment and Determination of Treatment Effects with Primary and Secondary Liver Tumors

W. Schreml

Kreiskrankenhaus, 8870 Günzburg, FRG

Introduction

Recent developments in operative und pharmacological techniques for locoregional treatment of liver malignancies have focused the interest of oncologists on this organ. With respect to indication for treatment and determination of treatment effects of systemic chemotherapy in liver tumors, a number of questions may be formulated:

1. Is there anything specific in malignant liver disease as compared with involvement of other organs?
2. Does liver involvement modify the indication or results of systemic treatment used in disseminated cancer?
3. Is the determination of treatment effects in disseminated cancer influenced by liver involvement?

These questions are formulated in a rather general form to avoid interference with the specific topics of this volume. They are applied primarily to metastatic liver disease, which represents a complex oncological problem; as far as primary liver tumors are concerned, the questions can be answered in a rather straightforward manner.

Are There "Specific" Aspects of Malignant Liver Disease?

"Magnitude of the Problem"

For the planning of systemic therapy, the liver is usually only one of several metastatic sites to be taken into consideration. Figure 1 shows the occurrence of liver metastases in more than 8,000 postmortem examinations [11]; in patients dying of malignant tumors, metastases restricted to the liver only constitute a rare event. The data of the Oncological Telephone Service of the Tumor Center Ulm probably represent the problems of everyday oncology [20]. Table 1 shows that less than 20% of the inquiries concerned patients with liver metastases; of these, one-half to two-thirds presented with metastases to the liver only except breast cancer. Therefore, systemic therapy is usually concerned with a broad range of problems of which liver involvement is only one aspect.

Recent Results in Cancer Research. Vol 100

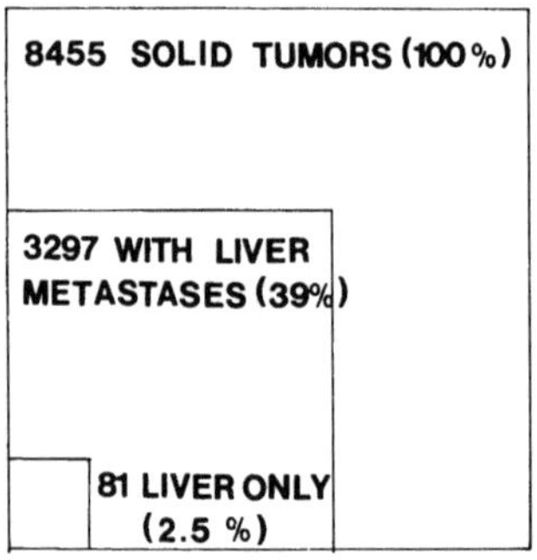

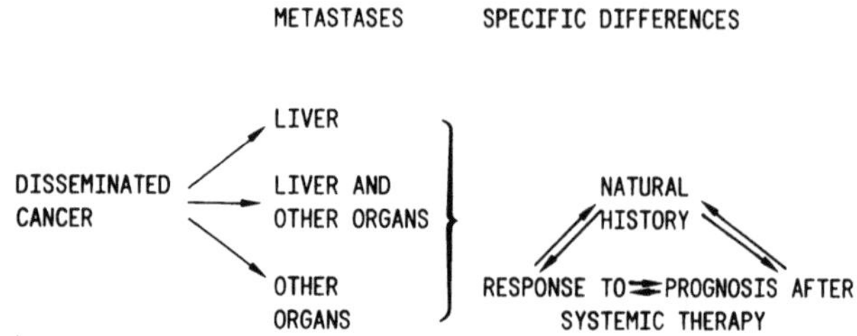

Fig. 1 *(Left).* Fraction of patients with liver metastases and metastases confined to the liver at autopsy [11]

Fig. 2 *(Right).* Diagram of interactions which may be relevant in evaluating metastatic liver disease

Table 1. Evaluation of the Oncological Telephone Service of the Ulm Tumor Center 1978–81 with respect to the prevalence of liver metastases

Patients with metastases			1540
Patients with liver metastases			274 (18%)
	n	Liver only	Combined
Colon/rectum	81	48 (59%)	33
Stomach	20	11 (55%)	9
Pancreas	15	9 (60%)	6
Breast	57	13 (23%)	44
Melanoma	16	9 (56%)	7
Lung	16	7 (44%)	9
TUP[a]	20	12 (60%)	8
Other	49	23 (47%)	26

[a] Metastases from tumor of unknown primary (TUP) site

Definition of "Specific" Problems

In patients with disseminated malignancies, metastases may be present in the liver only, in other organs, or in both liver and other organs (Fig. 2). Where could there be "specific" problems related to liver involvement? Metastases to the liver could influence the natural history of the disease, or could modify the response to systemic therapy, and thus alter the prognosis for the individual patient. Since these factors are closely interconnected, it is difficult to single out the contribution of an individual parameter such as liver involvement. Frequently, data reported in the literature do not concentrate on such specific questions. For some tumors, the data of the Ulm Tumor Center have been evaluated with respect to these questions and are included in the following section.

Evaluation of Malignant Tumors with Respect to Liver Metastases

Breast Cancer

It is now widely recognized that the evaluation of breast cancer is complicated by the influence of many prognostic factors which generate different subtypes of the disease. Therefore, reported data are sometimes difficult to compare. Reviewing the reports on systemic therapy of breast cancer in the journals of 1983 and 1984 [Brass B (1984) personal communication], 33 studies were screened for their information on liver involvement (Table 2). The prevalence of liver metastases within the various study populations ranges from less than 10% to over 40%. Very few studies reported on the occurrence of liver metastases in combination with other metastatic sites. The remission rate was specified in 25% of the patients with liver involvement, which represent only 4% of the total patient population. Thus, the difficulties in extracting the specific information useful for our subject become apparent. In a comprehensive review, Kemeny [8] has collected response rates in breast cancer studies (Table 3); the response rate in patients with liver metastases was slightly but significantly lower than in patients without liver involvement. Generally, liver metastases are considered an important indicator of poor prognosis. This fact has been brought into mathematical terms by applying a linear logistic regression model to the patient population of one institution [5]. Out of 25 tested covariates, only four were relevant for the equation describing the probability of response (Table 4); liver involvement contributed with a large negative coefficient.

In a regional study of the Ulm Tumor Center the therapeutic strategies for metastatic breast cancer are coordinated in cooperation with regional hospitals and practicing physicians [13]. The high-risk group is defined by the following criteria: liver or CNS involvement, inflammatory skin metastases, lymphangiosis carcinomatosa of the lungs, negative receptor status or rapid progression. This group receives primary chemotherapy with 5-fluorouracil + Adriamycin + cyclophosphamide (FAC) or cyclophosphamide + methotrexate + 5-fluorouracil (CMF), combined with hormonal treatment unless the receptor status is negative. At present, the high-risk group comprises 35 patients with and

Table 2. Evaluation of 33 recently published studies on systemic therapy of advanced breast cancer. (Brass B 1984, personal communication)

% with liver metastases	Number of studies		
No information	8		
<10%	9		
10%-19%	9		
20%-29%	1		
30%-39%	5		
>40%	1		
In these studies reported			
Total patients	3290	(100%)	
Patients with liver metastases	526	(20%)	100%
Information on combined metastases	30	(1%)	6%
Information on remission			
Rate in liver metastases	131	(4%)	25%

Table 3. Collected data on response of different metastatic sites in breast cancer [8]

	n	Response rate
Total	1083	51%
Liver metastases	304 (28%)	46% > $P=0.04$
No liver metastases		53%
Lung metastases		49%
Soft tissue		56%

Table 4. Linear logistic regression model to predict the response of patients treated for metastatic breast cancer [5]. Liver involvement has a high negative impact

$\ln p/(1\text{-}p) = 0.587 + 0.703\ Z + 0.011\ D - \mathit{1.045}\ L - 0.510\ P$

P, probability of response; *Z*, therapy (0 or 1, depending on therapy); *D*, diseasefree interval (in months); *L*, liver involvement (0 if not, 1 if present); *P*, performance status (0 if ambulatory, 1 if bedridden)

No influence
- Age
- Bone involvement
- Duration of metastatic disease
- Nodal involvement
- Number of involved sites
- SGOT levels
- Other 15 covariates

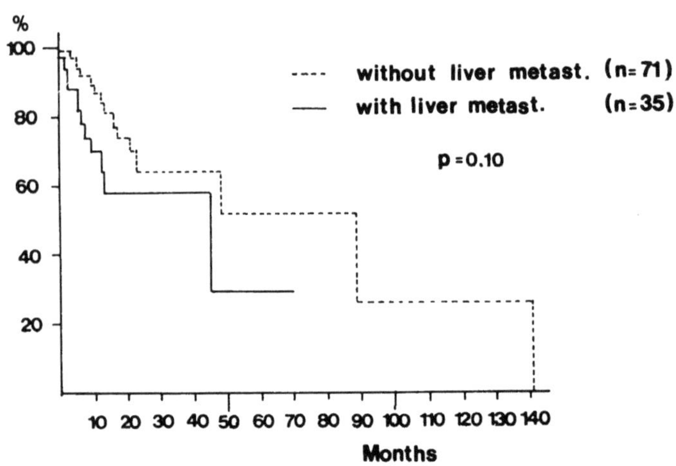

Fig. 3. Survival of patients with high-risk metastatic breast cancer treated within the regional study of the Ulm Tumor Center [13]

71 patients without liver involvement; the probability of survival (Fig. 3) is only slightly different with a marginally significant p value (0.10).

In summary, for breast cancer with liver metastases the following statements can be made:

1. Detailed data on the exact influence of liver involvement on natural history, response to systemic therapy, and prognosis are not available,
2. Liver metastases are one indicator of poor prognosis, probably a significant one
3. Liver involvement places patients into a "high-risk group," which is usually treated by initial chemotherapy, combined with hormonal therapy when indicated, but is considered not suitable for hormonal treatment only.

Chemotherapy - Sensitive Tumors

It could be expected that highly chemotherapy-sensitive tumors would more clearly show an influence of liver metastases on the outcome of systemic therapy if they were an important prognostic factor. Data on metastatic malignant teratoma (Table 5) show that liver metastases are a rare event, usually included within the stages of "bulky disease," which carries a more serious prognosis than early metastatic teratoma. In a large group of patients with bulky disease (E. D. Kreuser 1984, personal communication), only 7/84 had liver metastases. In view of the small fraction of patients a separate evaluation for the impact of liver metastases in malignant teratoma is difficult.

In small cell cancer of the lung (SCCL), about 22%-28% of the patients are diagnosed to have liver metastases by biopsy at presentation [4, 7]. Liver involvement places the patients into the "extensive disease" category, which still has a very short survival probability. The subgroup with liver metastases is usually not considered separately in clinical trials.

An evaluation of the patients treated at the Ulm Tumor Center with combination chemotherapy for extensive SSCL is presented in Fig. 4; in this group, patients with liver metastases have a much shorter median survival (25 vs. 250 days); the log rank test is significant ($P < 0.05$). Despite these differences, there is no consequence for the selection of systemic therapy since maximal aggressive treatment is indicated in all cases of SCCL in the stage of extensive disease.

Table 5. Data on the occurrence of liver metastases in testicular cancer

	n	Liver metastases	Comment
Samson et al. [16]	143	12 (8%)	Included in "bulky disease"
Reynolds [15]	74	6 (9%)	No CR
Seeber [21]	157	18* (11%)	*Stage IV D
Pontes [13]	93	13* (14%)	*"Visceral" = liver/bone; 31% long-term survival; at autopsy 18/33 = 54% liver metastases
Ulm Tumor Center[a]	84*	7 (8%)	*Bulky disease

[a] Kreuser ED (1984) personal communication

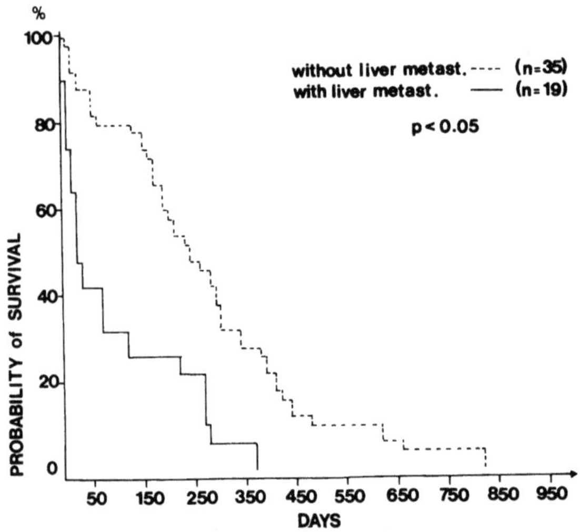

Fig. 4. Survival of patients with extensive small-cell carcinoma of the lung treated with combination chemotherapy at the Ulm Tumor Center

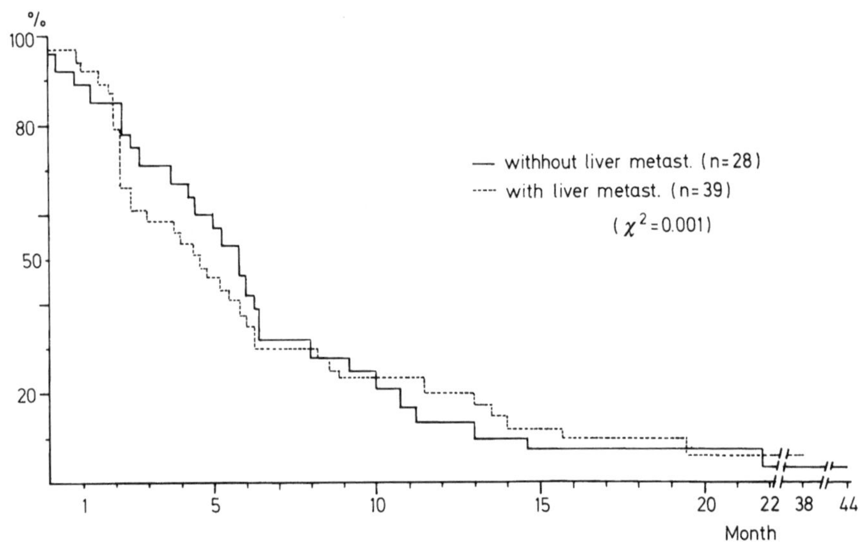

Fig. 5. Survival of patients with advanced gastric carcinoma treated at the Ulm Tumor Center

Tumors with Low Sensitivity to Systemic Treatment

Presently available chemotherapy regimens are still of limited value in disseminated gastrointestinal tumors, and it is still doubtful whether any combination chemotherapy is superior to 5-fluorouracil monotherapy in gastric and pancreatic cancer [3] or in cancer of the large bowel [1].

From the experience of the Ulm Tumor Center presence or absence of liver metastases does not significantly affect survival in disseminated gastric (Fig. 5) or pancreatic (Fig. 6) carcinoma.

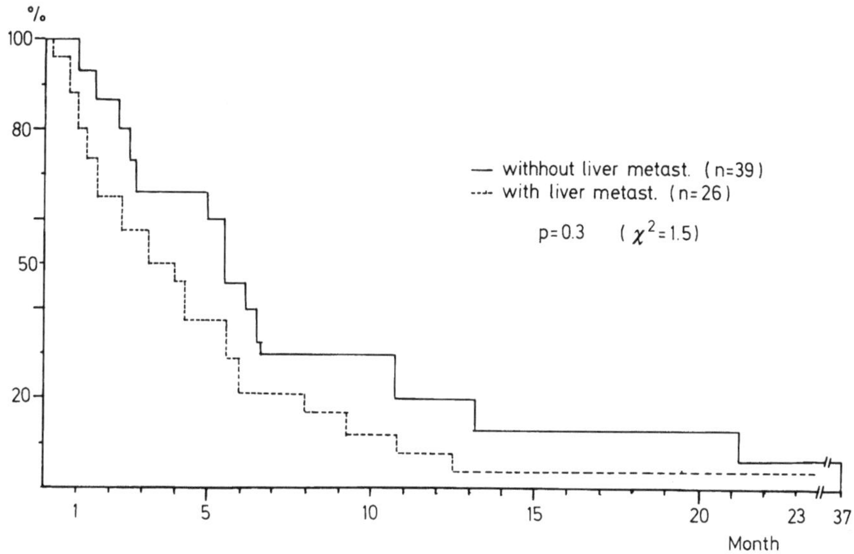

Fig. 6. Survival of patients with advanced pancreatic carcinoma treated at the Ulm Tumor Center

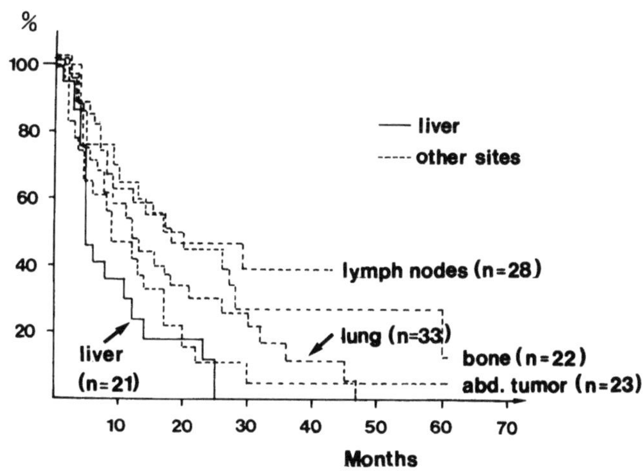

Fig. 7. Survival of patients presenting with metastases of tumor of unknown primary site at the Ulm Tumor Center. Log-rank test in comparison with liver metastases: abdominal tumor *p*, 0.7; lung *p*, 0.1; bone *p*, 0.02; lymph nodes *p*, 0.01

Metastases from tumors of unknown primary site represent an interesting group of neoplasms [22]. Figure 7 compares the survival patterns of 127 patients seen at the Ulm Tumor Center with respect to the metastatic site at presentation [17]. Although the patients presenting with liver metastases show the shortest survival, the log-rank test reveals significant differences ($p < 0.05$) only in comparison to bone and lymph-node metastases. Systemic therapy had no recognizable effect on progression of disease [17], indicated by similar survival for treated and untreated patients.

Therefore, there are only marginal differences in various tumors between disseminated stages with or without liver involvement with respect to survival. Considering another parameter, the overview of Kemeny [8] concentrates on response rates to systemic chemotherapy in hepatic metastases. For colorectal, gastric, pancreatic and non-small-cell-lung carcinoma, response rates are similar for the overall groups and for those with liver metastases. Patients with malignant melanoma have a lower response rate when liver involvement is present. In none of these tumors has the therapeutic regimen been specifically adapted to liver metastases.

Indication for Systemic Chemotherapy in Malignant Liver Disease

The various aspects of possible indications for systemic therapy in malignant liver disease are summarized in Table 6. In primary hepatocellular carcinoma, the indication is strictly palliative, since cure or significant prolongation of life cannot be obtained with presently available chemotherapeutic strategies (Falkson and Coetzer, pp. 103-110).

Portal type metastases are of special interest, since they represent the first step in the metastatic process and may occur "solitary" or restricted to this organ. On the other hand, systemic chemotherapy is of rather low potential in this group of tumors. Therefore, regional measures of treatment, as amply discussed during this symposium, e.g., intraarterial chemotherapy, may have priority if performed in carefully designed and conducted clinical studies. If no such treatment protocol is active, patients should be treated by systemic chemotherapy for palliation. If there are few symptoms and the progression of the metastases is slow, supportive measures should be given preference to avoid deterioration of quality of life.

In view of the promising results for adjuvant therapy by hepatic artery infusion [9, 21], it should be stated that there is no clear evidence that systemic adjuvant chemotherapy improves the cure rate in gastrointestinal tumors [18].

Liver metastases are frequently one of several manifestations of hematogenous metastases. As stated above, there is usually not much difference in response rate or survival between patients with liver metastases and those with other forms of disseminated disease.

Table 6. Indications for systemic chemotherapy in primary and metastatic liver cancer

Primary hepatocellular cancer	For palliation only
Portal-type metastases	Secondary to regional measures if available (?) For palliation No proof of effective adjuvant chemotherapy
Hematogenous metastases	Depending on effectiveness on specific tumors With curative aim in selected tumors (e.g., testicular carcinoma, Hodgkin's disease) For prolongation of survival/palliation of symptoms (e.g., in breast cancer) Usually not indicated in resistant tumors (e.g., hypernephroma)

Therefore, the indication is not "specific" for this type of metastases. In some tumors, liver involvement places the patient into a high-risk group which is subject to more aggressive chemotherapeutic regimens, e.g., in breast cancer or testicular tumors. However, the generally accepted indications are as applicable to liver involvement as to other forms of disseminated disease (Table 6). The curative aim will not be abandoned in testicular cancer, although liver involvement is a grave prognostic sign. The indication for palliative therapy or the decision not to use it in resistant tumors depends on the sensitivity of the different primary tumors and is not directly influenced by liver involvement.

Modifications of Systemic Therapy in Liver Involvement

The aggressiveness of chemotherapy and the probability of response depend on the performance status of the patient. Liver involvement frequently leads to a rapidly deteriorating clinical condition, which may be prohibitive against the institution of systemic treatment.

More specifically, there is a wide range of interactions between liver function and cytostatic agents (Table 7). Therefore, it is conceivable that liver metastases, by altering the functional state of the organ, will modify effectiveness and toxicity of cytostatic agents. Although several such interactions are described in experimental animal models [16], there are only limited and approximate guidelines that can be formulated in liver dysfunction (Table 8).

Table 7. Interaction of liver function with systemic therapy [16]

Impaired liver function may *decrease* effectivity of cytotoxic agents by	
Decreased activation	(DTIC, CCNU)
Increased metabolism	(Cyclophosphamide)
Increased excretion	(Adriamycin)
Impaired liver function may *increase* effectivity of cytotoxic agents by	
Increased activation	(6-MP, cyclophosphamide)
Decreased metabolism	(ARA-C, 5-FU, 6-TG, 6-MP, nitrosoureas, cyclophosphamide)
Decreased excretion	(MTX, vinca alkaloids, anthracyclines)

Table 8. Dose modification in liver dysfunction for anthracyclines and vinca alkaloids VP-16 and VM-26 [2]

1. Only approximate guidelines can be offered and are probably inaccurate
2. For bilirubin of > 1.5 mg/100 ml, reduce dose by 50%
3. For bilirubin of > 3.0 mg/100 ml, reduce dose by 75%

Determination of Treatment Effects

Sophisticated methods for imaging liver metastases and quantifying the extent of disease have been presented in this symposium. It has become possible to measure the rate of growth of intraabdominal metastases with surprising precision (Fig. 8). However, such sophistication does not usually contribute to the determination of treatment effects in oncological practice. Methods should be selected according to the aim of treatment.

In curative therapy, the achievement of a complete response is usually mandatory to reach the intended goal; therefore, thorough restaging is mandatory with reevaluation of all parameters of the initial staging. On the other hand, if the aim is palliation of symptoms, the clinical evaluation of these symptoms is the guiding parameter of evaluation.

For clinical studies, it may be important to define most precisely the change of tumor mass. Here, serial imaging of liver metastases may be helpful. However, the final test for effectiveness of a new treatment should be the comparison of the overall survival in prospective randomized trials [10]. Furthermore, emphasis should be placed on the development of methods suitable to measure the "quality of life" during systemic therapy.

Whenever systemic chemotherapy is instituted, the parameters which will be followed for definition of response should be determined before starting therapy. It is preferable to select only a limited number of parameters to reduce the inconvenience to the patient. For the follow-up of a palliative therapeutic trial, the complaints of the patient, palpation of liver size, and few laboratory parameters may be sufficient.

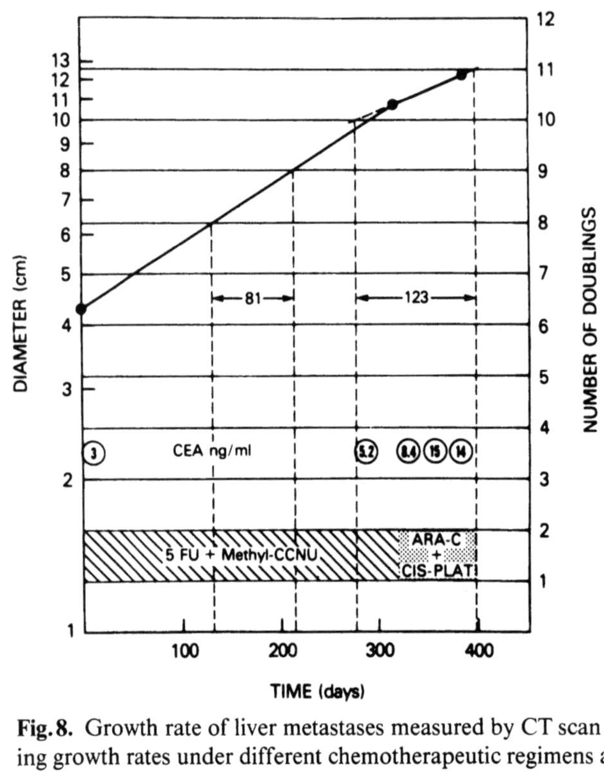

Fig. 8. Growth rate of liver metastases measured by CT scan and with EOE-13 contrast [6]. Changing growth rates under different chemotherapeutic regimens are postulated

Conclusion

The general rules of oncology for indication and evaluation of systemic chemotherapy are fully applicable to patients with liver malignancies, with only minor specific aspects as compared with other forms of disseminated disease.

References

1. Buroker T, Moertel C, Fleming T, Everson L, Cullinan S, Krook U, Foley J, Schutt A (1984) A randomized comparison of 5-FU containing drug combinations with 5-FU alone in advanced colorectal carcinoma. Abstract C-537. Proc Am Soc Clin Oncol 3: 138
2. Chabner BA, Myers CE (1982) Clinical pharmacology of cancer chemotherapy. In: DeVita VT, Hellman S, Rosenberg SA (eds) Cancer. Principles and practice of oncology. Lippincott, Philadelphia
3. Cullinan S, Moertel C, Fleming T, Everson L, Krook J, Schutt A (1984) A randomized comparison of 5-FU alone (F), 5-FU + adriamycin (FA) and 5-FU + adriamycin + mitomycin C (FAM) in gastric and pancreatic cancer. Abstract C-536. Proc Am Soc Clin Oncol 3: 137
4. Dombernowsky P, Hirsch F, Hansen HH, Hainau B (1978) Peritoneoscopy in the staging of 190 patients with small-cell anaplastic carcinoma of the lung with special reference to subtyping. Cancer 41: 2008-2012
5. George SL, Hoogstraten B (1978) Prognostic factors in the initial response to therapy by patients with advanced breast cancer. J Natl Cancer Inst 60: 731-736
6. Havelaar IJ, Sugarbaker PH, Vermess M, Miller DL (1984) Rate of growth of intraabdominal metastases from colorectal cancer. Cancer 54: 163-171
7. Ihde DC, Makuch RW, Carney DN, Bunn PA, Cohen MH, Matthews MJ, Minna JD (1981) Prognostic implication of sites of metastases in patients with small cell carcinoma of the lung given intensive combination chemotherapy. Am Rev Respir Dis 123: 500-507
8. Kemeny N (1983) The systemic chemotherapy of hepatic metastases. Semin Oncol 10: 148-158
9. Metzger U, Mermillod B, Aeberhard P, Egeli R, Laffer U, Martinoli S, Mueller W, Schroeder R, Cavalli F, Weber W (1984) Adjuvant portal liver infusion with 5-fluorouracil and mitomycin C following curative large bowel cancer surgery. In: Jones SE, Salmon SE (eds)Adjuvant therapy of cancer IV. Grune and Stratton, New York
10. Peto R (1978) Clinical trial methodology. Biomedicine 28: 24-36
11. Pikren JW, Tsukuda Y, Lane WW (1984) Liver metastases: analysis of autopsy data. In: Weiss L, Gilbert HA (eds) Liver metastases. Hall, Boston
12. Pontes JE, Wajsman Z, Beckley S, Williams P, Murphy GP (1983) The treatment of stage III nonseminomatous testicular tumors. Cancer 51: 1327-1331
13. Porzsolt F, Schreml W, Mende S, Buchelt L, Knöchelmann R, Brass B, Gerteis D, Stier R (1984) A phase IV protocol for treatment of metastatic breast cancer. Abstract 5/8 GL. J Cancer Res Clin Oncol [Suppl] 107: 12
14. Reynolds TF, Vugrin D, Cvitkovic E, Cheng E, Braun DW, O'Hehir MA, Dukeman ME, Whitemore WF, Golbey RB (1981) VAB-3 combination chemotherapy of metastatic testicular cancer. Cancer 48: 888-898
15. Samson MK, Fisher R, Stephens RL, Rivkin S, Opipari M, Maloney T, Groppe CW (1980) Vinblastine, bleomycin and *cis*-diaminodichloroplatinum in disseminated testicular cancer: response to treatment and prognostic correlations. Eur J Cancer 16: 1359-1366
16. Sauer H (1983) Beeinflussung der Wirkung von Zytostatika. In: Drings P, Schreml W (eds) Supportive Maßnahmen bei der Internistischen Tumorbehandlung. Zuckschwerdt, München, p 175-197
17. Schreiber C (1984) Metastasen bei unbekanntem Primärtumor. Dissertation, Ulm
18. Schreml W (1985) Adjuvante Therapie gastrointestinaler Tumoren - gegenwärtiger Stand. Der informierte Arzt (in press)

19. Schreml W, Porzsolt F, Brass B (1985) Telefonische Beratungsstelle des Tumorzentrums Ulm - Bericht über 6 Jahre Tätigkeit. Münch Med Wschr (in press)
20. Seeber S, Schütte J, Niederle N, Schmidt CG (1983) Neue Ergebnisse der Behandlung metastasierender Hodentumoren im Früh- und Spätstadium. Tumor Diagn Ther 4: 45-54
21. Taylor J, Mullee MA, Machin D (1984) Adjuvant therapy of colorectal cancer with portal vein cytotoxic perfusion. In: Jones SE, Salmon SE (eds) Adjuvant therapy of cancer IV. Grune and Stratton, New York
22. Ultmann JE, Phillips TL (1982) Management of the patient with cancer of unknown primary site. In: DeVita VT, Hellman S, Rosenberg SA (eds) Cancer. Principles and practice of Oncology. Lippincott, Philadelphia

Application and Results of Different Chemotherapy Regimens in Primary Liver Malignancies

G. Falkson and B. J. Coetzer

Department of Cancer Chemotherapy, University of Pretoria, Private Bag X 169, Pretoria 0001, Republic of South Africa

Introduction

The approach to treatment of patients with primary liver cancer has differed in different parts of the world. Where the difference in treatment approach is based on true pathological differences in the disease this is justified.

Until recently no systematic controlled trials of any treatment modalities had been performed. The clinician is faced with a rapidly growing tumour which would be expected (on preclinical grounds) to be sensitive to oncolytic chemotherapy and earlier studies claimed predictable results. Systematic investigations of "standard" forms of treatment and in depth studies of patients with primary liver cancer are dispelling many preconceived conceptions of both the disease and response to treatment. The good results claimed with 5-fluorouracil as a systemic treatment or surgery for "early" cases in the United States and Europe have been discredited.

The first attempt to treat systematically primary liver cancer in South Africa was made by Berman [2]; however, anecdotal reports date back to the end of the nineteenth century. Until the rapid increase in the incidence of oesophagus cancer made this the most common form of malignancy in the black man in South Africa, primary liver cancer was the leading cause of death from cancer.

In 1958 clinical trials in the treatment of primary liver cancer with cytostatics were started at the University of Pretoria. In 1966 the Primary Liver Cancer Research Unit of the National Cancer Association of South Africa was established with the prime aim of performing controlled clinical trials. Since 1973 South African patients have been entered into the propectively randomized clinical trials of the Eastern Cooperative Oncology Group of the United States of America so that data on South African patients could be compared with data on both white and black patients in the United States.

Throughout these studies clinical measurements, radiological measurements, biochemical measurements, markers and histological data have all been analysed so that response criteria are reliable. Anecdotal reports and reports in which the response criteria, duration and median survival (relative to patient and disease discriminants) are not set out continue to appear in the literature, causing false optimism.

Data from Eastern Cooperative Oncology Group (ECOG) studies indicate that histological grade of the tumour has a significant impact on the survival time. Data on this and other discriminants explain some of the clinically apparent differences between the clinical course of the disease in South Africa and in North America. The technique most often

Recent Results in Cancer Research. Vol 100

used to improve results is to exclude patients from analysis because of early death. As these patients met the criteria for entry on the study, it is of particular importance that they be included in analysis of for example survival time. This is particularly pertinent when intensive treatment that may play a role in early death is under investigation. Except for the publications of Berman, no publications have attempted to set out results relative to the total population of patients seen even at one institution on whom the diagnosis of primary liver cancer is made.

Oncolytic Chemotherapy

With the known clinical facts the hope of disease control and eradication for patients with primary liver cancer must lie with oncolytic chemotherapy. That the results achieved with various cytostatics in the treatment of patients with primary liver cancer remain unsatisfactory does not detract from this principle. The hope that better results could be achieved in future is supported by the fact that agents already available do occasionally change the course of the disease for individual patients.

Prospective controlled clinical trials have excluded from further consideration most of the usually used anticancer drugs. Patients with primary liver cancer can therefore be saved unnecessary toxicity from being exposed to agents that have toxic effects without adequate hope of therapeutic effect. It is therefore useful to list such agents not only so that they are not given to patients with primary liver cancer but also to exclude such agents from anticancer drug combinations given to patients with primary liver cancer. This principle is unfortunately often ignored.

There is no exception of the rule, known to the authors, where oncolytic effect in any type of cancer is improved by the addition of inactive agents.

The largest series of carefully studied patients where consistent criteria for response have been used (and where patient discriminants have been investigated prospectively to help judge results) is that of the ECOG and that of the University of Pretoria. Performance status at the start of treatment and the histological differentiation of the tumour are the major factors affecting prognosis and override most treatment differences [12, 13, 14, 15, 16, 17, 18, 22].

Placebo

In a prospective randomized study the median survival time for patients treated with placebo was 2 months.

Single Drugs

Alkylating Agents

No single alkylating agent has been shown to be of value in the treatment of patients with primary liver cancer. The most adequately investigated drug in this group, cyclophosphamide, has been tested at dosage ranges up to 70 mg/kg without therapeutic benefit being derived. The nitrosoureas, chloroethyl-cyclohexyl-nitrosourea (CCNU) and methyl-CCNU did not appear promising in a limited trial in South Africa.

Antimetabolites

The most extensively used antimetabolite is 5-fluorouracil. The response rates reported have varied very considerably and the optimistic response rates are all derived from uncontrolled studies. In the ECOG study EST 2273 none of 45 patients randomized to receive oral 5-fluorouracil showed objective response to treatment. The median survival time of North American white patients receiving this treatment was 7.3 weeks, while for North American black patients it was 14.7 weeks and for South African black patients it was 3.1 weeks. This is no better than placebo, so that the often quoted smaller, uncontrolled series, are best ignored.

Methotrexate, cytosine arabinoside, hydroxyurea, and 6-mercaptopurine are not of value.

Plant Alkaloids

Plant alkaloids tested in man and found not to be of value include vincristine, vinblastine and the podophyllin derivative SPG 827. In a trial of oral VP-16-213 (a semisynthetic epipodophyllotoxin) by the European Organisation for Research and Treatment of Cancer (EORTC), 26 patients were treated. Three achieved a partial remission status (for 12, 16 and 35 weeks) [4]. Short remissions (less than 2 months) were obtained in 3 of 14 patients initially treated with VP-16 compared with 5 of 21 initially treated with Adriamycin in a randomized crossover trial [28].

Diverse Agents

Agents that have been adequately investigated include dehydroemitine, procarbazine, cobaltiprotoporphyrin complex, and DL-serine bis (2-chloropropyl) carbamate ester. None of these are of value. Some response was observed with butyryloxyethylglyoxal dithiosemicarbozone. In the phase II trial of *m*-Amsa [4′-(9-acridinylamino)-methansulphon-*m*-anisidide, NSC 249992] one of 35 patients showed a partial response, indicating that a response rate would be significantly lower than 20% ($P=0.01$). The median survival time of these patients was 11 weeks. In this trial 31 of the patients were black [17]. In a subsequent randomized trial involving North American and European patients no response was observed among 26 patients treated with this agent (including 17 previously untreated patients). The median survival time of the previously untreated patients was 11.6 weeks [19]. Half of the patients suffered at least one severe period of toxicity. In a Southwest Oncology Group (SWOG) study partial response occurred in 2/14 previously treated patients and 1/9 previously untreated patients [3]. In a phase II trial of *m*-AMSA no reponse was seen in 16 patients with primary liver cancer at the Memorial Sloan Kettering Cancer Center in New York [5].

Electrophiles

Cis-diamino-dichloroplatinum has not received an adequate phase II trial in patients with primary liver cancer. Because of the activity shown by this agent in stomach cancer [4, 26], it is worthy of trial in primary liver cancer. Response has been reported in 1/13 patients with primary liver cancer previously treated with Adriamycin and VP-16-213 [27]. With the development of new platinum derivatives the testing of platinum becomes a high priority and has been incorporated as one of the treatment arms of the current ECOG primary liver cancer treatment protocol.

Antibiotics and Related Substances

Antibiotics that have been shown not to be of value include mitomycin-C, actinomycin-D, carzinophyllin and chromomycin-A_3. Neocarzinostatin showed some promise in a phase II ECOG pilot trial [16]. Partial response with a median duration of 12.7 weeks was seen in 7 of 30 evaluable patients. Twenty-two of the patients were black and 8 were white. The South African black patients had a median survival time of 5 weeks.

In a subsequent randomized clinical trial performed by ECOG, 2 of 36 patients were considered to have had partial response (10 and 30 weeks duration respectively). The median survival time of the 18 evaluable North American patients without prior treatment who received neocarzinostatin in this study was 10.7 weeks. Among all 31 South African patients treated with neocarzinostatin in two studies, the median survival time was 12 weeks. It can therefore be stated that this treatment has a response rate lower than 20% ($P = 0.058$) [19].

Anthracyclines and Anthracycline Derivates

In 1975 investigators in Uganda reported very good results in patients with primary liver cancer treated with Adriamycin [30]. These authors have recently reaffirmed good response in their patients with response claimed in 22 of 74 patients [31]. The median survival time of the 74 patients considered eligible for treatment with Adriamycin is not stated. In a prospectively randomized ECOG trial response was only seen in 3 of 31 previously untreated patients and the median survival time of the 16 North American white patients treated with Adriamycin was 15 weeks [15]. In a subsequent prospectively randomized ECOG trial 5 of 43 previously untreated patients with primary liver cancer (3 of 34 North American and European patients and 2 of 9 South African patients) responded to treatment and 2 of 46 previously treated patients responded [19]. In the ECOG trials 16 of 146 patients with primary liver cancer treated with Adriamycin responded (8 of 74 previously untreated patients). In the ECOG study EST 2273 the median survival time of NA/E patients on Adriamycin was 12 weeks, while for black South African patients it was 16 weeks. Of the 29 black South African patients treated with Adriamycin in the ECOG trials, the median survival time was 15 weeks, which is not statistically different from median survival time for South African patients treated with *m*-AMSA or neocarzinostatin (drugs rejected as ineffective).

Other workers in the United States have also reported low response rates to Adriamycin [7, 24, 33]. While these and other reports confirm some activity for this agent in patients with primary liver cancer it can be stated that, at least among North American patients and black South African patients, this agent gives too low a response rate and too short a survival time to justify its use as a single agent, while histological grading and other patient discriminants at the start of treatment further explain away much of the response claimed on the African continent.

Mitoxanthrone, an anthracycline derivative, showed preclinical promise and, following a limited phase II pilot study in Pretoria, is now being investigated in a prospective randomized study by ECOG. At present a median survival time of 12 weeks is estimated, but we will have to wait for the final analysis of the ECOG trial before drawing any conclusions concerning this drug.

Combination Chemotherapy

Throughout the field of clinical oncology there are no exceptions to the rule that nothing is gained by adding drugs that do not have single-agent activity to a drug combination regimen. On the contrary, the addition of agents whithout therapeutic activity can not only lead to increased toxicity but, by decreasing the amount of therapeutic agent administered, will decrease therapeutic response. The literature is peppered with small series of uncontrolled trials of drug combinations in patients with primary liver cancer where patient discriminants are ignored and the results claimed are best explained by variations in the natural history of the disease. These reports are best ignored and will not be referred to. Recent attention to prognostic variables in the pathology, especially the subset of young white men (who have a much better prognosis), are pertinent.

Among the chemotherapy combinations investigated and found not to be effective are (1) vincristine (VCR) plus methotrexate (MTX) plus 6-mercaptopurine (6-MP) plus prednisone (Pred); (2) BCNU plus cytosine arabinoside; (3) 5-fluorouracil (5-FU) plus thiotepa; (4) 5-FU + mitomycin-C; (5) 5-FU + cyclophosphamide + MTX + VCR [8, 14, 25].

In the largest prospectively randomized controlled studies performed [15, 18] the following response rates were documented: oral 5-FU + streptozotocin, 12%; oral 5-FU + MeCCNU, 5%; intravenous 5-FU + MeCCNU, 13% in North American and European patients and 0% in South African black patients; intravenous 5-FU + streptozotocin, 10% in North American and 0 in South African patients; and intravenous 5-FU plus MeCCNU plus Adriamycin (ADM), 19% in North American and European patients. Of particular significance was the severe toxicity encountered in the patients treated with intravenous 5-FU + MeCCNU + ADM. The most finite measurement is median survival time. The median survival times in these two ECOG studies are shown in Table 1.

Of importance is that analysis showed initial performance status to be of more prognostic significance than treatment differences but that, among North American/European patients, those treated with intravenous 5-FU + MeCCNU survived longer than those

Table 1. Median survival times on combination chemotherapy in patients with primary liver cancer

Agent combinations	North American/European		South African	
	No. of patients	Survival (weeks)	No. of patients	Survival (weeks)
Oral 5-FU + STZ	White 15	31.1	11	11.5
	Black 5	14.2		
Oral 5-FU + MeCCNU	White 21	26.1	13	6.3
	Black 9	15.1		
iv. 5-FU + MeCCNU	45	28.0	10	8.0
iv. 5-FU + STZ	40	22.0	9	8.0
5-FU + MeCCNU + ADM	32	17.0	6	13.0

treated with ADM (28 vs 12 weeks, $P < 0.01$). Among South African patients the differences between treatment arms were not statistically significant. In these two ECOG studies objective response was seen in 29 of 309 evaluable patients, giving an overall response rate of less than 10%. A performance status of 0 at the start of treatment resulted in a median survival time of 52 weeks in contrast to a 5-week median survival time for patients with an initial performance status of 3. Illustrative of the real state of the art at the present time is the time to treatment failure (TTF) data from the latter of these two large ECOG studies. The median TTF (in weeks) among North American and European patients by treatment were: ADM, 7; intravenous 5-FU + MeCCNU, 10; intravenous 5-FU + STZ, 10; and 5-FU + MeCCNU + ADM, 11. Among South African blacks the corresponding figures were 16, 7, 5 and 13 weeks respectively.

Following the initial reports of therapeutic effect of Adriamycin for patients in Africa, combination chemotherapy incorporating ADM has been tried by various investigators. The results of the prospectively randomized ECOG trial with 5-FU, MeCCNU + ADM have been referred to above. In a SWOG study of ADM and 5-FU, of 38 patients eligible for the protocol, 5 patients had objective remission (13%) [1]. Morstyn et al. [29] found ADM + STZ to have only modest activity (9% partial response, 2 of 23 patients, median survival time 3 months).

Objective response was reported in 3 of 21 patients (14%) treated with a combination of ADM and MeCCNU, the median survival time in this series being 87 days [6].

Response has been reported in one of nine patients treated with ADM plus dichloromethetrexate, one of six treated with ADM plus 5-azacytidine, one of six treated with ADM plus ICRF 159, and one of six treated with ADM plus CTX [31].

As recently as March 1983 the results of a four-drug combination (5-FU, ADM, Mitomycin-C and MeCCNU) in 12 patients with primary liver cancer were published [32]. Until such time as more predictable and worthwhile response has been adequately documented for single agents, or until such time as an adequate motivation can be found for combination chemotherapy in patients with primary liver cancer, it is not justifiable to treat small groups of patients with drug combinations.

Children with hepatoblastoma have a different response to treatment. The pathology is unfortunately seldom reviewed and in the literature is often referred to only as malignant hepatoma (thus including hepatocellular carcinoma). The children's cancer study group and the pediatric group of SWOG recently reported on 62 patients studied. The median survival time is not given for all the patients on the study nor is it given by histological classification. Nevertheless a high response rate and long median survival is given both with and without measurable residual disease after surgical resection. The chemotherapy employed was vincristine, cyclophosphamide, Adriamycin and 5-fluorouracil [10].

Hormones and Primary Liver Cancer

Differences in sex incidence, liver changes ascribed to oral contraceptive drugs and the relatively young age of many patients with primary liver cancer have focused attention on the possible role of hormonal imbalance in the etiology of this disease. In the 1950s before controlled clinical trials had become fashionable, sex hormones and alloxan were given to patients with primary liver cancer [11, 23]. More recently oestrogen receptors have been demonstrated in the tumours of some patients with primary liver cancer [21]. These authors claimed tumour regression in two of five patients treated with progestin. The ECOG is investigating the effect of the anti-oestrogen tamoxifen, prompted by research done at the Memorial Sloan Kettering Cancer Centre and the American Oncologic Hospital by E. Cheng (personal communication, 1982) and P. Engstrom (personal communication, 1982).

The Present Approach to Treatment

The present approach to treatment of patients with primary liver cancer is dictated by the various discriminants, the most important of which remains initial performance status. Data from the large ECOG studies of North American, European and South African patients reconfirms this. For patients with a performance status of 0, the median survival time is 52 weeks, while for those with a performance status of 3, it is 5 weeks. From these data it is quite clear that for patients with a performance status of 4 (that is, bedridden patients) the approach should be as for any patient with a terminal malignant disease. The approach to treatment of patients with terminal malignant disease is aimed at treatment of symptoms without intensive care procedures. There is evidence that primary liver cancer behaves differently in different parts of the world. Recent in depth studies have shown that the difference, though in part due to racial factors, is largely explained by other identifiable discriminants such as performance status (and the factors affecting this, such as nutritional status) and histological differentiation. The median life expectancy of North American and European patients who still have an adequate performance status is in the order of 19 weeks, while for South African black patients this is in the order of 10 weeks. Series giving better survival times seldom have had the pathology material reviewed by a panel. It is clear that there is no treatment that can be called the treatment of choice. For a highly selected, very small subgroup of patients where primary liver cancer is diagnosed when it is early and localized, surgery can be considered. There are no available techniques for diagnosing a larger number of patients at an earlier time, so that patients suitable for surgery are most likely to be diagnosed by serendipity.

Most patients with primary liver cancer are eligible for protocols studying the value of new oncolytic agents in this disease. This approach is more logical than administering treatments known to be of value for less than 20% of the patients treated. Furthermore, the first oncolytic drug given to a patient has a far better chance of helping the patient than subsequent treatments. If is therefore recommended that patients with primary liver cancer should be referred to a cancer centre so that the disease can be better delineated and so that the patient can be offered new cytostatics rather than older agents shown to have only minimal therapeutic potential in this disease. When patients cannot be referred to an academic centre the doctor involved must face the agonizing decision as whether only to use symptomatic treatment or to administer treatment that has predictable toxicity, little hope of helping the patient but makes the doctor feel that he is treating the tumour as well as the patient.

Based on preclinical studies there is a list of agents showing considerable promise that have not yet been adequately tried in this disease.

Furthermore, as our understanding of the disease process increases, new and more specifically designed chemotherapy treatments are being designed. An example of a new approach that offers hope is the synthesis of daunomycin-fatty acid complexes by Deutsch of Madison [9].

Acknowledgment. This study was supported in part by a grant from the National Cancer Association of South Africa.

References

1. Baker LH, Saiki JH, Jones SE, Hewlett JS, Brownlee RW, Stephens RL, Vaitkevicius VK (1977) Adriamycin and 5-fluorouracil in the treatment of advanced hepatoma: a Southwest Oncology Group Study. Cancer Treat Rep 61: 1595-1597
2. Berman C (1951) A study of incidence, clinical manifestations, pathology and aetiology in primary carcinoma of the liver. Lewis, London
3. Bukowski RM, Legha S, Saiki J, Eyre HJ, O'Brein R (1982) Phase II trial of *m*-amsa in hepatocellular carcinoma - a Southwest Oncology Group Study. Cancer Treat Rep 66 (8): 1651-1652
4. Cavalli F, Rosenzweig M, Renard J, Goldhirsch A, Hansen HH (1981) Phase II study of oral VP-16-213 in hepatocellular carcinoma. Eur J Cancer Clin Oncol 17: 1079-1082
5. Cheng E, Lightdale C, Young C, Yagoda A, Fortner J, Golbey R (1983) Phase II trial of (*m*-AMSA) 4'-9-(acridinylamino)methanesulfon-*m*-anisidide in primary liver cancer. Am J Clin Oncol 6: 211-213
6. Chlebowski RT, Chan KK, Tong MJ, Weiner JM, Ryden VMJ, Bateman JR (1981) Adriamycin and methyl-CCNU combination therapy in hepatocellular carcinoma. Cancer 48: 1088-1095
7. Chlebowski RT, Brzechwa-Adjukiewicz A, Cowden A, Block JB, Tong M, Chan KK (1982) Full dose adriamycin in hepatocellular carcinoma: clinical and pharmacokinetic results. Proc AACR 23: 110
8. Cochranc AMG, Murray-Lyon IM, Brinkley DM, Williams R (1977) Quadruple chemotherapy versus radiotherapy in treatment of primary hepatocellular carcinoma. Cancer 40: 609
9. Deutsch HF, Tsukada Y, Sasaki T, Hirai H (1982) The in vivo cytotoxic effects of daunomycin-fatty acid complexes on rat hepatomas. Cancer Res (in press)
10. Evans AE, Land VJ, Newton WA, Randolph JG, Sather HN, Tefft M (1982) Combination chemotherapy (vincristine, Adriamycin, cyclophosphamide and 5-fluorouracil) in the treatment of children with malignant hepatoma. Cancer 50: 821-826
11. Falkson G (1959) Chemotherapie van Primêre Lewerkarsinoom. Spekulum 3: 5-11
12. Falkson G (1975) Therapeutic approaches to hepatoma. Cancer Treat Rev 2: 73-76
13. Falkson G (1976) The treatment of liver cell cancer. In: Cameron HM, Lirisell DA, Warwick GP (eds) liver cell cancer. Elsevier, Amsterdam
14. Falkson G (1982) The management of tumours of the liver and biliary tract. In: Carter SK, Glatstein E, Livingston RB (eds) Principles of cancer treatment. McGraw-Hill, New York
15. Falkson G, Moertel CG, Lavin P, Pretorius FJ, Carbone PP (1978) Chemotherapy studies in primary liver cancer. Cancer 42: 2149-2156
16. Falkson G, Von Hoff D, Klaassen D, Du Plessis H, Van der Merwe CF, Van der Merwe AM, Carbone PP (1980) A phase II study of Neocarzinostatin (NSC 157365) in malignant hepatoma. Cancer Chemother Pharmacol 4: 33-36
17. Falkson G, Coetzer B, Klaassen DJ (1981) A phase II study of *m*-amsa in patients with primary liver cancer. Cancer Chemother Pharmacol 6: 127-129
18. Falkson G, Moertel CC, MacIntyre JM, Lavin P, Engstrom PF, Carbone PP (1981) The value of cytostatic agents in the treatment of patients with primary liver cancer. In: Friedman M, Ogawa M, Kisner D (eds) Diagnosis and treatment of upper gastrointestinal tumors. Excerpta Medica, Amsterdam, pp 455-459
19. Falkson G, McIntyre J, Coetzer B, Schutt AJ, Engstrom PF, Carbone PP (1983) Phase II-III trial of neocarzinostatin versus *m*-amsa or Adriamycin in hepatocellular carcinoma. Proc AACR 24: 139
20. Falkson G, McIntyre JM, Moertel CG, Johnson LA, Scherman RC (1984) Primary liver cancer: an ECOG therapeutical trial. Cancer 54 (6): 970-977
21. Friedman MA, Demanes JD, Hoffman PG (1982) Hepatomas: hormone receptors and therapy. Am J Med 73: 362-366
22. Geddes EW, Falkson G (1970) Malignant hepatoma in the Bantu. Cancer 25: 1271-1278
23. Gillman T, Hathorn M, Lamont NME (1957) Alloxan as a possible therapeutic agent for primary carcinoma of the liver. Lancet 272 (6970): 687-688

24. Ihde DC, Kane RC, Cohen MH, McIntyre KR, Minna JD (1977) Adriamycin therapy in american patients with hepatocellular carcinoma. Cancer Treat Rep 61: 1385-1387
25. Lee Yeu Tsu M (1977) Systemic and regional treatment of primary carcinoma of the liver. Cancer Treat Rev 4: 195-212
26. Leichman L, MacDonald B, Dindogin A, Samson M (1982) Platinum: a clinically active drug in advanced adenocarcinoma of the stomach. Proc AACR 23: 110
27. Melia WM, Westaby D, Williams R (1981) Diaminodichloride - platinum (*cis*-platinum) in the treatment of hepatocellular carcinoma. Clin Oncol 7: 275-280
28. Melia WM, Johnson PJ, Williams R (1983) Induction of remission in hepatocellular carcinoma. A comparison of VP-16 and Adriamycin. Cancer 51: 206-210
29. Morstyn G, Ihde DC, Eddy JL, Bunn PA, Cohen MH, Minna JD (1982) Combination chemotherapy with doxorubicin and streptozotocin (DXC/STZ) in hepatocellular carcinoma (HC). Proc AACR 23: 113
30. Olweny CLM, Toya T, Katongole-Mbidde E, Mugerwa J, Kyalwazi SK, Cohen H (1975) Treatment of hepatocellular carcinoma with Adriamycin: preliminary communication. Cancer 36: 1250-1257
31. Olweny CL, Katongole-Mbidde E, Bahendeka S, Otim D, Mugerwa J, Kyalwazi SK (1980) Further experience in treating patients with hepatocellular carcinoma in Uganda. Cancer 46: 2717-2722
32. Stein SH, Ajani JA, Karlin DA, Nelson RS (1983) Combination chemotherapy of hepatocellular carcinoma with 5-fluorouracil, Adriamycin, mitomycin-C and methyl-CCNU (FAMMe). Proc ASCO 2: 120
33. Vogel CL, Bayley AC, Brooker RJ, Anthony PP, Ziegler JL (1977) A phase II study of Adriamycin (NSC 123 127) in patients with hepatocellular carcinoma from Zambia and the United States. Cancer 39: 1923-1929

Systemic Therapies for Patients with Liver Tumors: Prospects for the Future

M. A. Friedman

Clinical Investigations Branch, Cancer Therapy Evaluation Program, Division of Cancer Treatment, National Cancer Institute, Landow Building, Room 4A04, Bethesda, MD 20892, USA

Attempts to identify effective chemotherapy for patients with liver metastases represent a specific aspect of the more general search for meaningfully beneficial systemic chemotherapy of primary and metastatic tumors.

For most adult malignant diseases, liver metastases have the biologic features of that cancer at the primary or nonhepatic metastatic site. Those cancers which are considered refractory to chemotherapy are as insensitive at an hepatic as any other site of metastases. Unfortunately, intravenous (i.v.) systemic chemotherapy is inadequate for most of the commonly encountered tumors, such as colon, pancreas, and non-small-cell lung cancers. Moreover, even for those disseminated malignancies somewhat more sensitive to chemotherapy, such as breast, gastric, small-cell lung, and ovarian cancers, the potential for cure is nearly nonexistent. This therapeutic intractibility, coupled with the frequency of liver metastases, defines the magnitude of this serious clinical problem.

Recently, Huberman [1] and Kemeny [2] have reviewed the published data on the effectiveness of systemic chemotherapy utilized in patients with a variety of cancers which metastasize to the liver. Their compilations and conclusions are frustratingly familiar to those of the clinical oncologic community. Fewer than 25% of patients with colorectal cancer metastatic to liver respond to any chemotherapy [either single-agent 5-fluorouracil (5-FU) or any other combination program]. Moreover, the median survival for this group of colorectal cancer patients is limited and usually ranges from 2 to 9 months. The clinical situation for melanoma and lung, gastric, and pancreatic cancer is no better. As expected, breast cancer metastases in the liver are more frequently palliated since this disese is inherently more responsive to chemotherapy. If more effective systemic treatment were uniformly available, there would be no need for whatsoever specific hepatic therapies. Special regional approaches to patients with Hodgkin's disease or testicular cancer in the liver are not considered reasonable since systemic therapy is so uniformly effective. Where such meaningfully efficacious intravenous therapy is lacking, clinical investigators have tried to exploit modestly active agents in focussed regional approaches.

Due to the large number of patients with liver metastases, the lack of effective "competing" therapies, and technologic advances (in catheters, radiologic imaging, infusion devices, etc.), there has been a renaissance or interest in locoregional therapy of liver metastases patients. This enthusiasm has been fueled by encouraging phase II trials. However, these data are not conclusive because of their uncontrolled nature (utilizing historical controls), small sample size, and possible patient-institution-investigator selection biases. To date, no prospective randomized phase III study has conclusively demonstrated the supe-

Recent Results in Cancer Research. Vol 100

riority of hepatic intraarterial (i.a.) therapy over i.v. therapy. In fact, the phase III trials so far support the opposite contention. These studies are, however, flawed in design (not ideal drug choices, dosages, and schedules) and cannot be considered definitive. There are in progress several studies which should answer this question, including those of the Northern California Oncology Group, North Central Cancer Treatment Study Group, Memorial Sloan-Kettering Institute, Piedmont Oncology Association, and the Ensminger consortium. It is possible that the benefits detected in the phase II studies are due to improved drug dosage and scheduling, rather than route of administration. Currently, there is no single BEST therapy for patients with hepatic metastases of colorectal cancer, and further careful investigation is warranted.

Even if focussed hepatic therapy is beneficial, is it appropriate for all cases with liver involvement? The answer is almost assuredly "no".

The design of therapeutic approaches to the patient with liver metastases is based on several simple, logical considerations, including:

Patient characteristics
1. Performance status
2. Hepatic organ dysfunction
3. Coexisting significant illnesses
4. Extent of disease (number of metastatic sites)
5. Overall tumor burden
6. Specific metastatic sites

Disease characteristics
1. Inherent sensitivity of tumors to chemotherapy
2. Proclivity for metastases
3. Virulence of tumor (median survival)

For example, the use of regional hepatic therapy for patients with disseminated pancreatic cancer is usually ineffective and inappropriate because liver metastases are only a portion of the metastatic burden (which often includes nodal, peritoneal, and other sites), the disease is notoriously chemotherapy refractory, and patients die within weeks of diagnosis. By contrast, some patients with colorectal cancer appear to have metastases confined only to the liver and a survival of many months. It is quite reasonable to consider a focussed hepatic therapy for palliation of some of these patients.

Arguably, the above features can be synthesized into the following schema:

Candidates for focussed hepatic therapy

I. Ideal - always appropriate
   None

II. Satisfactory - sometimes appropriate
   Colorectal
   Hepatoma
   Biliary

III. Unsatisfactory - rarely appropriate

Breast	Gynecologic
Gastric	Genitourinary
Pancreatic	Melanoma
Lung	Sarcoma

IV. Not to be considered - never appropriate
   Lymphoma
   Testicular

Awaiting the advent of strikingly effective new systemic single agents or combination chemotherapy, it is worthwhile to explore the opportunities that currently exist for palliating patients with hepatic tumors. This following discussion will focus primarily on new approaches to colorectal adenocarcinoma patients. This tumor type is probably the ideal model system for these investigations because of its frequency of liver metastases, survival times, and responsiveness to therapy.

Pharmacologic Exploitation of Systemic Drugs

If the principal clinical problem to be addressed is liver metastases, it is rational to employ an effective agent which, because of chemical characteristics, is preferentially concentrated in the liver. There are, currently, at least two drugs which have this pharmacologic feature. Both 5-fluoro-2′-deoxyuridine (FUdR) and dichloromethotrexate (DCMTX) have enhanced hepatic concentration and metabolism when administered either by the i.v. or i.a. route. Ensminger [3] has demonstrated that for a 2-hour i.v. infusion of FUdR the hepatic extraction ranged from 59% to 92% (average of 80%). The hepatic concentration of i.v. FUdR was inferior to its i.a. administration (94%-99% one-pass extraction), but was two to four times better than 5-FU given i.v. (22%-45%). It can, therefore, be persuasively argued that FUdR administered i.a. or i.v. is the pharmacologically preferred fluoropyrimidine for patients with liver metastases. The data for DCMTX are not as precisely known, but Ensminger and colleagues [4] have demonstrated a 40%-65% one-pass hepatic extraction of i.a.-administered drug (200 mg/m^2 over 2 h). A substantial proportion of DCMTX is hepatically metabolized and excreted in bile and feces (up to 50%) [5]. It is suspected, although not specifically determined, that i.v. DCMTX has a similarly favorable hepatic extraction ratio (almost certainly superior to methotrexate administered i.v. or i.a).

As i.v. single agents, both FUdR and DCMTX have been reported to induce partial responses in patients with hepatic metastases of colon and hepatocellular cancer [1, 5] but such benefits have been infrequent and transient. The enhanced localization of a minimally effective agent should not, of course, result in dramatic benefits. Moreover, it is not known if these drugs merely concentrated in the liver or preferentially in the hepatic metastases.

It is unlikely that single agents even with favorable physical-chemical characteristics, like FUdR or DCMTX, will result in dramatic antitumor effects. Therefore, the identification of a drug which has enhanced hepatic concentration is only the first step in designing combination programs.

Systemic Biochemical Modulation

In parallel with an enhanced understanding of the systemic and regional pharmacology of antitumor agents we are gaining greater appreciation of potentially useful biochemical interactions. There have been considerable efforts devoted to the elucidation of the interactions of antimetabolites, especially antifols and fluoropyrimidines, in order to try to improve clinical response rates.

In murine and human tumor cell lines, the sequenced use of methotrexate (MTX) preceding 5-FU (MTX→5-FU) results in synergistic cell kill superior to that of either drug used alone, the simultaneous use of both, or the reverse sequence (5-FU→MTX) [6-8]. Although the precise mechanism of action of this synergy is not known, one hypothesis is that MTX inhibits purine synthesis, resulting in increased phosphoribosyl pyrophosphate

(PRPP), and increases 5-FU incorporation in nucleic acid (DNA and/or RNA) [9]. In order to achieve synergistic cytotoxicity, careful attention to the MTX dosage (achieving adequate intracellular concentration) and interval between MTX and subsequent 5-FU is necessary. Cadman has suggested that $\geqslant 5\mu$-M or greater plasma MTX concentration might be required and that an interval of 8-24 h between the MTX and 5-FU (1 μM) might be optimal.

Based on this biochemical rationale, dozens of pilot studies employing various MTX doses (60-600 mg/m^2), 5-FU doses (600-1000 mg/m^2), intervals (1-24 h), and schedules (bolus and infusion) have been reported with various enthusiasm [10-19]. Objective response rates of 0%-50% have been reported with widely differing amounts of toxicity. Overall, relatively few biologically homogeneous patients have been carefully evaluated and therefore only broad confidence intervals of response are obtainable. To date no controlled phase III studies have been completed, and it is not currently possible to demonstrate the efficacy of this approach (see below).

At the same time, investigative interest in combinations of reduced folate cofactor (such as citrovorin) and 5-FU has been notable. Based on initial observations of Ullman, Santi, and others [20-22], it is now clear that intracellular-reduced folate cofactors encourage more avid binding of FdUMP to its target enzyme, thymidylate synthetase, and enhanced cytotoxicity in both murine and human tumor systems. Again, clinical trials have generally been uncontrolled phase II efforts with 5-FU and citrovorin factor (CF), but Machover [22], Bruckner [23-25], and others [26, 27] have demonstrated interesting preliminary antitumor and toxicity effects.

However, without large, well-structured definitive trials, it is not possible to determine if these attempts at biochemical modulation of antimetabolites will result in improved response rates and durations. To address these issues, there are at least three large phase III studies recently initiated in the United States. In these studies, 5-FU is the control (reference) therapy and is given by the i.v. route; the CF and MTX is given either parenterally or orally.

GITSG study 6384
Regimen
1. 5-FU 600 mg/m^2 q week
2. 5-FU 1000 mg/m^2 q 3 weeks
   +
   CF 25 mg/m^2
3. 5-FU 600 mg/m^2 q week
   +
   CF 500 mg/m^2
4. 5-FU 600 mg/m^2 q week
   +
   CF 25 mg/m^2

NCCTG study 83-46-52
Regimen

A	5-FU 500 mg/m^2/d × 5	q 5 weeks
B	MTX 200 mg/m^2 7 h + 5-FU 900 mg/m^2 + CF 14 mg/m^2	q 3 weeks

C	MTX 40 mg/m^2 24 h + 5-FU 600 mg/m^2	day 1, 8 q 4 weeks
D	CF 200 $mg/m^2/d \times 5$ + 5-FU 370 $mg/m^2/d \times 5$	q 4 weeks
E	CF 20 $mg/m^2/d \times 5$ + 5-FU 370 $mg/m^2/d \times 5$	q 4 weeks
F	CDDP 20 $mg/m^2/d \times 5$ + 5-FU 325 $mg/m^2/d \times 5$	q 5 weeks

NCOG Study 3C-83-1
Regimen

A	5-FU 12 $mg/kg/d \times 5$ then (4 weeks later) 15 mg/kg/week	
B	5-FU 400 $mg/m^2/d \times 5$ CF 200 $mg/m^2/d \times 5$	q 4 weeks
C	MTX 50 mg/m^2 q 6 h $\times$ 5 5-FU 500 mg/m^2 (24° later) CF 10 mg/m^2 q 6 h $\times$ 6	q week

Clearly, many different dosages and schedules are being explored but these represent only a small fraction of the possible permutations. If any of these studies proves positive (compared with standard 5-FU therapy) and the proposed MTX-5-FU ± CF hypotheses are in fact valid, there are additional experiments worthy of further investigation. Combining the hypotheses of the preferential pharmacologic localization of FUdR and DCMTX, and biochemical modulation concepts, an i. v. study of DCMTX→FUdR would be one of many worthwhile experiments.

Regional Aspects of Combination Chemotherapy, Biochemical, or Pharmacologic Modulation

Empirically, combinations of 5-FU and cis-diaminodichloroplatinum (CDDP) have been utilized in patients with metastatic colorectal cancer. Based on preclinical animal model systems, synergy of these agents can be demonstrated [28].

Despite relatively disappointing single-agent activity of i. v. CDDP, the combination of i. v. 5-FU and CDDP has been initially reported to be promising by Einhorn and colleagues at the University of Indiana [29, 30]. To date, no studies of FUdR + CDDP have been initiated and attempts to use i. a. CDDP + fluoropyrimidine have not been carefully explored.

In a similar way, a considerable body of in vitro data supports the synergistic activity of combinations of cytosine arabinoside (Ara-C) + CDDP. Dramatic and tumor synergy has been demonstrated with the simultaneous combination in LoVo human colon cancer cell line [31] and lymphoma cells [32]. The mechanism of action is thought to be Ara-C enhancement of DNA cross-linking by CDDP and diminished DNA repair [32]. However, in order to achieve this cytotoxic potentiation, relatively high intracellular concentrations of Ara-C are probably required. Initial trials with i.v. Ara-C at 20-60 $mg/m^2/d \times 3$ and 100 mg/m^2 CDDP have demonstrated hematologic toxicity without dramatic efficacy. However, it may be that Ara-C concentrations of 1000 µg/ml (and 10 µg/ml CDDP) may be required for synergistic cell kill [32].

Simultaneous doses of 1.5 g/m^2 Ara-C and 110 mg/m^2 CDDP have resulted in less marrow toxicity and some responses in squamous tumors. However, given the short serum half-time of Ara-C it is unknown whether i.v. administration provides adequate intracellular drug levels.

There are also data that Ara-C accumulation in L1210 cells can be enhanced by prior treatment with 5-FU and FUdR [33]. No single biochemical mechanism has been determined, but 5 *M* Ara-C for 4 h is an effective in vitro concentration when preceded by 5-FU or FUdR.

Recognizing the above data and to attempt to enhance the therapeutic ratio and exploit biochemical opportunities, specific combinations of i.v. and i.a. approaches could be considered.

Possible protocols for i.v. or i.a. routes to be considered for patients with metastatic colorectal cancer could include:

1. DCMTX → FUdR	Taking advantage of antifol-fluoropyrimidine interactions
2. Ara-C + CDDP	To achieve better intracellular CDDP cytotoxicity
3. FUdR → Ara-C + CDDP	Taking advantage of the inherent antitumor effects of FUdR and its ability to increase Ara-C intracellular concentration and thereby enhance CDDP effectiveness
4. DCMTX → FUdR → Ara-C + CDDP	All of the above

Obviously, phase II trials, no matter how carefully designed, carried out, or analyzed, do not substitute for phase III studies. Definitive comparison trials are required. However, important preliminary information can be obtained - especially for i.a. therapy in those patients who have a permanent catheter in place and who have failed a first-line single-agent approach (with FUdR for example). Preliminary toxicity and efficacy information can be gathered.

In comparative trials, there are many valid study end points besides response rates and durations. Analysis of the patterns of failure is crucial since an increased rate of extrahepatic metastases may negate the local hepatic benefits obtained by an i.a. approach. The quantity and quality of toxicity is important. The benefits of diminished hematologic toxicity may be negated by severe, irreversible hepatobiliary toxicity (as is seen with prolonged i.a. FUdR at 0.3 mg/kg per day × 14 q 28 days administration). Finally, the costs of i.a. therapy must be carefully assessed. The financial and morbidity consequences of i.a. therapy may outweigh favorable antitumor responses.

Finally, the clinical enthusiasm for biochemical modulation is appropriate, but must be tempered with some precautions. Prior to initiating a clinical study, careful attention should be paid to the preclinical biochemistry and pharmacology experiments. Misinterpretation of the in vivo and in vitro data leads to the design of poor clinical investigations. Also, it is necessary to identify and achieve the important biochemical goals (such as ↑-PRPP with MTX→5-FU) and pharmacologic end points ($\geqslant 5\ \mu M$ MTX→ $\geqslant 1\ \mu M$ 5-FU) of a study. Laboratory confirmation of the desired modulation assures the adequacy of the clinical trial. Testing of a biochemical modulation hypothesis is considerably more than a simple evaluation of clinical response and toxicity results.

Given our expanding understanding of biochemistry and pharmacology of antitumor agents there is cause for modest therapeutic optimism.

References

1. Huberman MS (1983) Comparison of systemic chemotherapy with hepatic arterial infusion in metastatic colorectal carcinoma. Semin Oncol 10, 2: 238-248
2. Kemeny N (1983) The systemic chemotherapy of hepatic metastases. Semin Oncol 10, 2: 148-158
3. Ensminger WD, Rosowsky A, Raso V, Levin DC, Glode M, Come S, Steele G, Frei E III (1978) A clinical-pharmacological evaluation of hepatic arterial infusions of 5-fluoro-2′-deoxyuridine and 5-fluorouracil. Cancer 38: 3784-3792
4. Ensminger W, Dakhil S, Doan K, Cho K, Wheeler R, Pollard HM (1981) Clinical pharmacology of dichloromethotrexate in hepatic arterial infusions. Proc AACR 22: 271
5. Tester WJ, Donehower RC, Eddy JE, Myers CE, Ihde DC (1982) Evaluation of weekly escalating doses of dichloromethotrexate in patients with hepatocellular carcinoma and other solid tumors. Cancer Chemother Pharmacol 8: 305-310
6. Bertino JR, Sawicki WL, Lindquist CA, Gupta VS (1977) Schedule dependent antitumor effects of methotrexate and 5-fluorouracil. Cancer Res 37: 327-328
7. Cadman E, Heimer R, Davis L (1979) Enhanced 5-fluorouracil nucleotide formation after methotrexate administration: explanation for drug synergism. Science 205: 1135-1137
8. Benz C, Cadman E (1981) Modulation of 5-fluorouracil metabolism and cytotoxicity by antimetabolite pretreatment in human colorectal adenocarcinoma HCT-8. Cancer Res 41: 994-999
9. Cadman E, Heimer R, Benz C (1981) The influence of methotrexate pretreatment on 5-fluorouracil metabolism in L1210 cells. J Biol Chem 256: 1695-1704
10. Weinerman B, Schacter B, Schipper, Bowman D, Levitt M (1982) Sequential methotrexate and 5-FU in the treatment of colorectal cancer. Cancer Treat, Rep 66: 1553-1555
11. Solan A, Vogl SE, Kaplan BH, Berenzweig M, Richard J, Lanham R (1982) Sequential chemotherapy of advanced colorectal cancer with standard or high-dose methotrexate followed by 5-fluorouracil. Med Pediatr Oncol 10: 145-149
12. Cantrell, Jr. JE, Brunet R, Lagard C, Schein PS, Smith FP (1982) Phase II study of sequential methotrexate-5-FU therapy in advanced measurable clorectal cancer. Cancer Treat Rep 66: 1563-1565
13. Herrmann R, Manegold C, Rittinghausen R, Fritze D, Schettler G (1981) Sequential methotrexate (MTX) and 5-fluorouracil (FU) in colo-rectal adenocarcinoma. Results of a pilot study. Proc ASCO/AARC 22: 457
14. Drapkin R, Griffiths E, McAloon E, Paladine W, Sokol G, Lyman G (1981) Sequential methotrexate (MTX) and 5-fluorouracil (5-FU) in adenocarcinoma of the colon and rectum. Proc ASCO/AACR 22: 453
15. Mehrotra S, Rosenthal CJ, Gardner B (1982) Biochemical modulation of antineoplastic response in colorectal carcinoma: 5-fluorouracil (F), high dose methotrexate (M) with calcium leukovorin (L) rescue (FML) in two sequences of administration. Proc ASCO 1: 100
16. Kemeny N, Michaelson R (1982) Phase II trial of low dose methotrexate and sequential 5-fluorouracil in the treatment of metastatic colorectal carcinoma. Proc ASCO 1: 95
17. Mahajan SL, Ajani JA, Kanojia MD, Bedikian AY (1983) Comparison of two schedules of sequential high-dose methotrexate (MTX) and 5-fluorouracil (5-FU) for metastatic colorectal carcinoma. Proc ASCO 2: 122
18. Ajani JA, Kanojia MD, Bedikian AY, Korinek JK, Stein SW, Espinoza EG, Bodey GP (1985) Sequential conventional dose methotrexate (MTX) and 5-fluorouracil (5-FU) in the primary therapy of metastatic colorectal carcinoma. Am J Clin Oncol 8(1): 69
19. Hansen R, Ritch P, Anderson T (1983) Sequential methotrexate (MTX), 5-fluorouracil (5-FU), and leukovorin (LCV) in colorectal cancer. Proc ASCO 2: 117

20. Ullman B, Lee M, Martin DW, Santi DV (1978) Cytotoxicity of 5-fluoro-2'-deoxyuridine: requirement for reduced folate cofactors and antagonism of methotrexate. Proc Nat Acad Sci USA 75: 980-983
21. Evans RM, Laskin JD, Hakala M (1981) Effect of excess folates and deoxyinosine on the activity and site of action of 5-fluorouracil. Cancer Res 41: 3283-3295
22. Machover D, Schwarzenberg L, Goldschmidt E, Tourani JM, Michalski B, Hayat M, Dorval T, Misset JL, Jasmin C, Maral R, Mathe G (1982) Treatment of advanced colorectal and gastric adenocarcinomas with 5-fluorouracil (5-FU) combined with high dose folinic acid (FA). Proc Am Soc Clin Oncol 1: 33
23. Bruckner HW, Ohnuma T, Hart R, Jaffrey I, Spiegelman M, Ambinder E, Storch JA, Wilfinger C, Goldberg J, Biller H, Holland JF (1982) Leucovorin (LV) potentiation of 5-fluorouracil (FU) efficiency and potency. Proc Am Assoc Cancer Res 23: 111
24. Bruckner HW, Storch JA, Holland JF (1981) Leucovorin increases the toxicity of 5-fluorouracil: phase I clinical pharmacological trials. Proc Assoc Clin Res 22: 192
25. Bruckner HW, Roboz J, Spigelman M, Ambinder E, Hart R, Holland JF (1983) An efficient leucovorin and 5-fluorouracil sequence: dosage escalation and pharmacological monitoring. Proc Am Assoc Cancer Res 23: 138
26. Byrne P, Smith F, Treat J, Bowers MW, McVie G, Hunink TB, Schein P (1983) 5-fluorouracil and higher dose for folinic acid treatment of colorectal carcinoma patients. Proc ASCO 474: 121
27. Cunningham J, Bukowski R, Budd T, Hewlett J, Purvis J (1983) Folinic acid (FA) combined with 5-flourouracil (5-FU): phase I-II clinical trial. Proc ASCO 167: 42
28. Schabel FM, Trader MW, Laster WR, Corbott TH, Griswold DP (1979) Cis-dichlorodiammine platinum (II): combination chemotherapy and cross resistance studies with tumors of mice. Cancer Treat Rep 63: 1459-73
29. Kovach JS, Moertel CG, Schutt AJ, O'Connell MJ (1983) Phase II study of *cis*-diammine dichloroplatinum (NSC-1119875) in advanced carcinoma of the large bowel. Cancer Chemother Rep 57: 357-358
30. Einhorn L, Williams SD, Loehrer PJ (1984) Combination chemotherapy with platinum (P) plus 5-FU in metastatic colorectal carcinoma. Proc ASCO 520: 133
31. Schilsky RL, Brown H, Monaghan G, Muscato J, Perry MC (1983) Phase I trial of cytosine arabinoside (Ara-C) and *cis*-platin (DDP) in patients with advanced cancer. Proc ASCO 2: 20
32. Bergerat J-P, Drewinko B, Corry P, Barlogie B, Ho DH (1981) Synergistic lethal effect of *cis*-dichlorodiammineplatinum and 1-μ-D-arabino-furanosylcytosin. Cancer Res 41: 25-30
33. Grant S, Cadman E (1982) Modulation of 1-μ-D-arabinofuranosylcytosin metabolism and cytotoxicity in L1210 cells by fluoropyrimidine pretreatment. Cancer Res 42. 3550-3556

Biochemical Basis for Improving Chemotherapeutic Regimens in Liver Malignancies

D. Keppler and A. Holstege

Biochemisches Institut, Universität Freiburg, Hermann-Herder-Strasse 7, 7800 Freiburg i. Brsg., FRG

Introduction

As long as it is impossible to prevent or to correct the altered expression of genetic information in malignant cells, tumor chemotherapy has to aim at the elimination of malignant cells by means of cytostatic or cytocidal drugs that are as selective as possible for a given tumor. The minimal difference in the sensitivity of normal and neoplastic cells remains a critical limitation in the use of effective agents, many of which are antimetabolites that inhibit enzymes of essential metabolic pathways on the basis of a structural similarity with physiological intermediates, interfering thereby with cellular growth and proliferation. This may be illustrated by the blockade of thymidylate synthetase induced by 5-fluoro-5′-deoxyuridinemonophosphate (FdUMP), a metabolite of the pyrimidine analog 5-fluorouracil (reviewed by Heidelberger [5]. The consequent depletion of deoxythymidine-5′-monophosphate (dTMP) and deoxythymidine-5′-triphosphate (dTTP) pools should result in DNA synthesis inhibition due to substrate deficiency. This is one of several mechanisms by which fluorinated pyrimidines preferentially inhibit proliferating cells. This effect may be circumvented, however, by dTMP formation from deoxythymidine on the salvage pathway, and this underlines the critical importance of quantitative metabolite-antimetabolite relationships in tumor chemotherapy.

Pyrimidine nucleotide formation on the salvage pathway is largely due to the pyrimidine nucleosides circulating in plasma (reviewed by Keppler and Holstege [12]) and to increased activities of pyrimidine salvage enzymes in many tumors [18]. Furthermore, activities of pyrimidine salvage enzymes are by far higher than those of the rate-determining enzymes of de novo pyrimidine synthesis as demonstrated in a large spectrum of tumors [18]. In this contribution the emphasis is put on antimetabolites that interfere with pyrimidine nucleotide metabolism in a combination that exploits some of the specific metabolic capacities and the enzyme pattern of hepatocyte-derived tumors. The experimental studies in rat hepatomas may serve to improve the chemotherapy of human hepatocellular carcinoma. An inhibition of pyrimidine nucleotide synthesis will not only affect the synthesis of DNA and RNA, but also syntheses of phospholipids, glycolipids, glycoproteins, and other glycoconjugates.

Recent Results in Cancer Research. Vol 100

Inhibition of Pyrimidine Synthesis De Novo

A classical approach has been the blockage of de novo synthesis by inhibitors of enzymes in the pathway of pyrimidine synthesis de novo including *N*-(phosphonoacetyl)-L-aspartate (PALA), a transition state analog in the aspartate carbamoyltransferase reaction, certain naphthoquinones interfering with the oxidation of dihydroorotate, and the inhibitors of orotidine-5′-phosphate (OMP) decarboxylase derived from 6-azauridine and pyrazofurin (Fig. 1). All these antimetabolites are effective and deplete the uridine triphosphate (UTP) pool of hepatoma cells in culture [15]. In vivo, however, their effect can be circumvented by pyrimidine nucleotide synthesis on the salvage pathway. Up to now, the means to interfere with salvage synthesis are limited. We have therefore introduced an additional approach in which the pool of UTP and related nucleotides in tumor cells is depleted by metabolic diversion [10, 15].

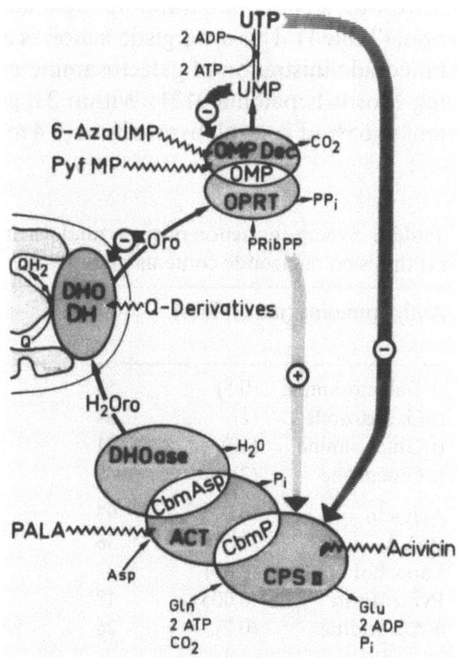

Fig. 1. Inhibitors, proteins, and regulation of de novo synthesis of UTP in mammalian cells. Glutamine-dependent carbamoyl-phosphate synthetase *(CPS II)*, aspartate carbamoyltransferease *(ACT)*, and dihydroorotase *(DHOase)* comprise the catalytic centers on the multifunctional protein pyr 1-3 that initiates de novo pyrimidine synthesis [8]. Dihydroorotate dehydrogenase *(DHODH)*, located on the outside of the inner mitochondrial membrane, produces orotate *(Oro)* from dihydroorotate *(H_2Oro)* and reduces ubiquinone *(Q)*. This enzyme is inhibited by Q-derivatives such as the 1,4-naphthoquinones dichloroallyl lawsone and lapachol [3]. The bifunctional UMP synthase, or multienzyme pyr 5,6, comprises orotate phosphoribosyltransferase *(OPRT)* and orotidine-5′-phosphate decarboxylase *(OMP Dec)* [8]. Potent inhibitors of the decarboxylase include the 5′-monophosphates of 6-azauridine *(6-AzaUMP)* and of pyrazofurin *(PyfMP)*. Allosteric effectors of the pathway include UTP as feedback inhibitor and 5-phosphoribose 1-diphosphate *(PRibPP)* as activator of carbamoyl-phosphate synthetase [17]

Synergistic Action of Uridylate-Trapping Sugar Analogs with Inhibitors of Pyrimidine Synthesis De Novo

Several sugar analogs lead to an accumulation of the respective UDP-hexose analog. As a consequence, the UTP pool is depleted, causing an inhibition of RNA synthesis due to substrate deficiency [13]. Among the hexose analogs that we have so far used as uridylate-trapping agents (Fig. 2), two are metabolized preferentially in hepatocytes and in hepatoma cells: D-galactosamine [4] and D-galactosone [14]. These galactose analogs are metabolized on the galactose pathway by the kinase, the transferase, and the epimerase, which are most abundant in liver and quite active in hepatomas [16]. In contrast to galactose metabolism, analogs such as galactosamine will not regenerate the UDP-sugar in a cyclic process, but will accumulate UDP-sugar analogs in a process continuously consuming UTP. Hepatoma cells, as well as other tumor cells, show high activities relative to hepatocytes of the enzymes of pyrimidine synthesis de novo [18]. This enables them to compensate for the uridylate-trapping action of the galactose analogs by an active formation of uridylate and UTP on the de novo pathway [9]. Combination of an inhibitor of pyrimidine synthesis de novo with an uridylate-trapping sugar analog results in a synergistic depletion of the UTP pool (Table 1). This synergistic action is also observed in vivo as exemplified by the combined administration of galactosamine and pyrazofurin in rats carrying the slowly growing Morris hepatoma 9121: Within 2 h galactosamine (1 mmol/kg) lowers the UTP content to 65% of control, pyrazofurin (0.4 mmol/kg) to 83%, and both agents deplete UTP to

Table 1. Synergistic action of sugar analogs and inhibitors of de novo UMP synthesis on nucleotide contents of hepatoma cells

Antipyrimidine (mmol/liter)		UTP	CTP	GTP	ATP
			(% of control)		
D-Galactosamine	(0.5)	53	47	79	71
D-Galactosone	(1)	64	64	95	86
D-Glucosamine	(10)	21	22	70	55
D-Glucosone	(2)	48	58	85	79
Acivicin	(0.075)	93	23	35	59
PALA	(1)	36	41	99	98
Lapachol	(0.01)	33	40	93	95
Pyrazofurin	(0.005)	18	21	117	110
6-Azauridine	(0.2)	26	35	34	103
D-Galactosamine + acivicin		18	19	28	46
D-Galactosamine + PALA		5	33	100	80
D-Galactosamine + lapachol		12	16	95	90
D-Galactosamine + pyrazofurin		4	37	113	76
D-Galactosamine + 6-azauridine		3	40	57	73
D-Galactosone + PALA		13	20	96	89
D-Glucosamine + 6-azauridine		5	30	58	71
D-Glucosone + PALA		12	36	93	81

AS-30D hepatoma cells were incubated for 3 h in the presence of antipyrimidines. Control contents were 0.65 ± 0.12, 0.39 ± 0.03, 0.44 ± 0.04, and 2.81 ± 0.32 mmol/kg AS-30D wet cells ± SD for UTP, CTP, GTP, and ATP, respectively [15]

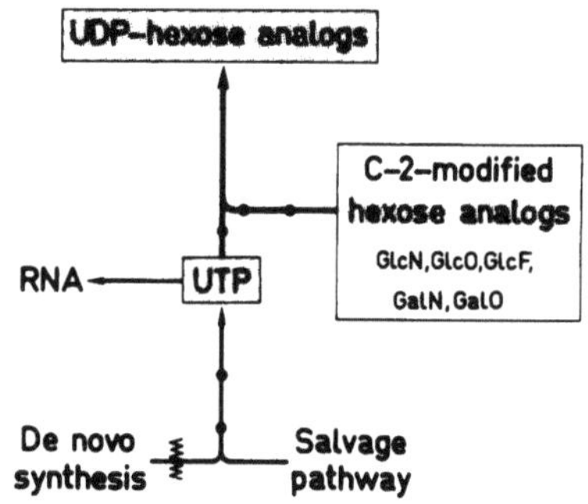

Fig. 2. UTP deficiency induced by the synergistic action of an inhibitor of UMP synthesis de novo and the carbon-2-modified analogs of D-glucose or D-galactose diverting uridylate and leading to an accumulation of UDP-hexose analogs. *GlcN,* D-glucosamine (2-amino-2-deoxy-D-glucose); *GlcO,* D-glucosone (D-*arabino*-hexos-2-ulose); *GlcF,* fluoroglucose (2-deoxy-2-fluoro-D-glucose); *GalN,* D-galactosamine (2-amino-2-deoxy-D-galactose); *GalO,* D-galactosone (D-*lyxo*-hexos-2-ulose)

17%. In non-hepatocyte-derived tumors, such as the solid TA3-mammary tumor line, glucose analogs, such as glucosamine, are more effective due to the different enzyme pattern in this tumor (Table 1).

Enhanced Uptake and Incorporation of 5-Fluorouridine in UTP-Depleted Tumor Cells

The synergistic action of an inhibitor of de novo pyrimidine synthesis together with uridylate-trapping sugar analogs can effectively inhibit cell proliferation [10], but the effect is transient in vivo. We have therefore used this cell-specific depletion of UTP for an increased uptake of 5-fluorouridine (FUrd) [2, 6, 11]. The rate-determing step in the formation of the active phosphorylated metabolites of FUrd is catalyzed by uridine kinase. This enzyme, which is more active in malignant than in normal cells [18], is under feedback control of the end products, and its activity can be raised by a depletion of UTP [1]. In exploiting this regulatory mechanism, it is essential to use the ribonucleoside FUrd, since 5-fluorouracil would not be a direct substrate for uridine kinase.

In cultured hepatoma cells, with depleted UTP and cytidine triphosphate (CTP) pools induced by D-galactosamine and an inhibitor of pyrimidine synthesis de novo, the uptake of FUrd was increased up to fourfold (Fig. 3). The predominant intracellular metabolite of FUrd was FUTP but considerable amounts of FUDP-amino sugars were formed as well [6, 19]. In rats carrying the Morris hepatoma 7777, the antipyrimidine treatment increased the incorporation of labeled FUrd into the isolated RNA of the tumor up to 3.5-fold, whereas incorporation of FUrd into host liver RNA was unchanged and low as compared with that into the tumor [2]. Tissue distribution of FUrd uptake in these rats demonstrates that pretreatment with D-galactosamine and 6-AzaUrd enhanced the uptake into the hepatoma more than twice, while liver, spleen, intestines, and brain were not affected significantly.

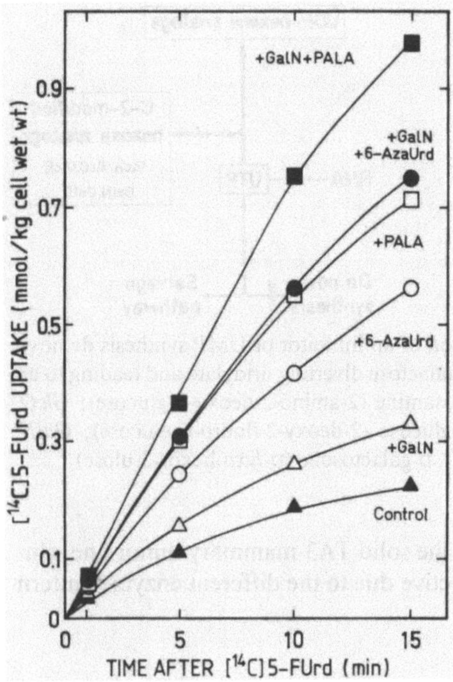

Fig. 3. Uptake of 5-fluoro[2-^{14}C] uridine into AS-30D hepatoma cells pretreated with antipyrimidines. Incubation in the presence of the inhibitors lasted for 3 h when labeled fluorouridine (0.23 mmol/liter; 1.2 Ci/mol) was added [6]

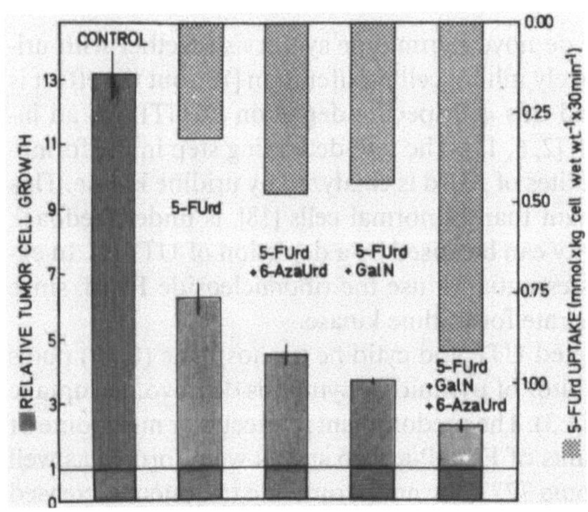

Fig. 4. Enhancement of 5-fluorouridine uptake and growth inhibitory action by antipyrimidine pretreatment in hepatoma cells. AS-30D cells were preincubated with D-galactosamine and/or 6-azauridine followed by 5-fluoro[^{14}C]-uridine treatment for 30 min. Washed hepatoma cells (5×10^7/rat) were injected i. p. and their in vivo growth measured after 54 h [7]

Growth Inhibition of Hepatoma Cells Induced by Combined Antipyrimidine Treatment

The inhibition of hepatoma cell growth in vivo correlated with the uptake of FUrd into the tumor cells (Fig. 4). The highest uptake, incorporation into RNA, and growth inhibitory action were induced when FUrd was administered after pretreatment of the cells with D-galactosamine, as uridylate-trapping sugar analog, and 6-azauridine, as inhibitor of pyrimidine synthesis de novo. In rats carrying the AS-30D ascites hepatoma, 80% cured survivors were obtained after sequential treatment with D-galactosamine, PALA, and FUrd [2]. Treatment of the same hepatoma line after its implantation into the liver extend-

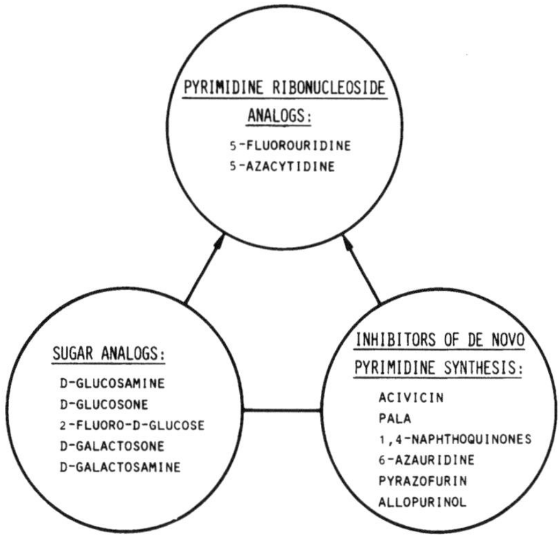

Fig. 5. Combination of antipyrimidines for tumor chemotherapy. UMP-trapping sugar analogs specify and intensify the effect of inhibitors of UMP synthesis de novo; the resulting depletion of pyrimidine nucleotide pools enhances the subsequent uptake and action of pyrimidine ribonucleoside analogs such as FUrd and 5-azacytidine [15]

ed the median survival time by 85% as compared with a 37% extension by FUrd alone; 70-day survivors were 29% of the rats treated with D-galactosamine, 6-azauridine, and FUrd, whereas 0% survived after treatment with FUrd alone [2]. These results indicate that the efficacy and selectivity of chemotherapeutic antipyrimidines can be increased by synergistic combinations. The dosage schedules may be further improved and optimal antipyrimidine combinations for a given tumor may replace D-galactosamine as the sugar analog; furthermore, the optimal inhibitors of pyrimidine synthesis de novo may not be 6-azauridine or PALA, but acivicin or an inhibitor of dihydroorotate dehydrogenase such as the 1,4-naphthoquinones (Fig. 5). Each combination would provide a rational approach for improving the chemotherapy of hepatocellular carcinoma and other malignant tumors.

Acknowledgments. The research outlined in this contribution was supported by grants from the Deutsche Forschungsgemeinschaft.

References

1. Anderson EP, Brockman RW (1964) Feedback inhibition of uridine kinase by cytidine triphosphate and uridine triphosphate. Biochim Biophys Acta 91: 380-386
2. Anukarahanonta T, Holstege A, Keppler D (1980) Selective enhancement of 5-fluorouridine uptake and action in rat hepatomas *in vivo* following pretreatment with D-galactosamine and 6-azauridine or *N*-(phosphonoacetyl)-L-aspartate. Eur J Cancer 16: 1171-1180
3. Bennett LL Jr, Smithers D, Rose LM, Adamson DJ, Thomas HJ (1979) Inhibition of synthesis of pyrimidine nucleotides by 2-hydroxy-3-(3,3-dichloroallyl)-1,4-naphthoquinone. Cancer Res 39: 4868-4874
4. Decker K, Keppler D (1974) Galactosamine hepatitis: key role of the nucleotide deficiency period in the pathogenesis of cell injury and cell death. Rev Physiol Biochem Pharmacol 71: 77-106

5. Heidelberger C (1975) Fluorinated pyrimidines and their nucleosides. In: Sartorelli AC, Johns DC (eds) Antineoplastic and immunosuppressive agents, part II. Springer, Berlin Heidelberg New York, pp 193-231
6. Holstege A, Herrmann B, Keppler D (1978) Increased formation of nucleotide derivatives of 5-fluorouridine in hepatoma cells treated with inhibitors of pyrimidine synthesis and D-galactosamine. FEBS Lett 95: 361-365
7. Holstege A, Herrmann B, Anukarahanonta T, Pausch J, Keppler D (1979) Die Wirkung von 5-Fluoruridin in Kombination mit Antipyrimidinen in Tumorzellen. Verh Deutsch Ges Inn Med 85: 1296-1300
8. Jones ME (1980) Pyrimidine nucleotide biosynthesis in animals: genes, enzymes, and regulation of UMP biosynthesis. Ann Rev Biochem 49: 253-279
9. Keppler D (1975) Consequences of uridine triphosphate deficiency in liver and hepatoma cells. In: Keppler D (ed) Pathogenesis and mechanisms of liver cell necrosis. MTP Press, Lancaster, pp 87-101
10. Keppler D (1977) Uridine triphosphate deficiency, growth inhibition, and death in ascites hepatoma cells induced by a combination of pyrimidine biosynthesis inhibition with uridylate trapping. Cancer Res 37: 911-917
11. Keppler D (1978) Approaches to the chemotherapy of hepatomas. In: Remmer H, Bolt HM, Bannasch P, Popper H (eds) Primary liver tumors. MTP Press, Lancaster, pp 485-492
12. Keppler D, Holstege A (1982) Pyrimidine nucleotide metabolism and its compartmentation. In: Sies H (ed) Metabolic compartmentation. Academic Press, London, pp 147-203
13. Keppler D, Pausch J, Decker K (1974) Selective uridine triphosphate deficiency induced by D-galactosamine in liver and reversed by pyrimidine nucleotide precursors. Effect on ribonucleic acid synthesis. J Biol Chem 249: 211-216
14. Keppler D, Schulz-Holstege C, Fauler J, Reiffen KA, Schneider F (1982) Uridylate trapping, induction of UTP deficiency, and stimulation of pyrimidine synthesis *de novo* by D-galactosone. Biochem J 206: 139-146
15. Keppler D, Fauler J, Gasser T, Holstege A, Leube K, Schulz-Holstege C, Weckbecker G (1985) Uridylate-trapping sugar analogs in combination with inhibitors of uridylate synthesis *de novo* and 5-fluorouridine. Adv Enzyme Regul 23: 61-79
16. Reutter W, Bauer C (1978) Terminal sugars in glycoconjugates: Metabolism of free and protein-bound L-fucose, *N*-acetyl-neuraminic acid and D-galactose in liver and Morris hepatomas. In: Morris HP, Criss WE (eds) Morris hepatoma. Plenum Publ., Amsterdam, New York, pp 405-437
17. Tatibana M, Shigesada K (1972) Two carbamyl phosphate synthetases of mammals: specific roles in control of pyrimidine and urea biosynthesis. Adv Enzyme Regul 10: 249-271
18. Weber G (1983) Biochemical strategy of cancer cells and the design of chemotherapy: G. H. A. Clowes Memorial Lecture. Cancer Res 43: 3466-3492
19. Weckbecker G, Keppler D (1984) Substrate properties of 5-fluorouridine diphospho sugars detected in hepatoma cells. Biochem Pharmacol 33: 2291-2298

Enhancement of the Effects of 5-Fluorouracil

R. Herrmann

Medizinische Klinik, Klinikum Charlottenburg der Freien Universität, Spandauer Damm 130, 1000 Berlin 19, FRG

5-Fluorouracil (5-FU) is one of the few anticancer agents that has been developed on a rational basis [10]. Although it has been clinically used since the late 1950s, 5-FU has recently attracted new interest because of two developments:

1. Methods have been developed which allow the detection of small amounts of 5-FU and most of its metabolites.
2. There has been a revival of regional drug administration, especially hepatic artery infusion. Since 5-FU is metabolized in the liver to a significant degree, it is one of the drugs used for this administration.

Despite these newer developments the mechanism of action of 5-FU is not yet clearly understood. Several actions have been described:

1. Binding to thymidylate synthetase (TS), consequently inhibiting DNA synthesis [9]
2. Incorporation into RNA, resulting in a false, malfunctioning RNA [6]
3. Incorporation into DNA [14]

The relative importance of these actions is not easy to determine in human tumors in vivo. The mechanism of action responsible for the inhibition of tumor growth may vary from

Table 1. Substances affecting fluoropyrimidine metabolism

Methotrexate[a]
Citrovorum factor[a]
Methyl-mercaptopurine-riboside (MMPR)[a]
N-(Phosphonacetyl)-*L*-aspartic acid (PALA)[a]
Pyrazofurine
Allopurinol[a]
Thymidine[a]
Uridine
Guanosine
Deoxyuridine
Ribose-1-phosphate
Deoxyribose-1-phosphate

[a] Compounds studied in combination with 5-FU in man

Recent Results in Cancer Research. Vol 100

tumor to tumor and should depend on the concentration and activity of anabolic enzymes and the availability of substrates and cosubstrates.

The recent advances in our understanding of the biochemistry of the fluoropyrimidines have led to several intriguing approaches to combination chemotherapy on a rational basis. Table 1 gives a still incomplete list of substances that affect pyrimidine metabolism and therefore influence the metabolism of 5-FU.

Among the antimetabolites interfering with 5-FU metabolism, methotrexate (MTX) is the one most intensively studied. There is a large number of experimental studies indicating synergism between MTX and 5-FU if MTX is given prior to 5-FU [1, 4, 17]. The mechanism of this interaction has been studied in vitro. Following MTX preincubation Cadman and coworkers have found increased levels of phosphoribosyl pyrophosphate (PRPP) facilitating formation of 5-FU ribonucleotides, and subsequent incorporation into RNA [4]. On the other hand increased binding of 5-fluoro-2′-deoxyuridylate (FdUMP) to TS has been found following MTX preincubation [8]. However, all these findings have been called into question since they are results of studies in nonphysiological culture conditions [16]. We have therefore studied this problem in an in vivo system to find out about:

1. The relevance of the time interval between MTX and 5-FU
2. The effect of varying MTX doses
3. The mechanism of action of this sequential combination

The results of these in vivo studies have been published [13] and can be summarized as follows:

1. For sarcoma 180 there is an optimum time interval in the range of 8–12 h.
2. High, purine-synthesis-affecting MTX doses are necessary to achieve sufficient synergism.
3. MTX pretreatment increases 5-FU in the TS fraction as well as in the RNA fraction.

The sequential combination of MTX and 5-FU has also been studied in several clinical trials. While pretreatment characteristics and drug dosage and scheduling differ widely the results can be summarized:

1. There is preliminary evidence (phase II trials) that this sequential combination is synergistic in colorectal and breast cancer
2. Drug dosage and scheduling seem to be very important determinants of efficacy

In colorectal cancer we found a 38% response rate in previously untreated patients. The results of this study have been published in detail [11]. A phase III trial comparing this approach with single-agent 5-FU is underway and will be completed soon. In far advanced breast cancer a 28% partial remission (PR) rate was found in patients who had received adriamycin and CMF previously (cyclophosphamide, MTX, 5-FU) [12]. From this study we feel that this combination adds something to or is superior to CMF. Many investigators have used a 1-h time interval and their results have been disappointing [2, 3, 5, 7, 15]. We have compiled the available data for previously untreated colorectal cancer and found a response rate of 16% for those studies using a 1-h time interval and a response rate of 38% for those using a 4- or more h time interval.

Unfortunately there is a number of variables that may influence the activity of antimetabolites in vivo. For example, it has been shown that there may be large differences in the quantity and quality of important enzymes and nucleotide pools in tumor cells. The metabolic situation of the patient may vary dependent on his or her general condition or diet.

There may be diurnal variations in the concentrations of important substrates and cosubstrates. Most of these problems have not been looked at in detail.

The introduction of the sequential MTX-fluoropyrimidine concept into the intraarterial treatment of liver metastases is now being advocated. It should, however, be kept in mind that the sequential combination of MTX and FUdR, the drug most commonly used for this approach, cannot be expected to act synergistically [4].

Theoretically, biochemical modulation of 5-FU metabolism can be achieved with many substances. A number of them improve 5-FU efficacy in vitro. These results, however, need to be tested in appropriate in vivo models, where efficacy as well as toxicity can be determined. For the treatment of human cancer, combinations are required that increase the therapeutic index compared with 5-FU single-agent treatment.

References

1. Bertino JR, Sawicki WL, Lindquist CA, Gupta VS (1977) Schedule-dependent antitumor effects of methotrexate and 5-fluorouracil. Cancer Res 37: 327-328
2. Blumenreich MS, Woodcock TM, Allegra M, Richman SP, Kubota TT, Allegra IC (1982) Sequential therapy with methotrexate and 5-fluorouracil for adenocarcinoma of the colon. Proc Am Soc Clin Oncol 18: 102 (Abstr)
3. Burnet R, Smith FP, Hoerni B, Lagarde C, Schein P (1981) Sequential methotrexate-5-fluorouracil in advanced measurable colorectal cancer: lack of appreciable therapeutic synergism. Proc Am Soc Clin Oncol 17: 370 (Abstr)
4. Cadman E, Heimer R, Benz C (1981) The influence of methotrexate pretreatment on 5-fluorouracil metabolism in L1210 cells. J Biol Chem 256: 1695-1704
5. Cantell JE, Burnet R, Lagarde C, Schein PS, Smith FP (1982) Phase II study of sequential methotrexate-5-FU therapy in advanced measurable colorectal cancer. Cancer Treat Rep 66: 1563-1565
6. Carrico CK, Glazer RI (1979) Effect of 5-fluorouracil on the synthesis and translation of polyadenylic acid-containing RNA from regenerating rat liver. Cancer Res 39: 3694-3701
7. Coates AS, Hedley D, Fox RM, Raghavan D, Tattersall MHN (1983) Randomised trial of sequential methotrexate (M) followed by 5-fluorouracil (F) versus F followed by M. Proc Am Assoc Cancer Res 74: 140 (Abstr)
8. Fernandes DJ, Bertino JR (1980) 5-fluorouracil-methotrexate synergy: enhancement of 5-fluorodeoxyuridylate binding to thymidylate synthetase by dihydropteroyl-polyglutamates. Proc Natl Acad Sci USA 77: 5663-5667
9. Hartman KU, Heidelberger C (1961) Studies on fluorinated pyrimidines. VIII. Inhibition of thymidylate synthetase. J Biol Chem 236: 3006-3013
10. Heidelberger C, Chandhuri NK, Danenberg P, Mooren D, Griesbach L, Duschinsky R, Schnitzer J, Pleven E, Scheiner J (1957) Fluorinated pyrimidines, a new class of tumor-inhibitory compounds. Nature 179: 663-666
11. Herrmann R, Spehn J, Beyer JH, von Franque U, Schmieder A, Holzmann K, Abel U (1984a) Sequential methotrexate and 5-fluorouracil. Improved response rate in metastatic clorectal cancer. J Clin Oncol 2: 591-594
12. Herrmann R, Manegold C, Schroeder M, Tigges FJ, Bartsch H, Jungi F, Fritze D (1984b) Sequential methotrexate and 5-fluorouracil in breast cancer resistant to the conventional application of these drugs. Cancer Treat Rep 68: 1279-1281
13. Herrmann R, Kunz W, Osswald H, Ritter M, Port RD (1985) The effect of methotrexate pretreatment on 5-fluorouracil kinetics in sarcoma 180 in vivo. Eur J Cancer Clin Oncol 21: 753-758
14. Kufe DW, Egan EM (1981) Enhancement of 5-fluorouracil incorporation into human lymphoblast ribonucleic acid. Biochem Pharmacol 30: 129-133

15. Panasci L, Margolese R (1982) Sequential methotrexate and 5-fluorouracil in breast and colorectal cancer. Results of increasing the dose of FU. Proc Am Soc Clin Oncol 18: 101 (Abstr)
16. Piper AA, Nott SE, Mackinnon WB, Tattersall MHN (1983) Critical modulation by thymidine and hypoxanthine of sequential methotrexate-5-fluorouracil synergism in murine L1210 cells. Cancer Res 43: 5701-5705
17. Wayss K, Herrmann R, Mattern J, Volm M (1985) Sequential methotrexate and 5-fluorouracil in human tumor xenografts. Med Oncol Tumor Pharmacother 2 (1): 27-32

Systemic Infusional Chemotherapy for Liver Metastasis: An Improved Schedule for 5-Fluorouracil

J. J. Lokich

Section of Internal Medicine, Hematology and Oncology, New England Deaconess Hospital, 110 Francis Street, Boston, MA 02215, USA

Regional chemotherapy, and particularly hepatic arterial chemotherapy, has had a resurgence of interest in the recent past because of the development of improved technology in the form of the implanted infusion pump. The history of this form of chemotherapy, however, over the past 2 decades has consistently demonstrated response rates which are superior to standard systemic chemotherapy and in fact hepatic arterial chemotherapy is effective in 25%-60% of patients not responding to the standard systemic delivery. The rationale for regional delivery relates to maximizing the dose delivery to the tumor and because of hepatic extraction minimizing host toxicity in spite of the maximal doses. However, in addition to the regional delivery of drug, there is another important distinction from standard chemotherapy, namely the infusion schedule.

The importance of drug scheduling in cancer chemotherapy has been largely ignored in that traditional systemic chemotherapy involves delivery of bolus drug based on maximizing the dose of delivery and as a consequence of associated toxicity an intermittent schedule is an essential necessity. However, drug pharmacology and tumor kinetics combine to suggest at least on theoretic grounds that continuous drug exposure over time might improve tumor cell kill. Experimental trials for the antipyrimidines which have an extraordinarily short half-life have demonstrated in in-vitro systems that for a fixed dose increasing exposure time increases tumor cell death.

This presentation will review the systemic chemotherapy of metastatic colorectal cancer in particular with a historical review of randomized trials employing 5-fluorouracil as a bolus and as an infusion and will develop the rationale and experience of a new infusion schedule for 5-fluorouracil. Finally, the relative role and practical application of hepatic arterial chemotherapy versus systemic chemotherapy will be addressed.

Bolus Schedule Trials for 5-Fluorouracil

The two major clinical trials which examine the role of schedule (as well as route of administration) for 5-fluorouracil (5-FU) were conducted by the Central Oncology Group (COG) and the Eastern Cooperative Oncology Group (ECOG) [1, 2]. Table 1 reviews the details of these two trials. Additional clinical trials have employed a 5-fluorouracil single-agent arm as a control arm for evaluating multi-drug regimens which have incorporated 5-FU. As a generality, such trials have not established a superior treatment regimen to that of 5-FU [3-6].

Recent Results in Cancer Research. Vol 100

In the COG study, four treatment regimens were employed in a prospective randomized experimental design. The response rates were comparable for the less intense treatment arms employing either weekly or oral 5-FU, but the response rate was doubled or greater in the arm delivering 5-FU in an intensive regimen and this arm was also associated with a longer median survival. The ECOG study which also employs a weekly schedule, either oral or intravenous, had a similar low response rate and modest median survival.

Infusion Schedule Trials for 5-Fluorouracil: Short-term Delivery

In contrast to 5-FU bolus schedules, the infusion schedule has been evaluated in a series of clinical trials with both antipyrimidines (Table 2) [7, 8, 9]. In the initial study of 5-fluorouracil for short-term 8-h infusion by Reitemeier et al. in 1962, the response rate was comparable in the two arms as it was also in the 1972 study reported by Moertel et al., in which the infusion time was shortened to 2 h. In the study by Moertel et al. in 1967, a longer duration of infusion was evaluated in a prospective comparative trial against the bolus schedule, in this instance employing the antipyrimidine (5-fluoro-2′-deoxyuridine (5-FUdR). In this particular study, it was emphasized that the pattern of toxicity was altered substan-

Table 1. Effectiveness of bolus 5-fluorouracil in advanced colorectal cancer

Study	Dose/schedule (route)	Number	Response (%)	Median survival (weeks)
COG [1]	12 mg/kg/day × 5 (i. v.)[a]	35	33	55
	15 mg/kg weekly (i. v.)	35	13	42
	500 mg × 4 (i. v.)[b]	36	14	42
	15 mg/kg × 6 (oral)	35	14	25
ECOG [2]	600 mg/m^2 weekly (i. v.)	39	15	30
	600 mg/m^2 weekly (p. o.)	28	18	33

[a] Following the loading course patients received 50% doses × 11 q. d. then weekly
[b] Following the loading course patients received weekly doses

Table 2. Clinical studies of antipyrimidines by infusion in colorectal cancer

Study	Design	Number	Response (%)
Reitemeier [7]	5-FU bolus	45	20
	vs		
	5-FU 8-h infusion	45	11
Moertel et al. [8]	5-FUDR bolus	63	17.5
	vs		
	5-FUDR 5-day infusion	65	6.2
Moertel et al. [9]	5-FU bolus	74	12
	vs		
	5-FU 2-h infusion	75	12

tially by the infusion schedule and, furthermore, the response rate was superior in the bolus schedule, with a statistically significant advantage.

In addition to these earlier studies, two more recent studies of 5-FU scheduling have been performed and in both a distinct advantage for the infusion schedule was established (Table 2). The initial study by Seifert et al. in colorectal cancer evaluated a bolus schedule for 5 days versus a short-term infusion schedule for 5 days [10]. The response rate was doubled in the group receiving the infusion and the median survival was extended by a factor of 4. In the study by Kish et al. [11] in head and neck cancer, a similar advantage for the infusion schedule was identified. In this study, all patients received platinum as well as 5-FU and the bolus schedule for the 5-FU was a day, 1,8 schedule as opposed to a daily times 5 days schedule. A response rate of 72% was achieved in patients with the infusion schedule compared with 20% for the bolus schedule, a difference which was statistically significant in favor of the infusion arm.

On the basis of the last two prospective randomized trials, the infusion schedule at least for the short term would appear to be the optimal schedule for the delivery of 5-fluorouracil. Additional clinical phase II studies without a prospective randomized design have also demonstrated higher response rates than usually associated with standard bolus 5-FU (Table 4). Nonetheless, there is an essential need to identify the optimal schedule for infusion in terms of duration, and in the presence of conflicting reports from various institutions it would appear prudent to expand these studies and confirm or deny the definitive role of schedule for delivery of the antipyrimidines.

Protracted Infusion Schedules for 5-Fluorouracil

In contrast to short-term infusion for up to 5 days, the rationale for a prolonged infusion is based on maximizing the duration of tumor cell exposure to drug. The fact that the half-life of most cytotoxic agents is relatively short as indicated earlier is complemented by the

Table 3. 5-FU schedule studies: bolus versus infusion

Study	Tumor	Infusion dose schedule	*N*	Response (%)	Bolus dose schedule	*N*	Response (%)	*P*
Kish et al. [11]	Head and neck	15 mg/kg/ day 96 h	20	72	600 mg/m^2	20	20	0.01
Seifert et al. [10]	Colon	30 mg/kg/ day 120 h	34	44	12 mg/kg/ day day 1-5	36	22	-

Table 4. Clinical studies of antipyrimidines by infusion

Study	Design	Number	Response (%)
Hartman et al. [13]	5-FU 5-day infusion (× 1 then bolus weekly)	36	23
Shah et al. [12]	5-FU 2-day infusion (weekly)	30	30

fact that tumors in general and gastrointestinal tumors in particular are slow-growing tumors with a small proportion of cells in the cycling phase reflected in a long tumor doubling time.

In the context of establishing a maximum duration of drug exposure, the optimal dose rate would be that which would permit prolonged exposure and would of necessity not be accompanied by toxicity which might interrupt the infusion or exposure time. In a series of phase I trials of protracted infusion chemotherapy, the optimal dose rate of eight cytotoxic agents covering the spectrum of drug classes has been established. This section will focus on the phase I and phase II trials which have involved protracted continuous infusion of the two antipyrimidine analogs, 5-FU and 5-FUdR [14, 15].

The practical logistics of such a treatment regimen have been previously reported. In brief, all patients have a central venous access established either by the use of a tunneled subclavian catheter or by the subcutaneous implantation of a venous access port with a silastic catheter in the subclavian vein. In the latter system, a right-angle Huber point needle is placed through the skin and into the venous access port (Fig. 1) and the needle is connected by catheter to an ambulatory infusion pump.

In the phase I trials of 5-FU, the goal was to establish an optimal daily dose rate in order to provide a minimum treatment duration of 30 days. A synopsis of that trial is given in Table 5. At the lower dose rates of 200 and 300 mg/m^2 per day, essentially no toxicity was observed, with the majority of the patients achieving the minimum treatment duration of 30 days. As a generality, the dose rate tolerated for 30 days could be tolerated for an extended interval without the development of limiting toxicity observed at the higher dose rates. At dose dose rates above 300 mg/m^2 per day the treatment duration was abbreviated to 3 or 2 weeks with all patients demonstrating toxicity primarily in the form of oral stomatitis and without marrow suppression. The optimal dose rate for delivery of protracted infusion of 5-FU is, therefore, 300 mg/m^2 per day, which represents an increase in the tolerated dose of approximately 400% over that delivered by a bolus schedule for a comparable period.

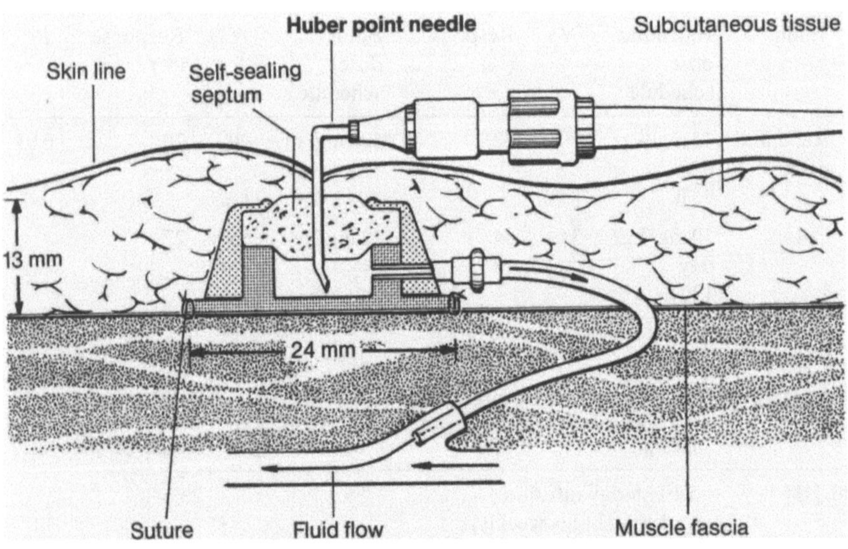

Fig. 1. Subcutaneous venous access disk indicating diagrammatically the component parts in situ

Table 5. Phase I study of continuous infusion 5-fluorouracil (5-FU)

Dose level (mg/m² day)	Number	Median treatment duration (days)	Toxicity
200	5	30	None
300	4	38	None
350	4	20	Stomatitis (4/4)
400	4	9	Stomatitis (4/4)
600	2	16	Stomatitis (2/2)

Table 6. Phase I study of continuous infusion 5-fluoro-2′-deoxyuridine (5-FUdR)

Dose level (mg/m² day)	Number	Median treatment duration (days)	Toxicity
0.1	4	30	None
0.125	2	34	None
0.15	5	16	Diarrhea 4/5 Stomatitis 1/5
0.175	4	9	Diarrhea 4/4
0.2	3	10	Diarrhea 3/3 Stomatitis 2/3

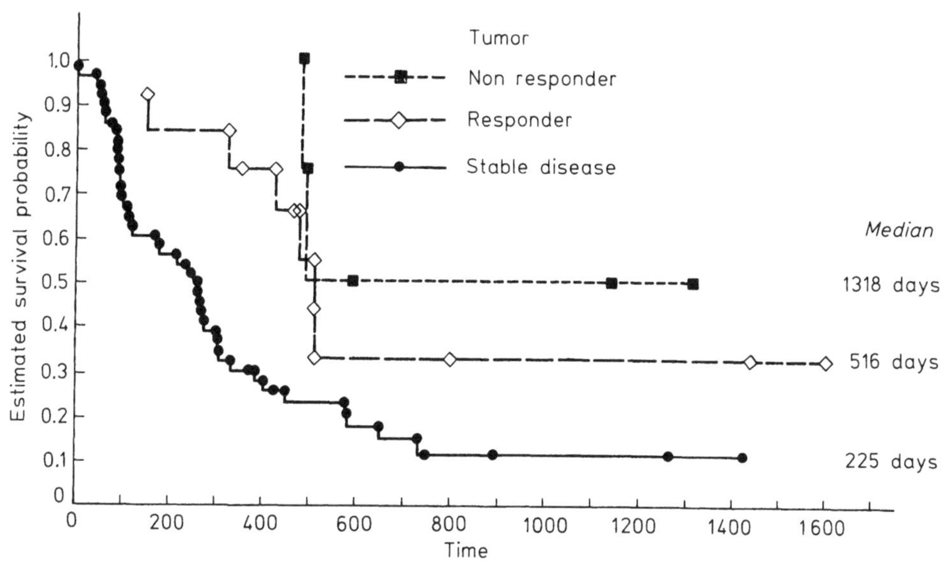

Fig. 2. Survival curves according to tumor response in 116 patients receiving protracted systemic infusion of 5-FU

The phase I trial of protracted infusion FUdR is given in Table 6. This study was initiated primarily to establish the optimal dose rate for this antipyrimidine in order that comparative trials of systemic and arterial delivery systems could employ a comparable drug since there is data which suggest that the clinical efficacy in terms of tumor response may be different for the two agents. In this phase I study the drug was delivered at doses of 0.1 mg/kg per day up to 0.2 mg/kg per day. There was no toxicity observed at the lower dose rates, with durations achieved of 4 weeks or more in most patients. At 0.15 mg/kg per day, dose-limiting toxicity was demonstrated in all patients, generally in the form of diarrhea and with durations of treatment that could not exceed 3 weeks. For this antipyrimidine, therefore, the dose deliverable on the infusion schedule decreased to one-tenth of that deliverable by the bolus schedule and is in distinct contrast to the 5-FU experience.

In the context of these phase I trials, a unique toxicity was observed with 5-FU but was not seen with 5-FUdR. The toxicity is manifest as a swelling and erythema of the palms and soles with periungual erythema as well. The cutaneous syndrome is associated with progressive pain in the distal extremities and recedes promptly over 4–5 days following interruption of the infusion with desquamation of the palms and soles. A summary review of the clinical manifestation of this syndrome has been reported [16].

Phase II trials with the protracted infusion schedule have been ongoing and in a series of 55 evaluable patients with advanced measurable colorectal cancer, tumor regression employing standard criteria was observed in 38% of 55 patients and the response rate was the same irregardless of prior treatment with bolus 5-FU. Survival data in an expanded group of 116 patients with colorectal cancer is indicated in Fig. 2. The median survival of the overall group is 400 days with responders and stable disease patients at 516 and 1318 days and nonresponders at 225 days. A statistical analysis of significance in these groups is not appropriate since the patient entries were heterogeneous and a number of factors may have contributed to the survival differences observed unrelated to tumor regression.

A New Perspective on 5-Fluorouracil?

Based on the previous discussion of infusion schedules for the two antipyrimidines, a reexamination of the clinical efficacy of these agents may be justified. Certainly, phase III trials should be expanded to evaluate the infusion schedule in relationship to traditional chemotherapy delivered as an intermittent bolus. Additional important issues, however, relate to the concern that infusion chemotherapy, particularly in the protracted schedule, may result in the earlier development of tumor cell resistance based upon selection or induction.

In addition, there may be practical advantages as well as theoretical advantages to employing shorter infusion intervals. Thus, for example, sequential administration of non-cross-resistant agents employing an infusion schedule may obviate the development of resistance. Similarly, the introduction of multiple agents in combination may restrict the evaluation of tumor cell resistance. Thus, phase III trials comparing short-term and protracted infusion are important.

Finally, short-term infusion 5-FU has become standard therapy for the treatment of anal cancer [18] and for esophageal cancer in conjunction with radiation [17], and in the prospective trial in head and neck cancer the infusion schedule was clearly superior. A phase III trial in colorectal cancer comparing protracted infusion 5-FU with standard bolus fluorouracil is in process under the auspices of the Mid-Atlantic Oncology Group in the United States. This study is designed to enter more than 200 patients and should definitively answer the question of the relative benefits of infusion and bolus schedules in terms of response rate as well as survival.

Hepatic Arterial Chemotherapy: Comparative Trials for Systemic Chemotherapy

The central issue in hepatic arterial chemotherapy is the question of whether the apparent advantage of hepatic artery infusion (HAI) is due not to the route of delivery but rather to the schedule of infusion. The limitations of hepatic arterial delivery systems for the treatment of liver metastasis are substantial, as indicated in Table 7. In addition, it is evident that the liver is the solitary site of metastasis in less than 30% of patients destined to develop metatasis from colorectal cancer. If indeed the infusion schedule is as effective systemically as in the liver, then the use of such therapy to treat all patients is expanded and the cost substantially decreased.

In order to address the question of route versus schedule the most appropriate vehicle would be a prospective comparative trial. The singular comparative trial of hepatic artery infusion and systemic chemotherapy reported in final form was marred by the experimental design as well as logistic issues [19]. In this trial by the Central Oncology Group, intravenous 5-FU delivered on a bolus schedule was compared with hepatic artery infusion 5-FU delivered on an infusion schedule as indicated in Table 8. Although the reported response rate was higher in the group receiving hepatic artery infusion, the median survival was in fact longer in the group receiving systemic 5-FU, although essentially there was no statistically significant difference in the two arms. More recent prospective trials comparing systemic FUDR delivered by infusion and hepatic arterial FUDR on a similar schedule will definitively answer the question of route versus schedule [20, 21].

Table 7. Limitations of hepatic arterial delivery for liver metastases (HAI)

1. Anomalous arterial vasculature
2. Inability to affect extrahepatic metastases
3. Toxicity related to biliary sclerosis and chemical hepatitis as well as gastritis
4. Cost and morbidity for procedures involving operatively placed systems particularly implanted pumps

Table 8. Details of prospective randomized comparative trial of systemic versus arterial chemotherapy for advanced colorectal cancer (COG-study)

Treatment	Schedule	Number	Response (%)	Median survival (months)
i.v. 5-FU	12 mg/kg/d × 4 bolus 6 mg/kg/d × 4 bolus 15 mg/kg/week bolus	30	23	13.3
HAI 5-FU	20 mg/kg/d × 14 infusion 10 mg/kg/d × 7 infusion 15 mg/kg/week bolus	31	34	10.0

Summary and Conclusions

The clinical studies of infusion schedules for cancer chemotherapy have established that this schedule substantially alters the pattern of drug toxicity without necessarily compromising therapeutic effectiveness. Although increased tumor cell killing has not been definitively established, in at least two prospective comparative trials of 5-FU the infusion schedule was superior to bolus delivery in terms of response rate. It is possible that the infusion schedule may be the primary determinant of the effectiveness of hepatic arterial chemotherapy, and preliminary reports of prospective trials comparing systemic infusion with hepatic infusion do suggest that response rates for both routes are similar. An important consideration with regard to infusion schedules is establishing whether or not tumor cell resistance is augmented by the continous exposure. Almost all chronic disease therapy necessitates maintaining adequate drug levels to ensure disease control including infections, seizure disorders, arthritis, and cardiovascular diseases. For cancer, the intermittent schedule of drug delivery has been dictated by the concept of the primacy of dose and the substantial toxicity associated with these agents. With the technological capability of providing an ambulatory setting for infusion chemotherapy and the substantial modification of toxicity, therapeutic regimens may be more cost effective with the constant infusion schedule.

Acknowledgment. This study was supported in part by the Carol A. Lewis Memorial Fund.

References

1. Ansfield F, Klotz J, Nealon T, Ramirez G, Minton J, Hill G, Wilson W, Davis H, Cornell G (1977) A phase III study comparing the clinical utility of four regimens of 5-fluorouracil. Cancer 39: 34-40
2. Lavin P, Mittelman A, Douglas H, Engstrom P, Klaassen D (1980) Survival and response to chemotherapy for advanced colorectal adenocarcinoma. An Eastern Cooperative Oncology Group Report. Cancer 46: 1536-1543
3. Engstrom PF, MacIntyre JM, Mittelman A, Klaassen DJ (1984) Chemotherapy of advanced colorectal carcinoma: fluorouracil alone vs two drug combinations using fluorouracil, hydroxyurea, semustine, dacarbazine, razoxane, and mitomycin. Am J Clin Oncol (CCT) 7: 313-318
4. Windschitl H, Scott M, Schutt A, McCormack G, Everson L, Cullinan S, Gerstner J, Krook J, Laurie J, Shreck R, Marschke R, Pfeifle D (1983) Randomized phase II studies in advanced colorectal carcinoma: North Central Cancer Treatment Group Study. Cancer Treat Rep 67 (11): 1001-1008
5. Engstrom PF, MacIntyre JM, Douglass HO, Muggia F, Mittelman A (1982) Combination chemotherapy of advanced colorectal cancer utilizing 5-fluorouracil, semustine, dacarbazine, vincristine, and hydroxyurea: a phase III trial by the Eastern Cooperative Oncology Group (EST: 4275). Cancer 49: 1555-1560
6. Presant CA, Denes AE, Liu C, Bartolucci AA (1984) Prospective randomized reappraisal of 5-fluorouracil in metastatic colorectal carcinoma. A comparative trial with 6-thioguanine. Cancer 53: 2610-2614.
7. Reitemeier RJ, Moertel CG (1962) Comparison of rapid and slow intravenous administration of 5-fluorouracil in treating patients with advanced carcinoma of the large intestine. Cancer Chemother Rep 25: 87-89
8. Moertel CG, Reitemeier RJ, Hahn RG (1967) A controlled comparison of 5-fluoro-2′-deoxyuridine therapy administered by rapid intravenous injection and by continuous intravenous infusion. Cancer Res 27: 549-552

9. Moertel CG, Schutt AJ, Reitemeier RJ, Hahn RG (1972) A comparison of 5-fluorouracil administered by slow infusion and rapid injection. Cancer Res 32: 2717-2719
10. Seifert P, Baker LH, Reed ML, Vaitkevicius VK (1975) Comparison of continuously infused 5-fluorouracil with bolus injection in treatment of patients with colorectal adenocarcinoma. Cancer 36: 123-128
11. Kish J, Ensley J, Weaver A, Jacobs J, Cummings G, Al-Sarraf M (1984) Superior response rate with 96 h 5-fluorouracil (5-FU) infusion vs 5-FU bolus combined with *cis*-platinum (CDDP) in a randomized trial for recurrent and advanced squamous head and neck cancer (HNC). Proc ASCO 3: 695
12. Shah A, MacDonald WC, Gudauskas GA, Sullivan B (1984) Weekly 48-hour 5-fluorouracil (5-FU) intravenous infusion in advanced colorectal cancer. Proc ASCO 3: 454
13. Hartman HA, Kessinger A, Lemon HM, Foley JF (1979) Five-day continuous infusion of 5-fluorouracil for advanced colorectal, gastric, and pancreatic adenocarcinoma. J Surg Oncol 11: 227-238
14. Lokich J, Bothe A, Fine N, Perri J (1981) Phase I study of protracted venous infusion of 5-fluorouracil. Cancer 48: 2565-2568
15. Lokich J, Sonneborn H, Paul S, Zipoli T (1983) Phase I study of continous venous infusion of floxuridine (5-FUdR) chemotherapy. Cancer Treat Rep 67: 791-793
16. Lokich J, Moore C (1984) Chemotherapy associated palmar-plantar erythrodysesthesia syndrome. Ann Int Med 101 (6): 798
17. Leichman L, Seydel HG, Steiger Z (1984) Pre-operative adjuvant therapy for squamous cell cancer (SCC) of the esophagus: SWOG and RTOG clinical Trials. Proc ASCO 3: 575
18. Leichman C, Leichman L, Migro N, Considine B, Vaitkevicius VK, Baker L (1984) Cancer of the anal canal: curative therapy without surgery. Proc ASCO 3: 529
19. Grage TB, Vassilopoulos PP, Shingleton WW, Jubert AV, Elias EG, Aust JB, Moss SE (1978) Results of a prospective randomized study of hepatic artery infusion with 5-fluorouracil versus intravenous 5-fluorouracil in patients with hepatic metastases from colorectal cancer: a Central Oncology Group Study. Surgery 86: 550-555
20. Kemeny N, Daly J, Oderman P, Chun H, Petroni G, Geller N (1984) Randomized study of intrahepatic vs systemic infusion of fluorodeoxyuridine in patients with liver metastases from colorectal carcinoma. Proc ASCO 3: 551
21. Stagg R, Friedman M, Lewis B, Ignoffo R, Goodnight J, Viele C, Hohn D (1984) Current status of NCOG randomized trial of continuous intraarterial (IA) versus intravenous (IV) floxuridine (FUDR) in patients with colorectal carcinoma metastatic to the liver. Proc ASCO 3: 577

Locoregional Chemotherapy

Pharmacologic Rationale for Hepatic Arterial Therapy

J. M. Collins

Pharmacokinetics Section, Clinical Pharmacology Branch, National Cancer Institute,
Bethesda, MD 20892, USA

Introduction

The use of intraarterial therapy is one of a series of strategies intended to provide selective targeting of drug delivery. Other approaches include intraperitoneal and intrathecal delivery [4], liposomes [9], and new drug design [6].

Pharmacokinetics and pharmacodynamics can provide a quantitative perspective. Some drugs are attractive candidates for intraarterial infusion while others are unattractive, and some sites of delivery are more favorable than others [1, 2, 3, 5, 7]. From a practical standpoint, one quick calculation can save months and years of clinical effort. Ideally, pharmacologic principles can focus resources into high-probability areas.

Pharmacokinetics is the description of drug concentrations during treatment, while pharmacodynamics is the description of drug effects, either therapeutic or toxic (Fig. 1). The relationship between these two domains is designated by a connecting arrow, since the drug must reach its site of action in order to exert an effect. To determine the potential advantage of intraarterial therapy, it is essential to consider both drug concentrations and drug effects.

For a general description of pharmacodynamics, we would expect response versus concentration curves such as those shown in Fig. 2. Until the maximum effect has been reached, increasing the drug concentration will increase the antitumor effect. Concurrently, host tissue toxicity will also be increased, which limits the maximum tolerable concentration.

Every anticancer drug has a narrow therapeutic index, i. e., the dose which must be given for efficacy is a dose which is close to the maximum tolerable concentration. The goal of intraarterial therapy is to provide selective changes in concentrations: to increase tumor concentrations without raising the host tissue concentrations, and/or to decrease host tissue concentrations without lowering tumor concentrations.

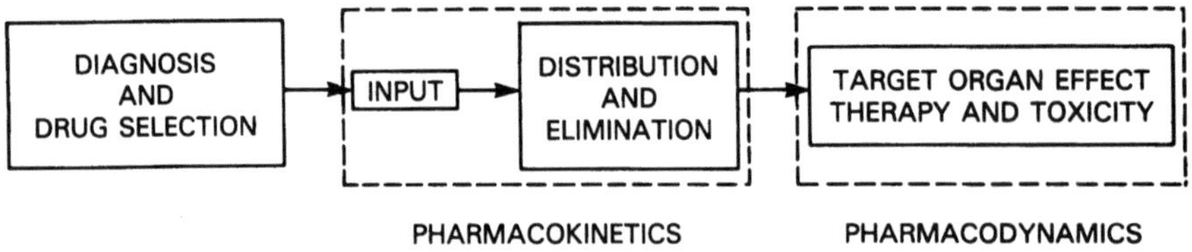

Fig. 1. The distinction between pharmacokinetics and pharmacodynamics [2]

Recent Results in Cancer Research. Vol 100

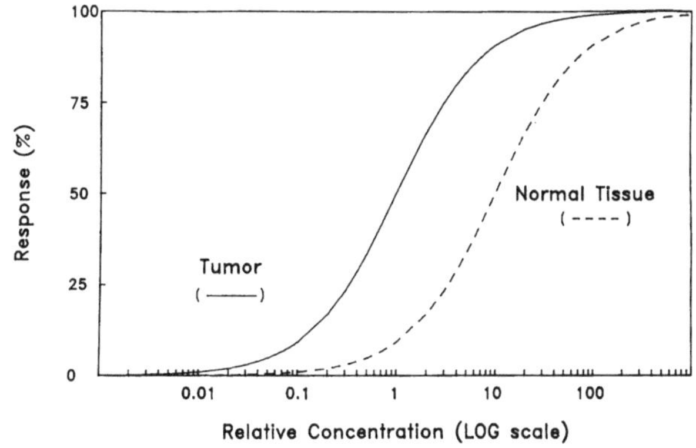

Fig. 2. Response versus concentration relationship for a typical drug. *Solid line,* tumor; *dashed line,* normal host tissue [3]

The complexity of intraarterial procedures has been a serious obstacle. Recently, the development of implantable pumps and other technical advances have made intraarterial infusions more widely available. Since the focus of this volume is on liver therapy, this paper deals primarily with hepatic arterial infusions. However, many of the principles in this paper can be applied to arterial infusions in other areas of the body.

Increased Local Drug Concentration

The potential to increase the drug concentration to which the tumor is exposed will be considered first. The increase in target concentrations for intraarterial versus intravenous delivery can be defined:

$$R_{\text{target}} = C_{\text{target}}\,(\text{i. a.})/C_{\text{target}}\,(\text{i. v.}) \tag{1}$$

Equation 1 is a general definition of the advantage of intraarterial delivery which can be used to evaluate experimental results. The next step in this analysis is to use pharmacokinetic modeling to develop formulas which can be used to calculate R_{target} for various intraarterial situations.

Both conceptually and from the viewpoint of mathematics, it is easier to describe the case for which there is no first-pass effect, that is, in which the liver does not metabolize the drug before it reaches the systemic circulation. Figure 3 is a simplified schematic representation of this case, assuming that the liver is supplied by a single blood vessel. For the same dose given intraarterially and intravenously, R_{target} is the ratio of target concentrations:

$$R_{\text{target}} = \frac{C_{\text{target}}\,(\text{i. a.})}{C_{\text{target}}\,(\text{i. v.})} = 1 + \frac{CL_{\text{TB}}}{Q} \tag{2}$$

CL_{TB} is total body clearance of the drug, which can be found in the literature or determined from intravenous doses. Q is blood flow in the infused artery (see next section). The ratio of CL_{TB} to Q is the sole determinant of drug delivery advantage. This advantage can be calculated *before* doing an experiment or clinical study. Such calculations should influence the selection of drugs, based upon CL_{TB} and the steepness of the dose-response curve. For intraarterial infusions at sites other than the liver, Q is an additional consideration.

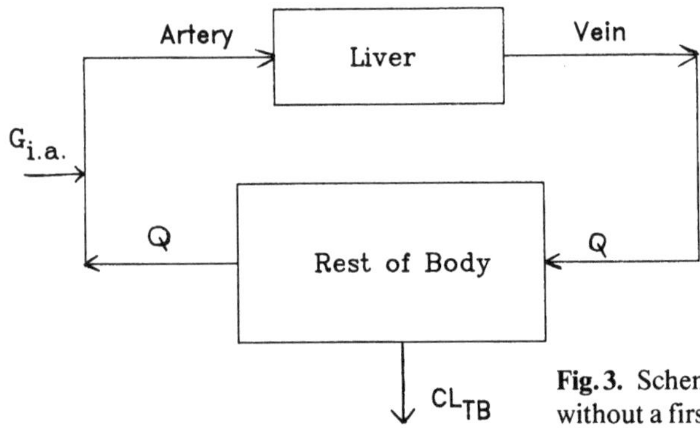

Fig. 3. Schematic diagram for intraarterial infusion without a first-pass effect. Modified from Collins [3]

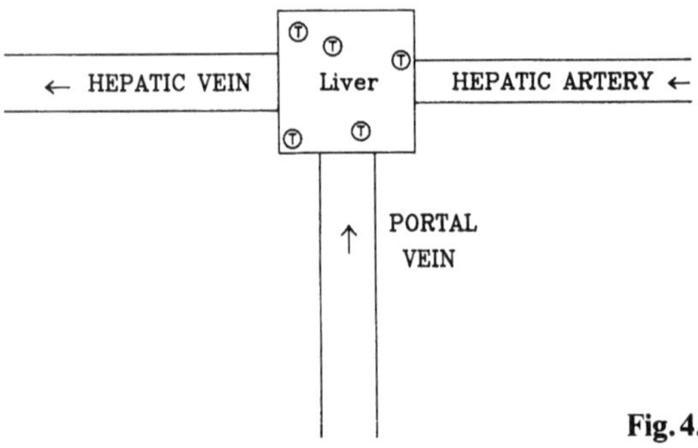

Fig. 4. Blood supply to small hepatic metastases [3]

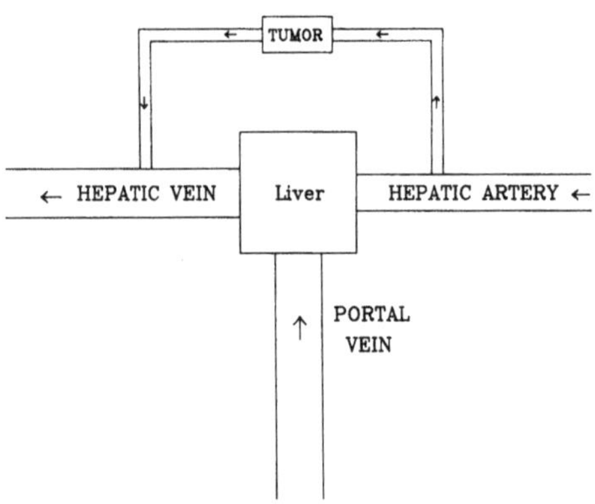

Fig. 5. Blood supply to large hepatic metastases [3]

One of the conditions for Eq. 2 (and many subsequent equations) is that the comparison between intraarterial and intravenous routes is based upon equal doses. This implies that the limiting host tissue is extrahepatic (e.g., bone marrow). If hepatic toxicity is limiting, then intraarterial administration of the same dose is not possible.

Anatomy of Liver Blood Supply

The simplified schematic in Fig. 3 must be modified to characterize the dual blood supply of the liver. The anatomy of the tumor blood supply is a critical determinant of tumor exposure. Tumor blood supply is mostly determined by the size of the metastases.

Small Metastases. When the metastases are small, they are mingled with normal liver tissue (Fig. 4) and derive their blood supply from the same sources as surrounding normal liver tissue [8]. Regardless of whether the drug is delivered into the hepatic artery or the portal vein, it is effectively diluted by the total liver blood flow (Q_{HV}) since small metastases are nourished by both the hepatic artery and the portal vein.

Large Metastases. As the hepatic metastases grow, they develop their own blood supply, chiefly from arterial vessels [8]. Large metastases can be modeled as a separate compartment in parallel with normal liver (Fig. 5). A fraction of the dose which is infused into the hepatic artery splits off to feed the tumor. The drug concentration in the tumor's branch of the hepatic artery should be the same as the drug concentration in the main branch of the hepatic artery. However, since the tumor cells are not nourished by the portal vein, the advantage of delivery via the hepatic artery is not diluted by the total liver blood flow. Although larger metastases are usually a poor prognostic indicator for response, the effective tumor concentration can be higher in a large metastasis than a small metastasis, since there is less dilution of drug by the blood supply. Isolation of the blood supply from the degradative enzymes of normal liver tissue can also enhance the therapeutic index for intraarterial delivery to large metastases. The effective tumor concentration can be higher than the concentration in normal liver tissue (or small metastases), since tumor tissue would not be expected to degrade the drug. These effects are not unique to intraarterial delivery, but would also occur for intravenous administration.

Examples of R_{target}. As discussed above, the blood supply of the tumor determines whether the infused drug is effectively diluted by hepatic arterial blood flow or by total blood

Table 1. Regional drug delivery advantage, R_{target} for selected anticancer drugs. Based upon Eq. 2

CL_{TB} (ml/min)	Drug	R_{target}	
		$Q_{HA}=250$ (ml/min)	$Q_{HV}=1000$ (ml/min)
25000	5-FUdR	101	26
5000	Teroxirone	21	6
4000	5-FU	17	5
3000	Ara-C	13	4
1000	BCNU	5	2
900	Adriamycin	4.6	1.9
400	AZQ	2.6	1.4
400	*cis*-DDP	2.6	1.4
200	Methotrexate	1.8	1.2
40	VP-16	1.2	1.04
–[a]	Cyclophosphamide	1	1

[a] Drugs which must be activated at a site other than the arterial infusion site have *no* drug delivery advantage

5-FUdR, 5-fluoro-2'-deoxyuridine; *5-FU,* 5-fluorouracil; *Ara-C,* cytosine arabinoside; *BCNU,* 1,3-bis(2-chloroethyl)-1-nitrosourea (carmustine); *AZQ,* diaziquone; *cis-DDP, cis*-diaminodichloroplatinum; *VP-16,* etoposide flow. The quantitative effect of the blood flow is expressed in the calculation of R_{target} (Table 1). A blood flow of 250 ml/min is used to approximate hepatic artery flow and 1000 ml/min is used for total hepatic blood flow.

Role of Liver Extraction

If a certain fraction, E, of the infused dose is eliminated by the liver, then $1\text{-}E$ is available to the systemic circulation. For equal doses:

$$R_{systemic} = \frac{C_{systemic}\ (\mathrm{i.a.})}{C_{systemic}\ (\mathrm{i.v.})} = 1 - E \tag{3}$$

If acute systemic toxicity is dose limiting, a larger dose can be given intraarterially than intravenously. If cumulative systemic toxicity is dose limiting, then a larger number of doses (or a longer infusion) can be given intraarterially.

The overall advantage of intraarterial administration, R_d, is composed of the increased local concentration and/or the decreased systemic concentration:

$$R_d = \frac{R_{target}}{R_{systemic}} = \frac{C_{target}\ (\mathrm{i.a.})/C_{target}\ (\mathrm{i.v.})}{C_{systemic}\ (\mathrm{i.a.})/C_{systemic}\ (\mathrm{i.v.})} \tag{4}$$

If $E=0$, $R_{systemic}=1$ and $R_d = R_{target}$. When $E \neq 0$, $R_{systemic}$ is less than 1, which generally increases the overall value of R_d. However, in some cases, R_{target} is adversely lowered by hepatic extraction. In fact, R_{target} can be reduced to 1 if the liver is the sole organ of drug elimination from the body. The specific details for the calculation of R_d are given in Appendix A.

Pharmacologic Response of Tumor and Normal Liver

It must be emphasized that the measurement (or prediction) of R_d is only the first step in the evaluation of the pharmacologic advantage of intraarterial infusions. The second step is a consideration of the concentration-response curve. A large value of R_d (e.g., 500) may appear to be more impressive than a small value (e.g., 3), but the therapeutic advantage depends upon the slope of the concentration-response curve.

Figure 6 illustrates the influence of the steepness of the concentration-response curve. The curves on the left half of the graph illustrate situations in which small changes in R_d

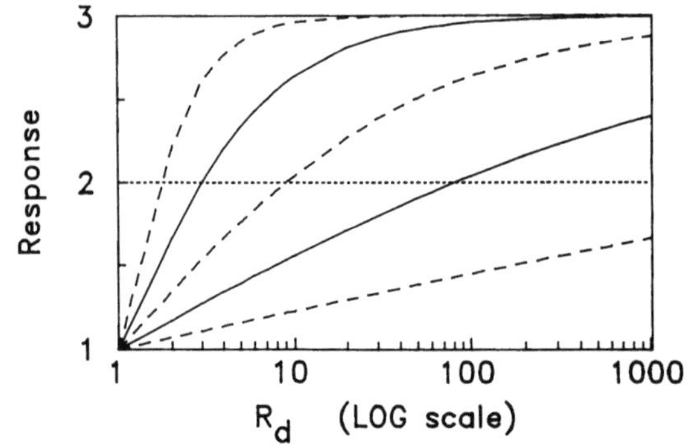

Fig. 6. Drug effect versus R_d. Different curves represent varying degrees of steepness for the dose-response curve

are expressed as large changes in target response. Moving toward the right half of the graph, very large changes in target drug concentration produce only small changes in target response.

One of the drugs with the most favorable pharmacokinetic properties for hepatic arterial infusion is 5-fluoro-2′-deoxyuridine (5-FUdR); yet the improvement in therapy for intraarterial versus intravenous delivery cannot be consistently demonstrated. One interpretation of the FUdR results is that the response versus concentration curve for FUdR must be very shallow. Also, the local toxicity, chemical hepatitis, limits the full exploitation of the potential advantage of 5-FUdR.

Conclusion

Pharmacokinetics offers a powerful tool for the prediction of concentrations which are achievable by use of the intraarterial route. However, a complete pharmacologic evaluation of the potential advantage of intraarterial delivery requires consideration of both the tumor response at higher concentrations and also the limits imposed by the chemosensitivity of normal liver tissue.

Appendix A. Effect of Liver Extraction on the Calculation of R_d

Small Metastases. For the schematic in Fig. 4:

$$R_{\text{target}} = \frac{C_{\text{target}}\,(\text{i.a.})}{C_{\text{target}}\,(\text{i.v.})} = 1 + \frac{CL_{\text{body}}}{Q_{\text{HV}}} \tag{A1}$$

Equation A1 is similar to Eq. 2, except that total body clearance (CL_{TB}) has been replaced by CL_{body}, i.e., the clearance in all areas of the body except the target area. Clearance within the target area (surrounding liver tissue) reduces the drug concentration delivered to the tumor for both intravenous and intraarterial routes. R_d is calculated from Eq. A1 divided by Eq. 3:

$$R_d = \frac{1 + \dfrac{CL_{\text{body}}}{Q_{\text{HV}}}}{(1-E)} \tag{A2}$$

Large Metastases. For the schematic in Fig. 5:

$$R_{\text{target}} = \frac{C_{\text{target}}\,(\text{i.a.})}{C_{\text{target}}\,(\text{i.v.})} = 1 + \frac{CL^*}{Q_{\text{HA}}} \tag{A3}$$

The value of the clearance parameter (CL^*) lies between CL_{body} and CL_{TB}:

$$CL^* = CL_{\text{body}} + Q_{\text{PoV}}\,E \tag{A4}$$

Q_{PoV} is the portal vein blood flow.

The first-pass effect (1-E) is still present for systemic tissues. Therefore, the overall advantage is:

$$R_d = \frac{1 + \dfrac{CL^*}{Q_{\text{HA}}}}{(1-E)} \tag{A5}$$

Liver as the Only Organ of Elimination: Small Metastases

If the liver is the *only* route of elimination ($CL_{\text{body}}=0$ in Eq. A1), the first-pass effect does not increase target concentrations:

$$R_{\text{target}}=\frac{C_{\text{target}}\ (\text{i.a.})}{C_{\text{target}}\ (\text{i.v.})}=1 \tag{A6}$$

We should not conclude from Eq. A6 that there is no advantage for intraarterial drug delivery in this circumstance. Systemic exposure will be lower as stated in Eq. 3, and R_{d} will equal Eq. A6 divided by Eq. 3:

$$R_{\text{d}}=\frac{1}{1-E} \tag{A7}$$

Liver as the Only Organ of Elimination: Large Metastases

Since part of the infused dose goes to the isolated tumor and part goes to the rest of the liver, there is some increase in target concentrations due to the first-pass effect:

$$R_{\text{target}}=\frac{C_{\text{target}}\ (\text{i.a.})}{C_{\text{target}}\ (\text{i.v.})}=1+\frac{Q_{\text{PoV}}}{Q_{\text{HA}}}E \tag{A8}$$

Systemic exposure will also be reduced, so that R_{d} will equal Eq. A8 divided by Eq. 3:

$$R_{\text{d}}=\frac{1+\frac{Q_{\text{PoV}}}{Q_{\text{HA}}}E}{1-E} \tag{A9}$$

All formulas are summarized in Table 2.

Table 2. Summary of formulas for R_{target} and R_{d} for small and large liver metastases

	Extrahepatic only	Hepatic plus extrahepatic		Hepatic only	
Size	$R_{\text{d}}=R_{\text{target}}$	R_{target}	R_{d}	R_{target}	R_{d}
Small	$1+\frac{CL_{\text{TB}}}{Q_{\text{HV}}}$	$1+\frac{CL_{\text{body}}}{Q_{\text{HV}}}$	$\frac{1+\frac{CL_{\text{body}}}{Q_{\text{HV}}}}{1-E}$	1	$\frac{1}{1-E}$
Large	$1+\frac{CL_{\text{TB}}}{Q_{\text{HA}}}$	$1+\frac{CL_{\text{body}}+Q_{\text{PoV}}E}{Q_{\text{HA}}}$	$\frac{1+\frac{CL_{\text{body}}+Q_{\text{PoV}}E}{Q_{\text{HA}}}}{1-E}$	$1+\frac{Q_{\text{PoV}}}{Q_{\text{HA}}}E$	$\frac{1+\frac{Q_{\text{PoV}}}{Q_{\text{HA}}}E}{1-E}$

References

1. Chen HSG, Gross JF (1980) Intra-arterial infusion of anticancer drugs: theoretic aspects of drug delivery and review of responses. Cancer Treat Rep 64: 31-40
2. Collins JM (1984) Pharmacologic rationale for regional drug delivery. J Clin Oncol 2: 498-504
3. Collins JM (1985) Pharmacokinetic rationale for intraarterial therapy. In: Howell SB (ed) Intra-arterial and intracavitary chemotherapy. Nijhoff, Boston, pp 1-10
4. Collins JM (1985) Pharmacokinetic rationale for intracavitary therapy. In: Howell SB (ed) Intra-arterial and intracavitary chemotherapy. Nijhoff, Boston, pp 41-51
5. Collins JM, Dedrick RL (1982) Pharmacokinetics of anticancer drugs. In: Chabner BA (ed) Pharmacologic principles of cancer treatment. Saunders, Philadelphia, pp 77-99
6. Driscoll JS (1984) The preclinical new drug research program of the National Cancer Institute. Cancer Treat Rep 68: 63-76
7. Eckman WW, Patlak CS, Fenstermacher JD (1974) A critical evaluation of the principles governing the advantages of intraarterial infusions. J Pharmacokinet Biopharm 2: 257-285
8. Ensminger WD, Gyves JW (1984) Regional cancer chemotherapy. Cancer Treat Rep 68: 101-115
9. Weinstein JN (1984) Liposomes as drug carriers in cancer therapy. Cancer Treat Rep 68: 127-135

Experiments on the Toxicity of Locoregional Liver Chemotherapy with 5-Fluoro-2'-deoxyuridine and 5-Fluorouracil in an Animal Model

M. R. Berger, T. H. Henne, J. L. A. Aguiar, R. Bartkowski, J. Dörsam, G. H. Geelhaar, P. Schlag, C. Herfarth, and D. Schmähl

Institut für Toxikologie und Chemotherapie, Deutsches Krebsforschungszentrum, Im Neuenheimer Feld 280, 6900 Heidelberg, FRG

Introduction

A major problem in the treatment of cancer are primary tumors and metastases of the liver. While hepatomas are rare in Western Europe, there is a high incidence of liver metastases, deriving mainly from colorectal cancer [25]. At the time of detection these metastases are mostly disseminated and therefore inoperable, in contrast to their primaries. Improvements in surgical technique and knowledge makes successful wedge resection and hemihepatectomy possible. However, this treatment mode is applicable to a limited number of patients only with certain surgical preconditions (isolated metastasis, general operability, and remaining liver tissue more than 20% [18]). Overcoming the immunological problems of organ transplantation enables successful liver transplantation to be performed today. However, this method in particular cannot be regarded as a routine treatment because of the lack of donors and remaining immunological problems [19]. Patients with disseminated liver metastases have therefore been candidates for systemic chemotherapy. Many cytotoxic single- and combination chemotherapy schedules have been tested over the years, but none of the combinations tested was superior to 5-fluorouracil (5-FU) monotherapy, resulting in up to 20% tumor response for 3–5 months [22]. Because of these disappointing results other approaches are currently under investigation.

Vascularization studies have demonstrated that normal liver parenchyma is mainly supported by the portal vein, whereas metastases receive up to 90% of their blood supply by the proper hepatic artery [1, 3, 6, 14]. It therefore seems advantageous to exploit this difference therapeutically.

For induction of tumor hypoxia, intermittent dearterialization of liver seems to avoid quick formation of collateral vessels, the unsolved problem of permanent dearterialization of liver [4].

Other experimental therapy modes are chemoembolization via the proper hepatic artery [21] and isolated perfusion of the liver with cytostatics [2, 13] aimed at higher drug concentrations within the tumor and reduced systemic drug levels. Since isolated liver perfusion does not permit long-term administration of drugs, liver infusion via the proper hepatic artery with a newly developed implantable infusion pump [11, 16] opens the possibility of long-term ambulatory treatment. The most frequently used agent in these investigations is 5-fluoro-2'-deoxyuridine (FUdR) because pharmacokinetic studies [10] indicate a higher retention in the liver (first-pass effect) in comparison with 5-FU.

Recent Results in Cancer Research. Vol 100

To test the significance of this difference between 5-FU and FUdR in a comparative study, we investigated the therapeutic efficacy together with systemic and local toxicity of both compounds at different routes and modes of administration in a standardized rat model.

Methods

Animals

Female Sprague-Dawley rats were obtained at an age of 50-80 days (Zentralinstitut für Versuchstierzucht, 3000 Hannover, FRG). The animals were kept under conventional conditions (temperature 22° +/−2 °C, relative humidity 55% +/−10%, dark-light rhythm of 12 h), one rat per size II Makrolon cage, had free access to Altromin 1320 laboratory chow and tap water, and were inspected twice daily.

In therapy experiments the animals were followed up until their natural death; all dead animals were dissected. Macroscopically changed organs were examined histologically. Animals used in toxicity experiments were killed at indicated time intervals after treatment (see below).

Tumor Inoculation

The rats were placed under ether anesthesia and 5×10^5 Novikoff-hepatoma cells were transplanted under the capsule of the left liver lobe.

Routes and Modes of Infusion

On day 7 after tumor inoculation polyethylene catheters (Portex PP10 or PP30) were inserted with the rats under ether anesthesia into one of the following vessels:

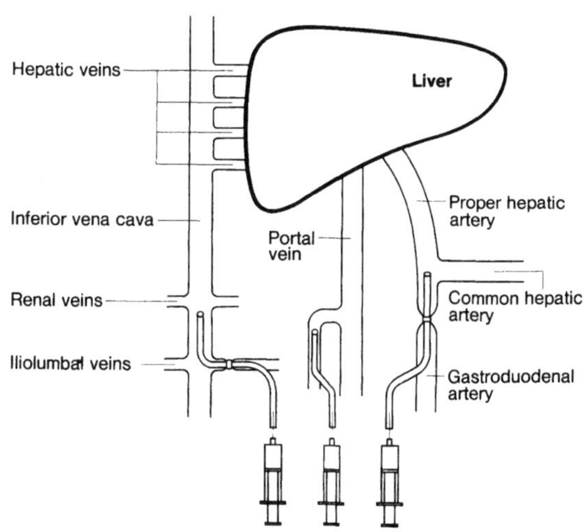

Fig. 1. Scheme of administration routes

1. The inferior vena cava via an iliolumbal vein
2. The portal vein via a mesenteric branch
3. The proper hepatic artery via the gastroduodenal artery [8]

All three routes are depicted in Fig. 1. To allow free movement of rats during infusion, catheters were exteriorized in the neck region, fixed, and secured by a coil of metal and connected with an infusion pump. For bolus injections catheters were connected with a small infusion port, which was fixed at the back of the rats. Injections were administered by percutaneous puncture of the port.

FUdR and 5-FU were given at equimolar daily doses of 60 mg/kg or 31.7 mg/kg, respectively, either as continuous infusion or as daily bolus injections on five consecutive days, starting on the day after the first relaparatomy (day 7). The total dose administered was 1220 μmol/kg of each compound.

Evaluation of Tumor Response

On days 7 (1 day before the start of therapy) and 21 (8 days after the end of therapy) laparotomy was performed to determine the tumor volume by measuring two vertical axes of the tumor according to the formula $V = a \times b^2/2$. For statistical analysis the Kruskal-Wallis test was used.

Evaluation of Toxicity

In toxicological experiments animals were killed 16 h after treatment. Then, femurs, tibias, and livers were removed and blood samples taken. Bone marrow cells were expelled under sterile conditions and washed in Hanks' solution. The livers were minced with scissors, incubated with collagenase (Sigma, Munich, FRG) for 45 min at 37 °C in a shaking water bath, and then passed through a sieve. The single-cell suspension obtained was washed with Hanks' solution and the erythrocytes were lysed in an osmotic buffer (0.155 M NH_4CL, 0.01 M $KHCO_3$, 0.1 mM Na_2EDTA; pH, 7.3).

Systemic Toxicity

The bone marrow cells were divided into three parts. A first aliquot was given on methylcellulose-agar plates in Petri dishes at decreasing concentrations according to the method described by Iscove and Sieber in 1975 [15] and incubated at 37 °C with 5% CO_2 atmosphere. After 6 days the colonies formed by committed bone marrow stem cells were counted and expressed as a percentage of the untreated control.

The second part of the cells was injected i. v. into lethally irradiated mice at decreasing concentrations. After 9 days the animals were killed and their spleens were removed and fixed in Bouin's solution. The colonies formed in the spleens by pluripotent bone marrow stem cells [24] were counted and expressed as a percentage of the untreated control.

The third aliquot was used to assess the rate of DNA single-strand breaks by means of a modified [5] alkaline elution technique [12, 17]. A controlled number of DNA single-strand breaks was introduced into cells of control and treated animals, using gamma irradiation. Aliquots of irradiated and nonirradiated cells of treated or untreated animals were layered onto polycarbonate filters (Nucleopore, Pleasanton, United States) and lysed with a detergent solution [2% w/v sodium dodecyl sulfate, 0.1 *M* glycine, 0.02 *M* Na_2EDTA, containing 0.5 mg protease IX/ml (Sigma, Munich, FRG) adjusted to pH 10]. After lysis the cells were washed and DNA was eluted from the filters with 20 ml alkaline buffer [0.02 *M* EDTA, acid form, adjusted to pH 12.2 with tetraethylammonium hydroxide (20% in water; Riedel de Haen, Hannover, FRG)]. Two-milliliter fractions were collected for 12 h. Then DNA was removed from the filters by mincing in alkaline elution buffer followed by shaking at 37 °C for 1 h. DNA was determined by reacting with Hoechst 33258 [7]. Single-strand breaks were quantitated in terms of radiation equivalents as previously described [17].

Liver Toxicity

To measure the local liver toxicity glutamic oxaloacetic transaminase (GOT), glutamic pyruvic transaminase (GPT), and total bilirubin (TB) were determined in the serum of blood samples. In isolated liver cells DNA single-strand breaks were assessed as described for the bone marrow cells.

Results

Mean tumor volumes of treated animals as percentages of the untreated control are given in Table 1. A significant decrease in tumor volume compared with controls was observed after continuous infusion of FUdR via the proper hepatic artery only ($P < 0.05$). However, no significant difference between the various routes and modes of administration could be ascertained. Treatment by equimolar doses with FUdR was somewhat more effective in terms of T/C% and induced lower mortality after bolus injection. Moreover, infusion via all routes seemed to induce higher tumor responses than corresponding bolus injections. Histologic examination of dead animals revealed all signs of malignancy (tumor cell

Table 1. Therapeutic efficacy of 5-fluoro-2′-deoxyuridine (FUdR) and 5-fluorouracil (5-FU) after systemic or locoregional infusion or bolus injection over 5 days at equimolar doses in Sprague-Dawley rats (total doses: 1220 μmol/kg each)

Administration		FUdR		5-FU	
Route	Mode	MTV ± SD[a]	T/C%[b]	MTV ± SD[a]	T/C%[b]
Vena cava	Infusion	1683 ± 930	24	8114 ± 3624	127
	Bolus	5111 ± 3854	74	-	+[c]
Portal vein	Infusion	3404 ± 3888	49	-	NT[d]
	Bolus	3594 ± 2590	52	-	NT[d]
Proper hepatic artery	Infusion	679 ± 1150	10	1647 ± 1430	26
	Bolus	2368 ± 2984	34		+[c]
Untreated control		6887 ± 3907	100	6364 ± 2873	100

[a] *MTV*, mean tumor volume (mm^3) ± standard deviation
[b] *T/C%*, mean tumor volume of treated rats as a percentage of untreated control
[c] +, all animals dead after 1 week
[d] *NT*, not tested

Table 2. Systemic toxicity of 5-fluoro-2′-desoxyuridine (FUdR) and 5-fluorouracil (5-FU) after systemic or locoregional infusion or bolus injection over 5 days at equimolar doses in Sprague-Dawley rats (total doses: 1220 μ*M*/kg each)

Administration		FUdR			5-FU		
Route	Mode	CFU-C ± SE[a]	CFU-S ± SE[b]	DNA-SSB ± SD[c]	CFU-C ± SE[a]	CFU-S ± SE[b]	DNA-SSB ± SD[c]
Vena	Infusion	43 ± 8.5	25 ± 6.6	159 ± 182	43 ± 40	25 ± 24	71 ± 19
cava	Bolus	29 ± 24	13.7	116 ± 15	14 ± 5	1.3 ± 0.9	68 ± 1
Portal	Infusion	75 ± 55	30 ± 8.5	101 ± 21	58 ± 26	39 ± 6	100 ± 80
vein	Bolus	27 ± 15.6	13.4	96 ± 52	44 ± 11	3.1 ± 0.6	137 ± 103
Proper	Infusion	115 ± 6.5	35 ± 9.5	48 ± 67	72 ± 5.3	66 ± 13	23 ± 25
hepatic artery	Bolus	33 ± 7.9	26 ± 14.6	208 ± 160	35 ± 15	10 ± 6.8	177 ± 9.2

[a] *CFU-C ± SE*, mean colony number (in cultures) of treated bone marrow cells as a percentage of control ± standard error
[b] *CFU-S ± SE*, mean colony number (in spleens) of treated bone marrow cells as a percentage of control ± standard error
[c] *DNA-SSB ± SD*, single-strand breaks (radiation equivalents) in DNA of treated bone marrow cells ± standard deviation

Table 3. Local toxicity of 5-fluoro-2′-desoxyuridine (FUdR) and 5-fluorouracil (5-FU) after systemic or locoregional infusion or bolus injection over 5 days at equimolar doses in Sprague-Dawley rats (total doses: 1220 μ*M*/kg each)

Administration		FUdR				5-FU			
Route	Mode	GOT ± SD[a]	GPT ± SD[b]	TB ± SD[c]	DNA-SSB ± SD[d]	GOT ± SD[a]	GPT ± SD[b]	TB ± SD[c]	DNA-SSB ± SD[d]
Vena	Infusion	74 ± 11.9	21 ± 6.4	0.31 ± 0.3	NT[e]	108 ± 24	40 ± 9.3	0.69 ± 0.08	43 ± 37
cava	Bolus	48 ± 2.5	20 ± 7	0.67 ± 0.1	NT[e]	35 ± 9.9	12 ± 4.2	0.86 ± 0.69	145 ± 37
Portal	Infusion	113 ± 100	34 ± 20	0.37 ± 0.21	NT[e]	69 ± 26	32 ± 6.8	0.36 ± 0.08	0
vein	Bolus	54 ± 22	29 ± 14	0.50 ± 0.1	NT[e]	40 ± 17	14 ± 7	0.14 ± 0.24	376 ± 277
Proper	Infusion	81 ± 44	25 ± 9.8	0.27 ± 0.22	NT[e]	78 ± 22	46 ± 8.2	0.97 ± 0.4	5 ± 4.9
hepatic artery	Bolus	43 ± 11.2	17 ± 8.3	0.15 ± 0.11	NT[e]	71 ± 60	19 ± 9.6	0.7 ± 0.7	270 ± 17

[a] *GOT ± SD*, GOT (units/l) ± standard deviation
[b] *GPT ± SD*, GPT (units/l) ± standard deviation
[c] *TB ± SD*, total bilirubin (mg-%) ± standard deviation
[d] *DNA-SSB ± SD*, single-strand breaks (radiation equivalents) in DNA of treated liver cells ± standard deviation
[e] *NT*, not tested

infiltration, elevated rates of mitoses, polymorph and hyperchromatic nuclei) of resting tumor tissue.

Inhibition of colony formation of bone marrow stem cells after administration of both compounds in terms of colony-forming unit-culture (CFU-C) and colony-forming unit-spleen (CFU-S) and DNA damage in bone marrow cells in terms of DNA single-strand breaks is shown in Table 2. CFU-C and CFU-S indicate equivalent remaining colony-forming capacity of bone marrow stem cells after infusion either of FUdR or 5-FU. In contrast to this observation a distinct difference was seen after bolus injections of both compounds, FUdR effecting less myelotoxicity, which was in turn partly responsible for death of 5-FU-treated animals. Comparison of the three administration routes shows highest systemic toxicity after administration into the vena cava, medium effect after administration into the portal vein, and lowest toxicity after administration into the proper hepatic artery; comparing the two administration modes, continuous infusion proved to be less toxic than repeated bolus injections.

DNA damage in terms of single-strand breaks after treatment with these uracil derivatives is a recent observation, since incorporation of FUdR into DNA was not observed until 1981 [9]. The results reflect a different incorporation of FUdR and 5-FU into DNA of rat bone marrow cells, the lowest values being observed after continuous infusion via the proper hepatic artery. For this mode of administration a negative correlation was found with regard to inhibition of bone marrow stem cell colony formation.

Reactions of liver enzymes, total bilirubin, and DNA damage in liver cells in terms of single-strand breaks are depicted in Table 3. Infusions of both compounds yielded higher increases of GOT and GPT than respective bolus injections. In contrast, total bilirubin displayed higher values after bolus injections except for administration via the proper hepatic artery. Few single-strand breaks could be observed in DNA of liver cells after infusion of 5-FU, whereas bolus injections caused more DNA damage.

Discussion

The rationale of locoregional chemotherapy is first to achieve higher drug concentrations in the tumor-bearing organ and second to lower systemic drug and/or metabolite levels. It is hoped that the pharmacokinetic advantages of locoregional drug administration will lead to pharmacodynamic improvements, i. e., higher tumor cell kill and reduced systemic toxicity, thus outweighing the risks and complications inherent in catheter implantation and probably elevated local toxicity [23].

In our model, locoregional therapy via the proper hepatic artery was somewhat more effective for both compounds, with best results after continuous infusion via this route; however, no significant differences with the other administration routes and modes could be ascertained. It can thus be concluded that locoregional administration of FUdR and 5-FU did not improve tumor cell kill significantly in the present model. This is not in agreement with theoretical considerations and might be due to shallow concentration-response curves of these compounds. Comparing 5-FU and FUdR the latter seemed to have a higher efficacy in terms of T/C%.

Systemic toxicity assessed in bone marrow cells was lowest for intraarterial infusion of both compounds, while the local liver toxicity was only moderately elevated. These findings correspond with the second argument for locoregional drug chemotherapy, predicting a reduced systemic toxicity in addition to a higher drug concentration at the tumor site.

Single-strand breaks in DNA of liver and bone marrow cells occurred at about the same order of magnitude after bolus injections. This is in contrast with assumed drug levels in both organs, but might be explained by recent findings, which indicate incorporation of substantial amounts of 5-FU into DNA of bone marrow cells in comparison with intestinal or mammary tumor cells [20]. The meaning of DNA single-strand breaks within mechanisms leading to cell death is still unclear and might be different in liver and bone marrow cells. While there is a good agreement between inhibition of colony formation and DNA damage in bone marrow, liver enzyme levels indicate low cell kill although considerable amounts of DNA single-strand breaks could be observed.

In conclusion only a continuous infusion via the proper hepatic artery proved to be effective with respect to tumor inhibitory efficacy. Systemic toxicity was significantly decreased, while local toxicity was only slightly elevated. These data indicate that fluorinated pyrimidines are limited in their therapeutic value in our model, whereas reduction of systemic toxicity could be ascertained. Other drugs that might satisfy toxicologic and therapeutic expectations for locoregional application are presently under investigation.

References

1. Ackerman NB, Lien WM, Kondi ES, Silverman NA (1969) The blood supply of experimental liver metastases. I: The distribution of hepatic arterial and portal vein blood to "small" and "large" tumors. Surgery 66: 1067
2. Aigner K, Walther H, Tonn J, Wenzel A, Hechtel R, Merker G, Schwemmle K (1983) First experimental and clinical results of isolated liver perfusion with cytotoxics in metastases from colorectal primary. Recent Results Cancer Res 86: 99-102
3. Ariel IM (1956) The treatment of primary and metastatic cancer of the liver. Surgery 39: 70
4. Bengmark S, Nobin A, Jeppson B, Tranberg KG (1983) Transient repeated dearterialisation combined with intra-arterial infusion of oncolytic drugs in the treatment of liver tumors. Recent Results Cancer Res 86: 68-74
5. Bolognesi C, Cesarone CF, Santi L (1979) Standardization of the alkaline elution procedure using X-ray-damaged nuclear DNA. Tumori 65: 511-516
6. Breedis C, Young G (1954) The blood supply of neoplasms in the liver. Am J Pathol 30: 969-986
7. Cesarone CF, Bolognesi C, Santi L (1979) Improved microfluorometric DNA determination in biological material using 33258 Hoechst. Anal Biochem 100: 188
8. Cotino HH, Zwaveling A (1976) Treatment of experimental liver tumors by continuous intraarterial chemotherapy. Eur J Cancer 12: 177-180
9. Danenberg PV, Heidelberger C, Mulkins MA, Peterson AR (1981) The incorporation of 5-fluoro2'-deoxyuridine into DNA of mamalian tumor cells. Biochem Biophys Commun Res 102: 654-658
10. Ensminger WD, Roskowsky A, Raso V, Levin DC, Glode M et al. (1978) A clinical-pharmacological evaluation of hepatic arterial infusions of 5-fluoro-2'-deoxyuridine and 5-fluorouracil. Cancer Res 38: 3784-3792
11. Ensminger WD, Niederhuber Y, Dakhil S, Thrall Y, Wheeler R (1981) A totally implanted drug delivery system for hepatic arterial chemotherapy. Cancer Treat Rep 65: 393-400
12. Ewig RAG, Kohn KW (1977) DNA damage and repair in mouse leukemia L 1210 cells treated with nitrogen mustard, 1,3-bis(2-chloroethyl)-1-nitrosurea and other nitrosureas. Cancer Res 37: 2114-2122
13. Ghussen F, Nagel K, Isselhard W (1983) Isolated liver perfusion in dogs. Recent Results Cancer Res 86: 93-98
14. Hanjo J, Matsumura H (1965) Vascular distribution of hepatic tumors: an experimental study. Rev Int Hepatol (Paris) 15: 681-690

15. Isove NN, Sieber F (1975) Erythroid progenitors in bone marrow detected by macroscopic colony formation in culture. Exp Hematol 3: 32-43
16. Kempf P, Olberman M, Fischer J (1983) Improved quality of life with an implantable pump for liver perfusion. Recent Results Cancer Res 86: 87-90
17. Kohn KW, Ewig RAG, Erickson LC, Zwelling LA (1981) In: Frieberg E, Hanawalt P (eds) DNA repair: a laboratory manual of research procedures. Dekker, New York, p 379-401
18. Pettavel J, Meyer A (1979) Indication selective a l'exerese chirurgicale des metastases hepatiques. Schweiz Med Wochenschr 109: 794-796
19. Pichlmayr R, Brölsch C, Tidow G, Neuhaus P (1981) Indikation zur Lebertransplantation bei Lebertumoren. In: Zelder O, Röher HD, Fischer M, Bode JCH (eds) Experimentelle und klinische Hepatologie. Schattauer, Stuttgart, pp 53-58
20. Sawyer RC, Stolfi RL, Martin DS, Spiegelman S (1984) Incorporation of 5-fluorouracil into murine bone marrow DNA in vivo. Cancer Res 44: 1847-1851
21. Schultheiss K-H (1983) Chemoembolisation: new treatment for malignant tumors. Recent Results Cancer Res 86: 46-47
22. Silverberg E (1982) Cancer statistics 1982. Cancer 32: 15-31
23. Stephens FO (1983) Pharmakokinetics of intra-arterial chemotherapy. Recent Results Cancer Res 86: 1-12
24. Till JE, McCulloch EA (1961) A direct measurement of the radiation sensitivity of normal mouse bone marrow cells. Radiat Res 14: 213-222
25. Union Internationale Contre le Cancer (1982) Hepatocellular carcinoma. In: Okuda K, Mackay I (eds) Report no 17. UICC, Geneva

Phase II Study of Hepatic Artery Infusion with 5-Fluorouracil, Adriamycin, and Mitomycin C (FAM) in Liver Metastases from Colorectal Carcinoma

J. Wils, J. Schlangen, and A. Naus

Department of Internal Medicine, St. Laurentius Hospital, Mgr Driessenstraat 6, 6043 CV Roermond, The Netherlands

Introduction

The liver may be the predominant organ of involvement in more than 50% of patients with colorectal carcinoma who develop metastatic disease. Once colorectal carcinoma metastasizes to the liver, prognosis becomes ominous. Median survival for untreated patients can be expected to be about 6 months [8, 13, 17] and it has been stated that the length of survival depends on the extent of hepatic metastases even if bones, lungs, and liver are all involved [8]. Systemic 5-fluorouracil (5-FU) is of limited value, median survival being approximately 8 months [15]. Because hepatic metastases receive their main blood supply from the hepatic artery, one way of approach has been ligation of the hepatic artery. In nonrandomized studies a median survival of about 11 months has been reported with this technique [1, 10]. Another treatment modality has been the infusion of cytostatic drugs into the hepatic artery. 5-FU (F), 5-fluoro-deoxyuridine (FUdR), and mitomycin C (M) are extracted by the liver; hence intraarterial administration of these drugs allows for a greater concentration into the tumor-bearing organ with less systemic toxicity. It has also been shown that the systemic Adriamycin (A) level during hepatic artery infusion (HAI) is 25% lower than the corresponding systemic level with peripheral venous infusion, while hepatic venous anthracycline levels, which are one measure of intrahepatic drug concentration in the hepatic and tumor capillary bed, are consistently higher when the drug is given by the hepatic artery route [5]. Employing the FAM combination systemically a response rate of only 17% has been reported in measurable advanced colorectal carcinoma [7]. HAI with a combination of five drugs including FAM yielded a response rate of 56% in patients with liver metastases from colorectal carcinoma [2]. In a pilot feasibility study in our institution 34 patients with liver metastases from colorectal carcinoma were treated by HAI with FAM. Results in a smaller series of patients with a shorter follow-up have already been reported [16]. In this report results are summarized after a median follow-up of 28 months.

Materials and Methods

Thirty-four consecutive patients with liver metastases from histologically proven colorectal carcinoma, not amenable to surgery, were treated from January 1979 to January 1984. Eligibility criteria were: age <75 years, Karnofsky index ≥70%, primary excised, no

Recent Results in Cancer Research. Vol 100

(73%) or minor (27%) extrahepatic disease, bilirubin <30 μmol/liter, and no previous treatment with radiotherapy or chemotherapy. A catheter was introduced into the femoral artery and placed selectively into the common or proper hepatic artery. Drugs were infused for 76 h. Dosages were: Adriamycin 70 mg/m^2 during 24 h, mitomycin C 10 mg/m^2 during 4 h, and 5-FU 1500 mg/m^2 during 48 h. Courses were repeated every 10 weeks. This time interval was chosen because each treatment cycle required at least 5 days of hospitalization and it was thought that a shorter recycling would seriously impair patients' quality of life. Liver involvement was judged by the surgeon during laparotomy (64%) or by angiography if metastases were detected after resection of the primary (36%). Stage I was less than 30% involvement, stage II 30%-60%, and stage III more than 60% invasion of the liver.

A complete response was defined as a complete disappearance of all signs of tumor and confirmed by CT scan. A partial response was defined as a ⩾50% reduction in tumor mass, judged by angiography by the sum of the products of the two longest perpendicular diameters of the lesions, in combination with a ⩾50% decrease in carcinoembryonic antigen (CEA) if elevated, an amelioration of liver function tests, and a subjective improvement in symptomatic patients. Stable disease was defined as unchanged lesions (<50% decrease or <25% increase) for at least 2 months. Responses were evaluated after the first infusion at the start of the second one and subsequently at each next cycle and had to be agreed upon by the three authors. Survival was measured from the start of the first infusion.

Results

In 30 out of the 34 patients (88%) the catheter could be placed correctly into the common or proper hepatic artery. In four patients this was not possible due to anatomical variations. In these four cases only one liver lobe could be infused at one time or parts of the gastrointestinal tract or the spleen were also in the infused area. In one patient a thrombosis of the hepatic artery occurred after the first infusion; this patient was considered not

Table 1. Patient characteristics (33 evaluable patients)

Median age (range)	58 years (34-74)
Male/female	21/12
Median Karnofsky index	80
Stage I (<30% invasion)	9 patients
Stage II (30%-60% invasion)	12 patients
Stage III (>60% invasion)	12 patients
Symptomatic status	
Symptomatic	18 patients
Asymptomatic	15 patients
Rectosigmoid	25 patients
Colon	8 patients
Liver plus minor extrahepatic metastases	9 patients
Metastases confined to the liver	24 patients

Table 2. Results (33 evaluable patients)

Not evaluable for response	3/33	
Evaluable for response	30 patients	
Complete remission	2/30	30%
Partial remission	7/30	
Stable disease	15/30	
Primary progression	6/30	
Median time to progression		
All patients	16 months	
Responders	26 months	
Median survival		
All patients	19 months	
Responders	28 months	

Table 3. Median survival in subgroups

	Number of patients	Median survival (months)	
Asymptomatic	15	20	$P<0.03$
Symptomatic	18	14	
Stage I	9	33	$P<0.03$
Stage II + III	24	15	
Stage I + II	21	20	$P<0.03$
Stage III	12	14	
Rectosigmoid	25	18	NS
Colon	8	22	
Metastases confined to liver	24	20	NS
Liver and minor extrahepatic metastases	9	16	

NS, not significant

evaluable. Table 1 lists the characteristics of the remaining 33 patients. Eighteen of them were symptomatic (pain, anorexia, malaise, or weight loss). Three patients did not have an angiography at the start of the second infusion and were not evaluable for response, only for survival.

Table 2 shows the results in 30 evaluable patients. There were two complete responders and seven partial responders. Stage of the disease had no significant influence upon response rate (three patients, stage I; four patients, stage II; two patients, stage III). All responses were noted after the first course and further regression was noted after successive courses. One of the complete responders died of lung metastases; the other is alive with no evidence of disease at 60+ months. Median time to progression for all patients was 16 months (responders 26 months; stable disease 13 months), only slightly less than medi-

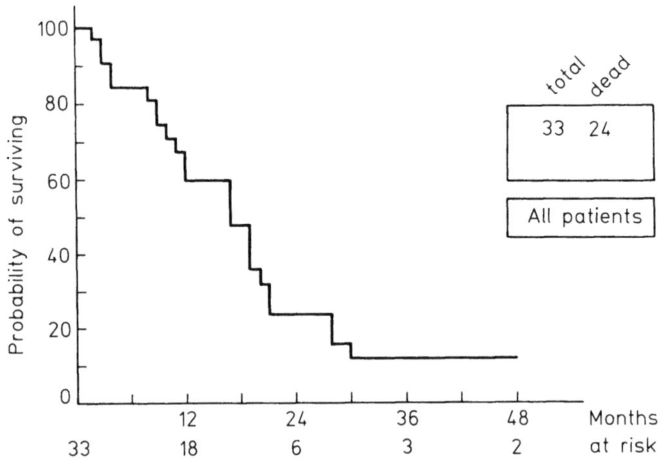

Fig. 1. Kaplan-Meier survival curve for all patients

Table 4. Toxicity of HAI with FAM

Number of courses	132	
Median number of courses per patient (range)	4	(1-9)
Median white cell count day 14 (range)	Grade[a] 2	(0-4)
Median thrombocytes day 14 (range)	Grade 0	(0-4)
Median grade nausea/vomiting per cycle	1	(0-2)
Median grade alopecia per patient	3	(1-3)
Granulocytopenic sepsis	2 patients	
Severe febrile reaction without sepsis (tumor necrosis)	4 patients	
Ulcus duodeni	2 patients	

[a] Gradations according to WHO criteria

an survival. In 68% of the patients, including all patients who had minor extrahepatic disease at the start of treatment, the main site of progression was extrahepatic and 32% had primary progression of the hepatic metastases. Once progression occurred, this was rapidly followed by death. In some patients secondary treatment was given (systemic chemotherapy or embolization of the hepatic artery) but in none of them a response was noted. After a median follow-up of 28 months, median survival for all patients was 19 months (range 2-66+ months) (Fig. 1). Table 3 shows the survival data for subgroups of patients. A significant difference in median survival was found in patients with stage I versus stage II + III and in patients with stage I + II versus stage III disease ($P < 0.03$; log rank test). Also asymptomatic patients had a significantly better median survival than symptomatic patients.

In two patients a stenosis of the hepatic artery occurred, which was reason for stopping treatment in one of them after three courses. A thrombosis of the hepatic artery occurred in another two patients, in one after one course (not evaluable) and in one after the fourth course. These events had no significant influence upon survival. In Table 4 a summary of toxicity is given. Two patients developed a granulocytopenic sepsis after the sixth course; after recovery HAI was stopped. In four patients a severe febrile reaction without granulocytopenia was seen after the first course, which was thought to be due to tumor necrosis. In two patients a duodenal ulcus was found; in both the gastrointestinal tract had been in the infused area. In one of these two patients, dying with progressive peritonitis carcinomatosa, the ulcus was found only at autopsy; in the other it was diagnosed by endoscopy and treated successfully with cimetidine. Catheter-related problems were not observed.

Discussion

Despite the lengthy experience with HAI, there has been no properly randomized study to define its place in comparison with systemic treatment. The only randomized study of HAI is inadequate in a number of critical respects. This study, conducted by the Central Oncology Group (COG), is commonly cited as demonstrating no benefit from HAI [6]. The 30 patients in this study randomized to receive 5-FU via HAI had either surgically or percutaneously placed catheters. In the majority of patients surgical staging of extrahepatic disease was not undertaken, so the comparability of both treatment groups was unknown in the critical area of the presence of extrahepatic disease.

In recent years HAI has undergone a rebirth especially since the introduction of a subcutaneously implanted infusion pump. A high response rate using continuous infusion with FUdR has been reported [3, 4], with a median survival from time of diagnosis for patients with metastases confined to the liver at operation of 24 months and a median survival from time of pump implantation of 18 months [12]. Toxicity with this technique, however, seems to be rather high, erosions and ulcerations of the gastrointestinal tract having been documented in 68% of cases [9]. Using the Seldinger technique and infusing a combination of drugs at regular intervals, response rates of 46%-53% have been reported, median survivals ranging between 11 months (overall) and 17 months (responders) [2, 14].

In this study the median survival for all patients was 19 months, toxicity being moderate. We like to stress the importance of looking at the overall survival for the whole group of treated patients and not mainly at the survival of responders. The comparison of responders versus nonresponders is only of limited value. The fact that responders live longer than nonresponders is all too frequently interpreted to mean that treatment itself prolongs survival. Response to therapy, however, may simply be a feature of the fact that these patients have an inherently better prognosis. In other words patients who respond to treatment might have done better than nonresponders even without treatment. Clear-cut evidence for survival benefit from treatment can only be obtained by comparing a treated group of patients with a matched nontreated or otherwise treated group, ideally in a randomized trial. Colorectal cancer patients with metastases confined to the liver may be a highly selected group with a substantially better prognosis. In such patients, treated with systemic 5-FU, a median survival has been reported of 11.5 months [11]. No conclusion can be drawn regarding the impact on survival of HAI as used in this study. Nevertheless we like to emphasize that more than half of our patients were symptomatic and the majority had more than 30% liver involvement.

In conclusion we think HAI remains an area for further therapeutic research with potential benefit for patients with colorectal carcinoma with metastases confined to the liver.

References

1. Almersjö O, Bengmark S, Rudenstam CM, Hafström LO, Nilsson LAV (1972) Evaluation of hepatic dearterialization in primary and secondary cancer of the liver. Am J Surg 124: 5
2. Douglass CC (1979) Improved survival in liver metastases from colorectal carcinoma following periodic arterial infusions with mitomycin C, 5-fluorouracil, adriamycin, velban and vincristin. Proc ASCO 20: 431
3. Ensminger WD, Niederhuber J, Gyves J, Trall J, Cozzi E, Doan K (1982) Effective control of liver metastases from colon cancer with an implanted system for hepatic arterial chemotherapy. Proc ASCO 1: 94
4. Ensminger WD, Gyves JW (1983) Regional chemotherapy of neoplastic disease. Pharmac Ther 21: 277
5. Garnick MB, Ensminger WD, Israel M (1979) A clinical-pharmacological evaluation of hepatic arterial infusion of Adriamycin. Cancer Res 39: 4105
6. Grage TB, Vassilopoulos PP, Shingleton WW, Jubert AV, Elias EG, Aust JB, Moss SE (1979) Results of a prospective randomized study of hepatic artery infusion with 5-fluorouracil versus intravenous 5-fluorouracil in patients with hepatic metastases from colorectal cancer: a Central Oncology Group study. Surgery 86: 550
7. Haller DG, Woolley PV, MacDonald JS, Smith LF, Schein PS (1978) Phase II trial of 5-fluorouracil, adriamycin and mitomycin-C in advanced colorectal cancer. Cancer Treat Rep 62: 563
8. Jaffe BM, Donegan WL, Watson F, Spratt JS (1968) Factors influencing survival in patients with untreated hepatic metastases. Surg Gynecol Obstet 127: 1
9. Kemeny N, Daly JM, Oderman P, Shike M (1983) Hepatic infusion chemotherapy for metastatic colorectal carcinoma, results and complications. Proc ASCO 2: 123
10. Koudahl G, Funding J (1972) Hepatic artery ligation in primary and secondary hepatic cancer. Acta Chir Scand 138: 289
11. Levine AW, Donegan WL, Irwin M (1982) Adenocarcinoma of the colon with hepatic metastases. J Am Med Assoc 247: 2809
12. Niederhuber JE, Ensminger W, Gyves J et al (1984) Regional chemotherapy of colorectal cancer metastatic to the liver. Cancer 53: 1336
13. Oxley EM, Ellis H (1969) Prognosis of carcinoma of the large bowel in the presence of liver metastases. Br J Surg 56: 149
14. Patt YZ, Wallace S, Freireich EJ, Chuang VP, Hersh EM, Mavligit GM (1981) The palliative role of hepatic arterial infusion and arterial occlusion in colorectal carcinoma metastatic to the liver. Lancet 2: 349
15. Schein PS, Kisner D, MacDonald JS (1975) Chemotherapy of large intestinal carcinoma: current results and future prospects. Cancer 35: 1074
16. Wils J, Schlangen J, Naus A (1984) Phase II study of hepatic artery infusion with 5-fluorouracil, adriamycin and mitomycin C (FAM) in liver metastases from colorectal carcinoma. Cancer Chemother Pharmacol 13: 215
17. Wood CB, Gillis CR, Blumgart LH (1976) A retrospective study of the natural history of patients with liver metastases from colorectal cancer. Clin Oncol 2: 285

Indication and Rationale for the Use of Implantable Devices for Arterial Regional Chemotherapy

R. M. Barone

School of Medicine, University of California, San Diego, CA 92103, USA

Hepatic arterial infusion chemotherapy for metastatic liver cancer has been used for over 20 years. The reason that intraarterial chemotherapy has not gained universal popularity has been the technical problems associated with such therapy. The therapy was carried out by the placement of angiographic catheters using the percutaneous Seldinger technique. This required hospitalization of the patient for each treatment cycle, for 7-10 days, every 4-6 weeks. Oberfield et al. [1] reported significant complications in 48 patients at the Lahey Clinic treated with prolonged continuous percutaneous intraarterial chemotherapy and metastatic liver adenocarcinoma from colorectal primary. These complications included complete or partial thrombosis of the common hepatic artery or celiac artery in 18.6% and 20.8% of the patients, respectively, and 30% had dislodgement of the catheter. Bleeding not controlled by pressure, stenosis of the common hepatic artery, pseudoaneurysms of the common hepatic artery, and the catheter breaking off in an artery were also reported. Minor complications, such as displacement of the catheter, occurred in 43.8% of the patients, cracked catheter in 31.3%, clotted catheter in 14.6%, infection in 4.2%, and diminished or lost pulse in 12.5%.

Complications experienced by the Lahey Clinic Group were similar to those of others employing percutaneous hepatic artery catheters [2-5].

Direct surgical placement of catheters into the hepatic artery, when compared with the response rates, duration of response, and duration of survival from the treatment using the percutaneous method were superior, as reported by Oberfield [6]. Although the response rates, duration of response, and survival appear superior, there were still significant complications associated with this method of chemotherapy delivery. Surgically placed catheters had to be externalized through the abdominal wall and connected to some type of external pumping device. Termination of treatment, using the operatively placed catheter, was almost always secondary to catheter malfunction [1, 7].

In December 1978 we began implanting an implantable continuous perfusion system for use in delivering regional chemotherapy [8, 9]. We used the Model 400 Infusaid pump produced by the Infusaid Corporation in Norwood, Massachusetts (Figs. 1, 2). The other implantable system involves the use of portal devices, which allows repeated access through a catheter placed into the liver attached to the portal. These ports are presently marketed in the United States by three companies (Figs. 3-5). We prefer using the Porta-cath if prolonged continuous infusion is planned because the port has a thicker silicone septum which holds the needle more securely in place during continuous infusions. This is especially important if the patient is being infused with vesicant drugs. External pump-

Recent Results in Cancer Research. Vol 100

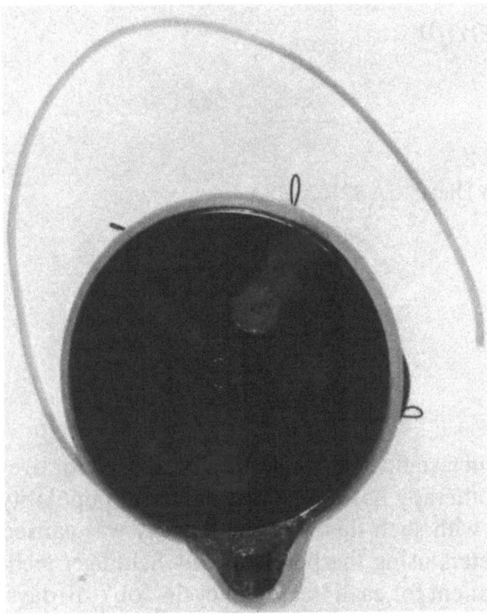

Fig. 1. Model 400 "Infusaid" pump produced by the Infusaid Corporation, Norwood, Massachusetts. The pump weighs 200 g and has overall dimensions of 3 × 9 cm. The sideport has an auxiliary system which bypasses the pumping mechanism for direct catheter injection. This model is a modification of an earlier model developed by Blackshear et al. [8] for continuous heparin infusions

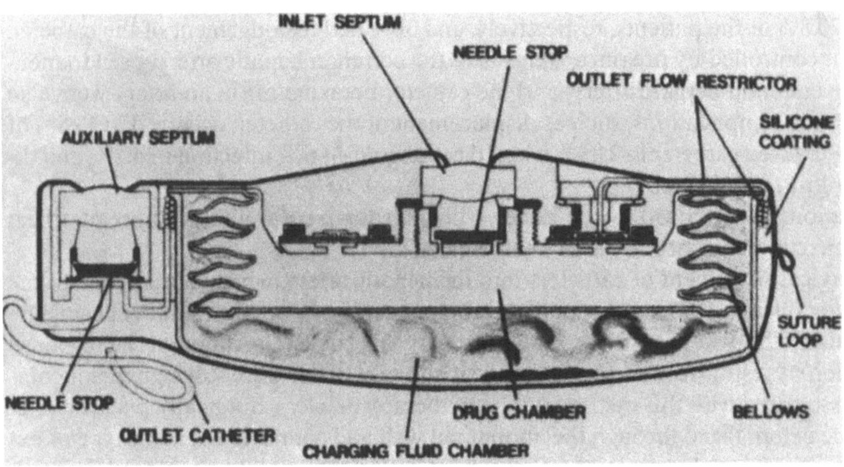

Fig. 2. Schematic of model 400 "infusaid" pump. The disk-shaped pump is separated into two chambers by a titanium bellows. The inner chamber contains the solution to be infused, and the outer charging chamber contains the fluorocarbon freon in equilibrium with its vapor phase. At 37 °C the vapor pressure exerted by the substance is approximately 300 mmHg greater than atmospheric pressure. This vapor pressure provides the power source, exerting pressure on the bellows and forcing the infusate through the 0.22-µm bacterial filter and a flow-regulating resistance element. The pump is placed beneath the skin and subcutaneous tissues and the inner drug chamber is refilled by percutaneous injection through a self-sealing septum. The pressure of this injection condenses the driving vapor, thus simultaneously filling the pump and recharging the power source. The pump has a 50-ml capacity and flow rates of individual pumps are factory calibrated to deliver a constant set rate as desired in the range of 1.5-6 ml/day

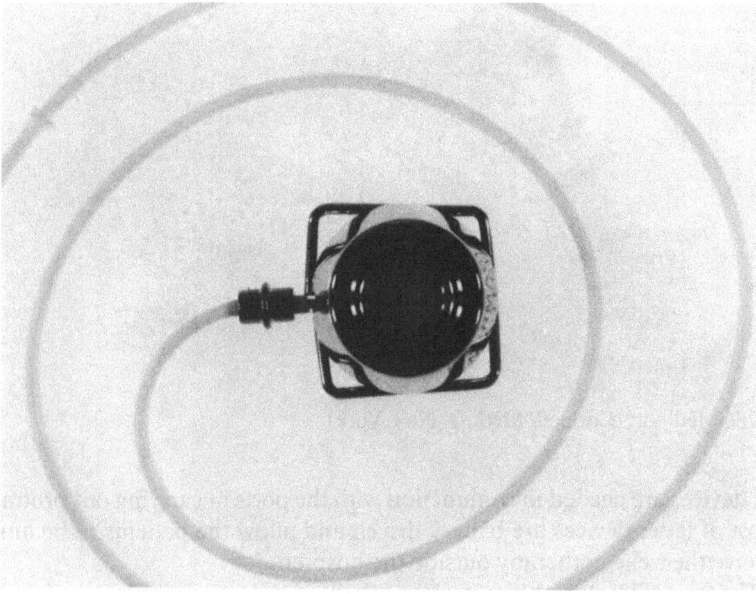

Fig. 3. Port-a-cath (Pharmacia Nu Tech, Walpole, Massachusetts)

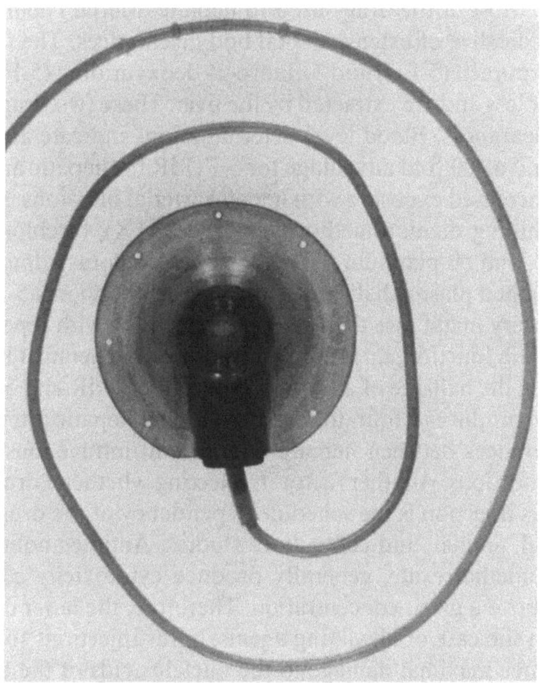

Fig. 4. Infusaport (Infusaid, Norwood, Massachusetts)

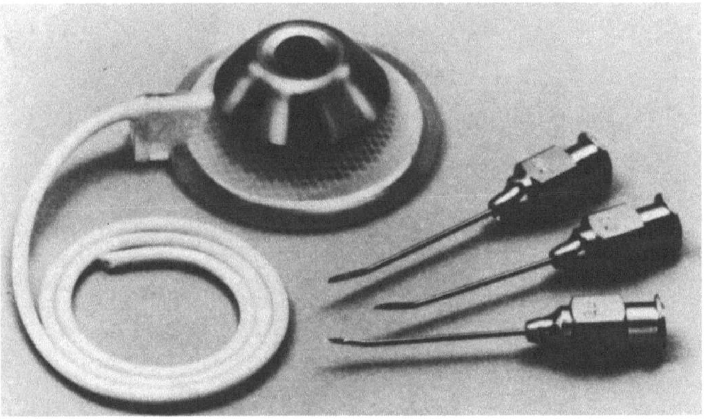

Fig. 5. Mediport (Cormed, Medina, New York)

ing devices are needed in conjunction with the ports in carrying out protracted perfusions. Most of latter devices are battery driven and allow the patients to be ambulatory and to receive their chemotherapy outside the hospital.

The type of implantable system one should implant in a patient undergoing intraarterial chemotherapy is dependent on the drug to be used for the infusion and the tumor type to be treated. At the present time, only FUdR and dichloromethotrexate are drugs compatible for use in the Infusaid implantable pump.

Most of the drugs used in hepatic arterial chemotherapy have short plasma half-lives indicative of extensive total body clearances. The two most commonly used drugs, 5-fluorouracil (5-FU) and 5-fluoro-2′-deoxyuridine (5-FUdR), have serum half-lives of 10 min or less and are extracted by the liver. These two drugs have even more extensive total body clearances. Blood level determinations indicate an eight- to tenfold advantage for 5-FU and a 400-fold advantage for 5-FUdR for hepatic artery infusions over systemic infusions. Increased exposure with hepatic arterial infusions is seen for a number of other agents, including dichloromethotrexate (DCMTX), bischlorethylnitrosurea (BCNU), mitomycin-C, and *cis*-platinum (CDPP). Repeated bolus administration of 5-FU will result in a prolonged plasma half-life. This suggests that bolus 5-FU injections directly into the hepatic artery might lose their regional selectivity with repeated daily administration. Altered hepatic function, underlying cirrhosis, and chemical hepatitis can all contribute to prolonging the half-life of all drugs, especially FUdR and 5-FU. *Cis*-platinum, given intraarterially, produces a four- to sevenfold higher hepatic arterial level of free drug. However, no differences between hepatic arterial and intravenous administration are noted with bolus injections. Another factor in selecting whether a drug is given as a slow infusion versus bolus injection is the schedule dependency of the drug. These usually are based on preclinical, animal, and cell culture studies. Antimetabolites, such as FUdR, 5-FU, and dichloromethotrexate, generally produce cytotoxicity as a function of duration of exposure above a given concentration. Therefore, the latter drugs are best given as a slow infusion. In the case of alkylating agents, bolus injections for short-term peak exposures may produce maximal damage to the nucleic acids of the cell. Lower drug concentrations might allow more of the reparative process to occur and thereby prevent lethal damage to the cell. Therefore, drugs such as mitomycin-C and BCNU are best given as a bolus, or a short infusion over several minutes. It is not known whether Adriamycin, an intercalating agent, or *cis*-platinum are best given as a slow infusion or as a short bolus infusion. Other drugs

Table 1. Mechanism of action and schedule for hepatic arterial drugs

Drug	Half-life (min)	Mechanism of action	Best probable schedule
5-FU	10	Antimetabolite	Prolonged infusion (5-14 days)
FUdR	<10	Antimetabolite	Prolonged infusion (7-14 days)
DCMTX	-	Antimetabolite	Prolonged infusion (14 days)
Mitomycin C	<10	Alkylating agent	Bolus/short (30 min-3 h) infusion
BCNU	< 5	Alkylating agent	Bolus/short (min) infusion
cis-Platinum	20-30	Alkylating agent	Short infusion (1-3 days)
Streptozotocin	15	Alkylating agent	Short infusion (3-8 h)
Adriamycin	10	Intercalating agent	Unknown
Vinblastine	180	Vinca alkaloid	Prolonged infusion (5 days)
DTIC	180	Miscellaneous	Short infusion (1-24 h)

that have been used for intraarterial infusion are the vinca alkaloid vinblastine and streptozotocin. The extraction ratios of these drugs are not known. Velban can be utilized as a slow intraarterial infusion while streptozotocin is best given intraarterially as a bolus or short infusion. Dimethyl-triazeno-imidazole-carboxamide (DTIC) has also been used as an intraarterial infusion for the treatment of melanoma; it is best administered as a short 1-h-infusion (Table 1).

When one is considering a patient for surgical implantation of a hepatic artery catheter, and some type of implantable device, the following patient evaluations should be performed prior to implantation. Some of these are to be considered as major contraindications for surgical exploration:

Severe malnutrition (>10% weight loss 1 month prior to surgery)
Malignant ascites
Portal systemic encephalopathy
Portal vein thrombosis
Prolonged prothrombin time (fails to correct with vitamin K)
Acute or chronic acute hepatitis
Serum bilirubin >4.0 mg/dl
Severe cardiovascular disease or renal disease
Karnofsky status <60%

Patients with severe malnutrition who have lost more than 10% of their body weight in the month preceding surgery, malignant ascites, portal systemic encephalopathy, prolonged prothrombin time with failure to correct within 3 s of normal with vitamin K, acute hepatitis or possible previous history of hepatitis with positive hepatitis antigen, serum bilirubin greater than 4.0 mg/dl, coexistent medical problems such as severe cardiovascular disease and renal disease, and a Karnofsky status of less than 60% are poor candidates for surgical exploration. When surgical implantation is attempted in these situations, the mortality and morbidity are quite high. Patients who have previously had infusional chemotherapy and radiation to the porta hepatis and liver are also poor surgical candidates since the fibrosis within the periportal area may make identification of the hepatic arterial anatomy impossible. Patients who have had previous major surgical hepatic resections, total gastrectomies with creation of gastric pouches, and pancreatectomies are also poor candidates from the standpoint that the arterial anatomy is distorted and there may be significant adhesions to make identification of the hepatic anatomy impossible.

Patients with colorectal cancer who have systemic extrahepatic metastases are also poor candidates for an implantable infusion pump, although these patients could be considered for possible percutaneous placement of hepatic artery catheter or a port. In our small series of patients who had implantable pumps who had extrahepatic disease within the peritoneum, as well as significant hepatic disease, the median survival was only 4 months. Therefore, it is difficult to justify the expense of the implantable pump for such a short survival time. Niederhuber and Ensminger [10] also reported significant decreases in the median survival in patients who had extrahepatic disease (9 versus 18 months). It appears that those patients who have metastatic intraabdominal disease or bone disease, in addition to hepatic disease, are poor candidates for pump placement. However, if the primary extrahepatic disease is pulmonary but the symptomatic disease is hepatic, then one could consider placement of an implantable pump or port, since a significant number of patients will have prolonged survival from treating their hepatic disease, despite having limited pulmonary disease. In general, then, patients with major extrahepatic disease, regardless of the extent of liver involvement, should not routinely receive intraarterial chemotherapy, because the extrahepatic disease may be or become the primary problem, especially if they have intraabdominal disease. In patients with major hepatic disease with minimal extrahepatic disease, intraarterial therapy may be of benefit, using the percutaneous technique. In the latter situation, patients may need a combination of systemic therapy, together with intraarterial chemotherapy. However, the results of this combination therapy are unknown. Patients found to have intraabdominal extrahepatic disease at the time of surgery should have port and catheter placed. If there is minimal extrahepatic disease to periportal or paraaortic lymph nodes, one can consider pump placement.

There may be anatomic reasons for surgical implantation, as opposed to percutaneous placement, such as if one was unable to perfuse the entire liver or if there was thrombosis or stenosis at the origin of the primary artery supplying the liver. The latter is commonly seen in patients who have had multiple percutaneous placements of hepatic artery catheters into the common hepatic artery. If there are multiple arteries supplying the liver, it may be impossible to perfuse the entire liver using one percutaneously placed catheter. Percutaneous placement with connection to a pump or port can be performed for poor-risk patients or those with significant extrahepatic disease, but with life-threatening hepatic disease. Other relative contraindications for the placement of the implantable pumps may be the differentiation of the tumor, especially in the case of colon or rectal cancer. Poorly undifferentiated rectal or colon cancer appears to have a poorer prognosis than the other two tumor types, mainly well and moderately well differentiated adenocarcinomas. Patients with poorly differentiated tumors are more prone to intraabdominal and other visceral metastases. The results of the Hepatic Tumor Study Group will help delineate whether intraarterial infusion is useful in this histologic type. Another relative contraindication is portal vein thrombosis. These patients are usually poor candidates for surgical exploration.

The following tumor types should be considered for possible implantable pump placement. These include the tumor types that are responsive to FUdR:

Colorectal carcinoma	Islet cell carcinoma
Gastric carcinoma	Carcinoid tumors
Hepatoma	Unknown primary

Colorectal carcinoma is the primary tumor type for use of the implantable pump. Gastric carcinoma, islet cell carcinomas, and carcinoid tumors confined to the liver and hepatoma are the other tumor types where one can use the implantable pump. Very few patients with breast carcinoma are candidates for pump placement since most of these patients have significant extrahepatic disease. Most of these patients have received systemic chemotherapy and the hepatic response rate for intraarterial chemotherapy following systemic chemotherapy is low. Those patients with unknown primaries are best treated with surgical placement of a pump and catheter. In our series, we have seven patients who were thought to have unknown primaries and six of them, at the time of surgery, were found to have gastrointestinal primaries, five of whom had carcinoid tumors of the small bowel and one, an islet cell carcinoma of the pancreas. All of these patients had placement of the implantable pump for infusion of FUdR with sideport bolus infusions of streptozotocin.

The patients who should be considered for portal implantation are those with extrahepatic colorectal disease; those with renal cell carcinomas who are to receive vinblastine or Adriamycin; those with melanoma where a combination of DTIC and hyperthermia or irradiation is to be used; those with breast carcinoma where multiple drugs may be used; and those with gallbladder carcinoma, pancreatic, and cholangiocarcinoma where 5-FU infusion is to be combined with irradiation. Lung carcinomas and sarcomas are best treated with ports since multiple-drug chemotherapy is used:

Colorectal carcinoma - extrahepatic disease	Pancreatic carcinoma
Melanoma	Cholangiocarcinoma
Breast carcinoma	Lung carcinoma
Gallbladder carcinoma	Sarcomas

In general, when multiple-drug infusions given over short periods are planned, it is best to use a port. The major advantage of the implantable Infusaid pump is that it allows the patient to carry on a relatively normal life style without any external pumping devices. However, they have their limitation in that the only drugs that are compatible with the pump at the present time are FUdR and dichloromethotrexate.

Surgical placement has the advantage of identifying those patients with extrahepatic disease. One can then determine whether a port or pump should be implanted depending on the extent of disease. Percutaneous placement, although it avoids a major operation, does not allow adequate staging for intraabdominal disease. However, in poor-risk patients or those with massive hepatic disease, percutaneous placement should be tried first and, if the patient responds, he or she can be considered for surgical placement at a later date.

It must be remembered that there has yet to be published the results of any prospective randomized study demonstrating the efficacy of intraarterial chemotherapy over systemic chemotherapy. Randomized studies are now under way which may give us answers to these questions. Obviously, newer pumps with greater versatility with adjustable flow rates and multiple drug compatibilities are needed. Newer techniques, using the biodegradable starch microspheres or monoclonal antibodies, labeled with radioactive agents or drugs may increase the need for ports, as opposed to implantable infusion pumps.

References

1. Oberfield RA, McCaffrey JA, Polio J, Clouse ME, Hamilton T (1979) Prolonged and continuous percutaneous intra-arterial hepatic infusion chemotherapy in advanced metastatic liver adenocarcinoma from colorectal primary. Cancer 44: 414-423
2. Ansfield FJ, Ramirez G, Skibba JL, Bryan GT, Davis HL, Wirtanen GW (1971) Intrahepatic arterial infusion with 5-fluorouracil. Cancer 28: 1147-1151
3. Ansfield FJ, Ramirez G, Davis HL Jr, Wirtanen GW, Johnson RO, Bryan GT, Manalo FB, Borden EC, David TE, Esmaili M (1975) Further clinical studies with intrahepatic arterial infusion with 5-fluorouracil. Cancer 36: 2413-2417
4. Ansfield FJ, Ramirez G (1978) The clinical results of 5-fluorouracil intrahepatic arterial infusion in 528 patients with metastatic cancer to the liver. In: Ariel I (ed) Progress in clinical cancer, vol 7. Grune and Stratton, New York, pp 201-206
5. Barone RM, Byfield JE, Goldfarb PB, Frankel S, Ginn C, Greer S (1982) Intra-arterial chemotherapy using an implantable infusion pump and liver irradiation for the treatment of hepatic metastases. Cancer 50: 850-862
6. Oberfield RA (1983) Intra-arterial hepatic infusion chemotherapy in metastatic liver cancer. In: Lokich JJ (ed) Primary and metastatic liver cancer. Semin Oncol X: 206-214
7. Cady B (1973) Hepatic arterial patency and complications after catheterization for infusion chemotherapy. Ann Surg 178: 156-159
8. Blackshear PJ, Rodhe TD, Varco RL, Buchwald H (1975) One year of continuous heparinization in the dog using a totally implanted infusion pump. Surg Gynecol Obstet 141: 176-178
9. Ensminger WD, Niederhuber J, Dakhil S, Thrall J, Wheeler R (1981) A totally implanted drug delivery system for hepatic arterial chemotherapy. Cancer Treat Rep 65: 393-400
10. Niederhuber JE, Ensminger W, Gyves J, Thrall J, Walker S, Cozzi E (1984) Regional chemotherapy of colorectal cancer metastatic to liver. Cancer 53: 1336-1343

Preliminary Results of a Randomized Study of Intrahepatic Infusion Versus Systemic Infusion of 5-Fluoro-2′-deoxyuridine for Metastatic Colorectal Carcinoma

N. Kemeny and J. Daly

Solid Tumor Service, Department of Medicine, Memorial Sloan-Kettering Cancer Center, 1275 York Avenue, NY 10021, USA

Development of a totally implantable infusion pump produced a renewed interest in hepatic infusional therapy. An initial study employing this pump by Ensminger and associates and the continuous hepatic infusion of 5-fluoro-2′-deoxyuridine (FUdR) observed an 83% response rate [1]. However, further work with this method brought the mean response rate down to 59% (Table 1) [2], which, however, is still higher than the mean response rate obtained with systemic chemotherapy.

Although surgical and technical complications with the use of an implantable pump have been minimal, chemotherapy-related complications have been substantial. In the study at Memorial Sloan-Kettering Cancer Center (MSKCC) on 45 patients using the dose of 0.3 mg/kg per day FUdR for 2 weeks alternating with 2 weeks of saline, 30% had endoscopically documented gastrointestinal ulceration. If severe gastritis and duodenitis are included, 50% had significant gastrointestinal disease. Hepatic toxicity was also seen frequently; an elevation of serum bilirubin level above 3 mg/dl was observed in 20% of the patients, and an elevation of serum glutamic oxaloacetic transaminase (SGOT) level three times above baseline values in 46%. Two patients developed strictures of their bile duct resembling sclerosing cholangitis [2].

The most useful laboratory test to help monitor and avoid some of these side effects is SGOT (Fig. 1). If one were to obtain SGOT values every 4 weeks, these spikes at 2 weeks, at the end of the infusion, would be missed. In reevaluating our first group of patients, we

Table 1. Result of hepatic artery infusion via infusaid pump

	Number of patients	% response
Ensminger	60	83
Balch	50	83
Barone	18	56
Cohen	26	53
Kemeny	41	41
Johnson	17	36
Levin	31	30
Weiss	17	29

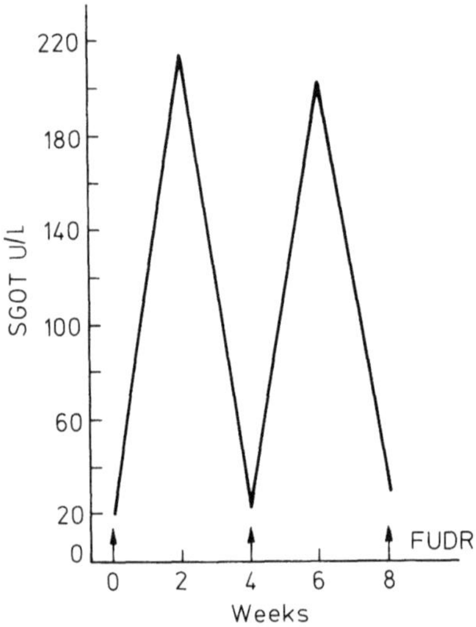

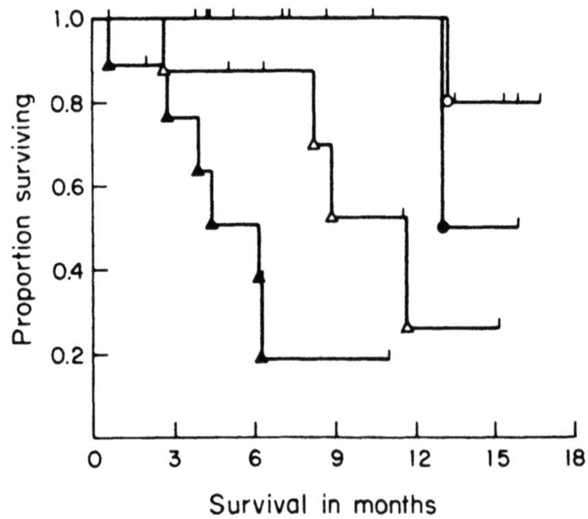

Fig. 1 *(Left).* Hepatic artery pump study: effect of FUdR on SGOT. Patient L. F.

Fig. 2 *(Right).* Effect of hepatic involvement on survival. Survival of patients according to extent of liver disease as assessed at laparotomy: ○, ⩽20%; ●, 21%–40%; △, 41%–60%; ▲, ⩾61%; *tick mark* indicates fast follow-up

noted that this pattern of SGOT elevation had occurred earlier in 11 out of 12 patients with ulcer disease and in all patients who had an increase in bilirubin.

In order to see the true impact of hepatic infusion therapy on response and survival, one needs a prospective randomized study with stratification for important parameters such as liver involvement and certain indicative laboratory values.

Many investigators have shown the extent of liver involvement by tumor is an independent prognostic factor influencing survival [3, 4, 5]. Figure 2 demonstrates the relationship of the surgeon's estimation of tumor involvement of the liver and of survival for our first 45 patients. Patients with less than < 20% involvement had a median survival of > 13 month while those with > 60% involvement had a 6 month median survival.

The influence of certain laboratory parameters on response and survival was evaluated in a study at MSKCC in 220 patients with advanced metastatic colorectal carcinoma. The most significant factor affecting both response and survival was the initial lactic dehydrogenase (LDH) level. Patients whose initial LDH and carcinoembryonic antigen (CEA) levels were normal had a median survival of 32 months versus only 8 months for those who originally had abnormal values of LDH and CEA [6].

This prospective randomized study will compare intrahepatic infusion to systemic infusion applying the same chemotherapeutic agent (FUDR), schedule, and method of administration. Patients with measurable metastatic colorectal carcinoma to the liver, without extrahepatic disease, are eligible. Patients with a Karnofsky performance status (PS) of less than 60% and a serum bilirubin greater than 4.0 mg/dl are excluded.

After stratification by LDH level (< 300 U/liter versus ⩾ 300 U/liter) and percentage liver involvement (< 50% versus ⩾ 50%), all patients are randomized to either intrahepatic or systemic therapy prior to surgery. The extent of liver involvement is assessed medically by an evaluation using computed tomography (CT) and/or radionuclide liver scans. The information is placed in a sealed envelope and opened only after the extent of liver in-

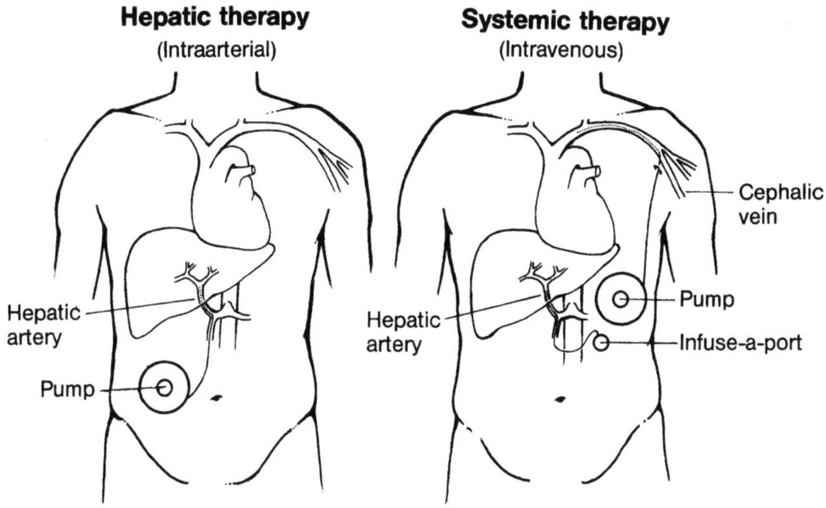

Fig. 3. Placement of catheter and Infusaid pump

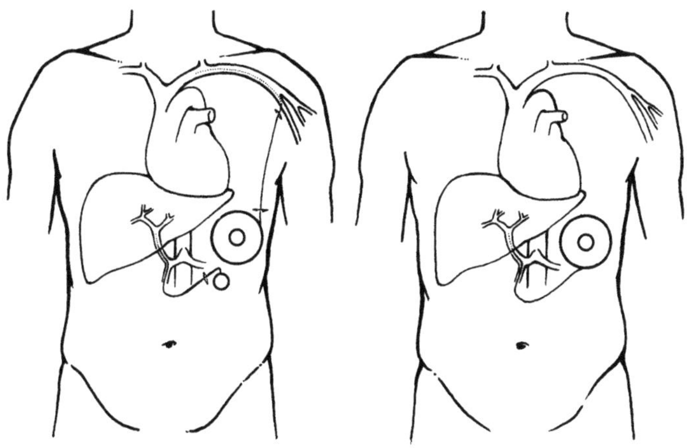

Fig. 4. Conversion of systemic to hepatic infusion therapy

volvement is assessed by a surgeon during exploratory laparotomy. If there is a disagreement between preoperative and surgical assessment of the extent of liver involvement, the patient is rerandomized.

All patients undergo exploratory laparotomy not only for the placement of a hepatic artery catheter and Infusaid pump but also to ensure that two arms of the study are comparable, by accurately defining the extent of liver involvement and assuring that there is no disease outside the liver. Any patients with a resectable hepatic lesion or extrahepatic disease is considered ineligible for the protocol.

Patients randomized to intrahepatic therapy have the hepatic artery catheter connected to the pump. In the systemic group, the hepatic catheter is connected to an Infuse-a-port, and the pump is connected to an additional catheter placed in the cephalic vein (Fig. 3). If the disease progressed in a patient in the latter group, a minor surgical procedure would allow a crossover to the intrahepatic therapy (Fig. 4), thereby also allowing further evaluation of the efficacy of regional therapy.

The drug FUdR is administered by continuous infusion for 14 days via an Infusaid pump in both groups. However, the starting dose is 0.3 mg/kg per day for the intrahepatic group and 0.15 mg/kg per day for those receiving systemic infusion.

Eighty-nine patients have been referred for entry into the study. Six patients refused randomization, and three were excluded because of anomalous arterial blood supply, i. e., more than three vessels perfused the liver. Therefore, 80 patients were randomized preoperatively (Table 2).

Table 2. Intrahepatic versus systemic FUdR infusion

Referred			89
Refused randomization		6	
Two or more arterial supply		3	
Randomized			80
Excluded		30	
Resected	13		
Extrahepatic disease	14		
Infection	1		
No tumor	2		
Entered			50

Table 3. Intrahepatic versus systemic FUdR infusion: patient characteristics

	Intrahepatic ($n=25$)	Systemic ($n=25$)
Age (years)[a]	61	62
Karnofsky PS (96)[a]	80	80
% liver involvement	40	45
Sex (M/F)	20/5	14/11

[a] Median

Table 4. Intrahepatic versus systemic FUdR infusion: initial laboratory data

		Intrahepatic ($n=25$)	Systemic ($n=25$)
LDH	> 500 units/liter	7	12
CEA	> 100 ng/ml	11	15
WBC	> 10000 cells/mm^3	3	6
Albumin	< 4.0 g/dl	9	9
Alkaline phosphatase	> 300 units/liter	8	7

Thirty patients were excluded from the study after surgical exploration for the following reasons: resectable disease in 13 patients, extrahepatic disease in 14, no tumor in 2, and intraabdominal infection in one. Fifty patients, therefore, have had the pump placed in the randomized study. The two groups were comparable (Table 3); they were well matched with respect to percentage liver involvement, initial laboratory values, performance status (PS), age, and unfavorable prognostic factors (Table 4). Sex was the only parameter by which they were not well matched; there were only 5/20 females in the intrahepatic group, while 11/25 patients were women in the systemic group. When the data were analyzed to see if gender influenced response rate, this appeared not to be the case.

Responses are assessed in the following manner: a complete response denotes the disappearance of all evidence of disease by CT, liver scan, physical examination, and CEA levels. A partial response (PR) is defined as a greater than 50% reduction in the size of measurable disease by CT or liver scan. If the liver is palpable, a 50% reduction in liver measurements is also required. A minor response (MR) is 25%-50% reduction in the size of measurable disease. CEA reductions are noted but are not used to define a response.

To date, 9 PRs in 21 evaluable patients were seen in the intrahepatic group and 7 PRs in 21 evaluable patients in the systemic group. The median duration of response is 7 months for both groups. There was one MR in each group. In the systemic group, five patients have had stable disease for 4-13+ months. Twelve patients in the intrahepatic group and 9 patients in the systemic group have had more than 50% reduction in CEA level (Table 5).

In evaluating the patients who had a crossover, there seems to be some relationship between initial response and the chance of getting a response from the crossover (Table 6). Five patients who responded and then failed systemic treatment have been crossed-over to the intrahepatic treatment. Three patients responded and one had a transient improvement which was followed by thrombosis of the hepatic artery and progression of disease. Six of seven patients who originally failed systemic infusion also failed intrahepatic infusion (Table 6).

The toxicity has been quite different between the two groups (Table 7). In the intrahepatic group, the toxicity has been mainly gastrointestinal and hepatic. Four of 25 patients developed significant gastrointestinal ulcers documented by endoscopy, and a fifth patient had severe gastritis. Fifteen patients developed an elevation of SGOT greater than 100% over baseline value, and five developed a significant elevation of serum bilirubin (as high as 10.0 mg/dl in one patient). Two of the five went on to develop biliary sclerosis. In the systemic group, the major toxicity has been diarrhea, seen in 16 patients. In two patients, sigmoidoscopy revealed sigmoid ulcerations suggestive of colitis. Both patients required hospitalization for supportive care including hydration.

Another significant difference between the two groups was the development of extrahepatic disease. In the intrahepatic group, 13 patients have already developed extrahepatic disease (7 lung, 3 intraabdominal and 1 bone). At the present time, four patients in the systemic group have developed extrahepatic disease (Table 10).

Although the starting dose for the intrahepatic therapy was twice as high as that for the systemic therapy, doses in both arms were quite similar after the third cycle of treatment (Tables 8, 9). In the systemic arm, the starting dose was 0.15 mg/kg per day × 14 days in the first 9 patients. After two patients developed severe diarrhea, the dose was reduced to 0.125 mg/kg per day.

There has been no difference in survival between the two treatment groups. The median survival, at the present time, for the intrahepatic group is 11 months, while it has not been reached for the systemic group because of limited follow-up thus far and very few deaths.

Table 5. Intrahepatic versus systemic FUdR infusion

	Intrahepatic	Systemic
Total entered	25	25
Too early	3	2
Inadequate trial	1	2
Evaluable	21	21
Partial response	9	7
Minor response	1	1
Stable	3	5
Reduction of CEA (> 50%)	12	9

Table 6. Results of crossover from systemic to intrahepatic FUdR infusion ($n = 12$)

Response to systemic FUdR	PR (5)		NR (7)	
Response to intrahepatic FUdR	PR (3)	NR (2[a])	NR (6)	Too early (1)

[a] One patient had progressive disease after thrombosis of hepatic artery; intraarterial treatment therefore had to be stopped

Table 7. Intrahepatic versus systemic FUdR infusion: toxicity in evaluable patients

	Intrahepatic ($n = 25$)	Systemic ($n = 25$)
Ulcer	4	0
Diffuse gastritis	1	1
SGOT ≥ 2 × baseline	15	1
Bilirubin > 3.0 mg/dl	5	0
Diarrhea	1	16
Colitis	0	2

Table 8. Dose adjustments for intrahepatic chemotherapy ($n = 25$)

		No. patients
Reduction after	1st treatment[a]	6
	2nd treatment	8
	3rd treatment	4
Median dose after	3rd treatment	0.2 mg/kg per day

[a] Starting dose 0.3 mg/kg per day

Table 9. Dose adjustment for systemic chemotherapy ($n = 25$)

	No. patients	Reduction	Escalation
Original dose FUdR 0.15 mg/kg per day	9	5	–
Subsequent starting dose FUdR 0.125 mg/kg per day	16	1	9

Median dose after third treatment 0.15 mg/kg per day

Table 10. Intrahepatic versus systemic FUdR infusion: development of extrahepatic disease

	Intrahepatic ($n = 25$)	Systemic ($n = 25$)	Crossover ($n = 12$)
Lung	7	2	3
Abdomen	3	0	0
Bone	3	0	0
Pelvis	0	2	0
Adrenal	1	0	0
Spinal	1	0	0
Total number of patients	13[a]	4	3

[a] Two patients had more than one extrahepatic site of disease

Conclusions

Although it is still too early to reach definite conclusions, the following observations on the infusional chemotherapy in hepatic metastases from colorectal carcinoma can be made:

1. The development of extrahepatic disease is significantly more common with intrahepatic infusion than with systemic infusion.
2. Gastrointestinal toxicity is common with both types of infusion; upper gastrointestinal ulceration is observed with intrahepatic infusion, whereas diarrhea is observed with systemic infusion. Hepatic toxicity is seen with intrahepatic therapy but not with systemic therapy.
3. Response rates for the intrahepatic and systemic groups (43% and 32%, respectively) are similar, although it is premature to draw any conclusions.

References

1. Ensminger W, Niederhuber J, Gyves J, Thrall J, Cozzi E, Doan K (1982) Effective control of liver metastases from colon cancer with an implanted system for hepatic arterial chemotherapy. Proc ASCO 1: 94
2. Kemeny N, Daly J, Oderman P, Shike M, Chun H, Petroni G, Geller N (1984) Hepatic artery pump infusion: toxicity and results in patients with metastatic colorectal carcinoma. J Clin Oncol 2: 595-600
3. Wood CB, Gillis CR, Blumgart LH (1976) A retrospective study of the natural history of patients with liver metastases from colorectal cancer. Clin Oncol 2: 285-288
4. Pettavel J, Morgenthaler F (1978) Protracted arterial chemotherapy of liver tumors: an experience of 107 cases over a 12-year period. In: Ariel IM (ed) Progress in clinical cancer. Grune and Stratton, New York, pp 217-233
5. Nielsen J, Balslev I, Jensen HE (1971) Carcinoma of the colon with liver metastases. Acta Chir Scand 137: 463-465
6. Kemeny N, Braun DW (1983) Prognostic factors in advanced colorectal carcinoma. Importance of lactic dehydrogenase level, performance status and white blood cell count. Am J Med 74: 786-798

Surgical Treatment

Surgical Anatomy of the Liver

H. Bismuth

Hepatobiliary Research and Surgery Unit, Paul Brousse Hospital, 14 Avenue P.V. Couturier, 94800 Villejuif, France

Morphological Anatomy

The first description of the anatomy of the liver is what we can term the morphological anatomy, based on the surface features of the organ (Fig. 1). On the anterior surface, the round ligament and the falciform ligament divide the liver into two lobes: the left and right lobes. On the inferior surface, the umbilical fissure, the gallbladder bed, and the hilus limit the quadrate lobe. Behind the hilus is the spigelian lobe. In total, there are two main lobes and two accessory lobes corresponding to the true definition of a lobe: "part of the parenchyma limited by fissures or grooves" *(Stedman's Medical Dictionary)*. However, this morphological description of the liver is inadequate to guide the surgeon in performing anatomical surgery.

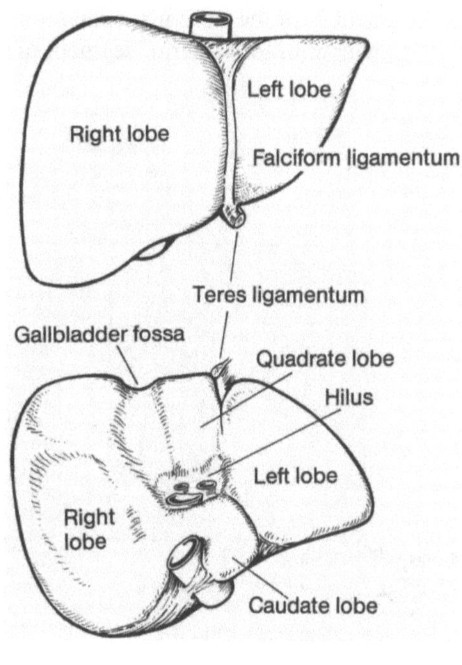

Fig. 1. Morphology of the liver

Recent Results in Cancer Research. Vol 100

Functional Anatomy

Based on the distribution of vessels in the liver, a second anatomy can be described: the functional anatomy. The three hepatic veins divide the liver into four sectors, each receiving a portal pedicle. There are three scissurae: the middle scissura in which runs the middle hepatic vein, the right scissura, and the left scissura. Figure 2 shows the four sectors separated by the three hepatic veins and receiving the four portal pedicles. Figure 3 shows, less schematically, the functional division of the liver. The main fissura divides the liver into two parts: the right hemi-liver or more simply the right liver and the left hemi-liver or the left liver. Each of these two livers receives one of the two branches of the portal vein and is drained by one of the two branches of the bile duct. Distribution of the hepatic artery does not strictly follow this division. The right liver is divided into two sectors by the right hepatic vein: the posterior and the anterior. The left liver is also divided into two by the left scissura: a medial sector and a lateral one.

It is possible according to the secondary divisions of the portal branches to divide the liver further. This has been done by the French anatomist and surgeon Claude Couinaud [3], who described the segments. Each of the two sectors of the right liver is divided into two segments: an inferior segment and a superior segment. The medial left sector is divided into two by the umbilical fissura: a medial segment and a lateral segment. The left lateral sector is only one segment. The spigelian lobe, which has independent hepatic veins and portal pedicles, is an autonomous segment. In total the liver is divided into eight segments. Numbers have been assigned to these segments:

The spigelian lobe is segment one; then, moving clockwise, we find:

- Segment 2 for the lateral segment (or sector) of the left liver.
- Segment 3 for the lateral segment of the medial sector of the left liver.
- Segment 4 for the medial segment of the left medial sector.
- Segment 5 for the inferior segment of the anterior sector of the right liver.
- Segment 6 for the inferior segment of the posterior sector of the right liver.
- Segment 7 for the superior segment of the posterior sector of the right liver.
- Segment 8 for the superior segment of the anterior sector of the right liver.

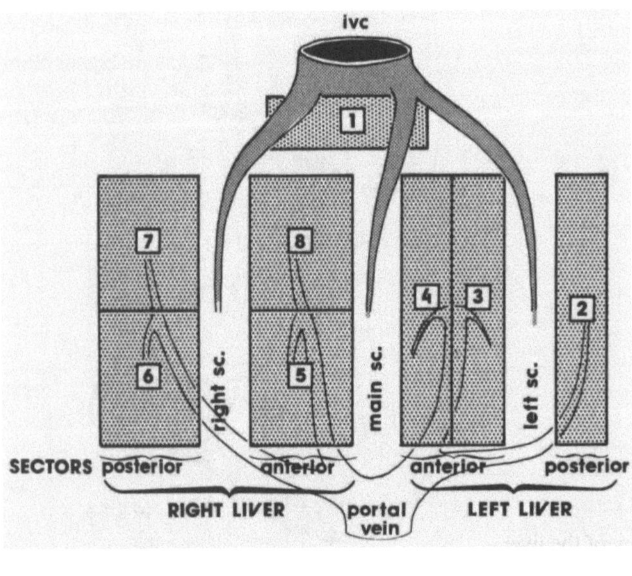

Fig. 2. Schematic representation of the functional anatomy of the liver

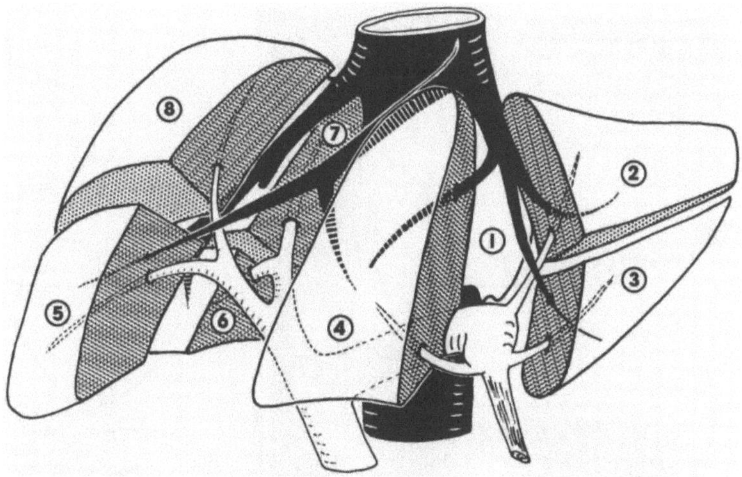

Fig. 3. The functional division of the liver and the hepatic segmentation (in vivo position of the liver)

We notice:

1. That the morphological left lobe, to the left of the umbilical fissura, comprises segments 2 and 3.
2. The anterior part of segment 4, which is anterior to the hilus, is the quadrate lobe (segment 4 is not equivalent to the quadrate lobe, which is only its anterior part).
3. The segments are usually described on an ex vivo liver placed on a table, and in this setting the posterior sector seems to be lateral to the anterior sector. In vivo, the posterior sector is almost completely behind the anterior sector and is not seen at the anterior surface of the liver.

In most countries, the segments and their numbers have become very popular among surgeons. This definition of the segments according to Couinaud's [3] nomenclature is different from that of Goldsmith and Woodburn [4]: according to the latter authors a sector of Couinaud is called a subsegment. This is a cause of confusion in the world literature as Goldsmith and Woodburn's nomenclature is usually used in the English-written literature.

Real Anatomy

Recent progress has been made in *operative ultrasound,* which gives the surgeon a precise picture of the anatomy of the liver being operated on [5].

Tracing the vascular distribution inside the liver is the first step in liver resection (Figs. 4, 5). By locating precisely the three main hepatic veins, the portal scissurae can be identified and their projections on the anterior surface of the liver marked by small incisions on Glisson's capsule. Operative ultrasound is even more useful for segmental resection as division inside the liver of the main portal branches can be easily located.

Segments can be more precisely defined by injection of dye under ultrasound guidance in the segmental portal branch or by balloon catheter occlusion.

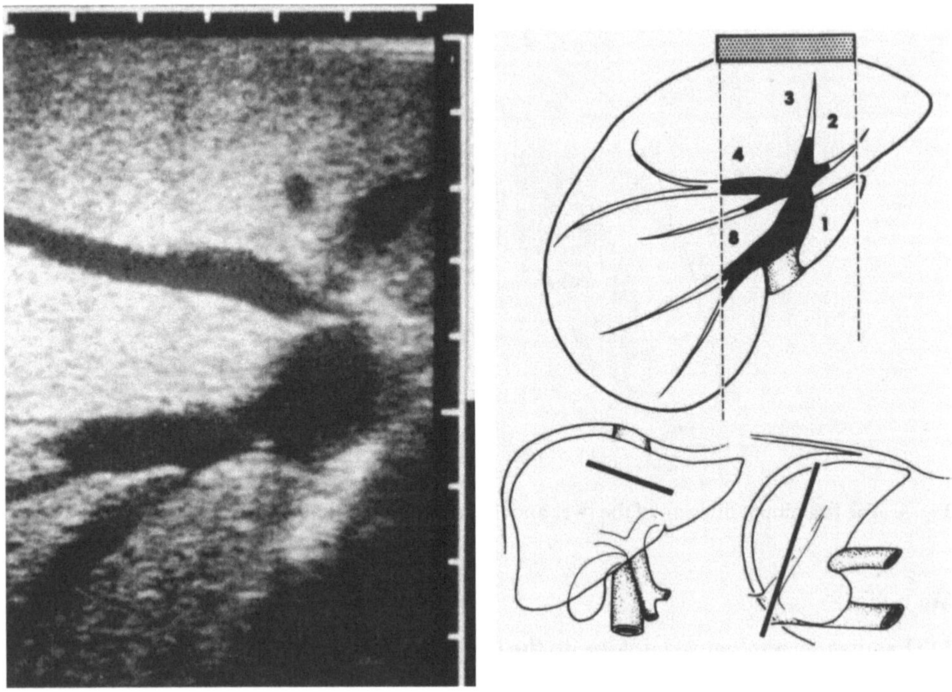

Fig. 4. Operative ultrasound anatomy: the three main hepatic veins

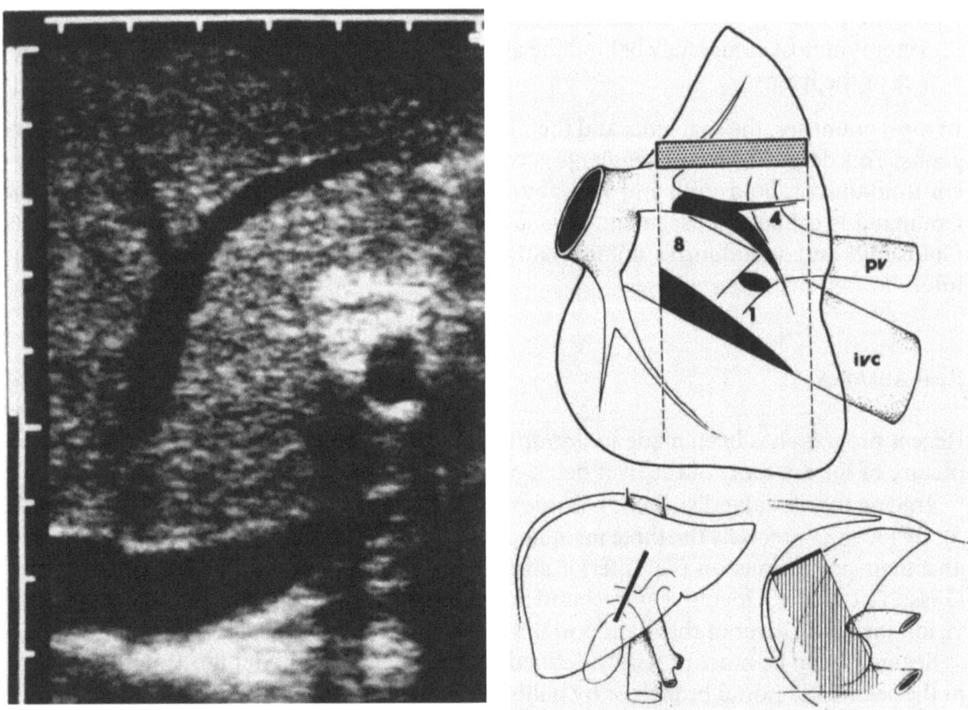

Fig. 5. Operative ultrasound anatomy: the main scissura and the middle hepatic vein

Anatomical Surgery

Anatomical liver resections, also called typical hepatectomies or *hepatectomies réglées,* are made by the resection of a portion of liver parenchyma following one or several anatomical scissurae. In contrast, resection of a portion of parenchyma not limited by anatomical scissurae, such as wedge resection, is an atypical hepatectomy [1].

Common Typical Hepatectomies

There are four common typical hepatectomies: right and left hepatectomies, in which the line of transection is the middle portal scissura separating the right and the left livers; and right and left lobectomies, in which the line of transection is the umbilical fissure. In our classification, right lobectomy corresponds to an extended right hepatectomy including segment 4: it covers the real right lobe according to the morphological description of the liver. The terms left and right lobectomy are frequently used in the literature to define what is in fact a left or right hepatectomy. This is the source of confusion and in our opinion it is preferable to avoid referring to as "lobectomy" the resection of a part of the liver which does not fit with the anatomical definition of the lobe.

Segmentectomies

Single or multiple segmentectomies are other types of anatomical hepatectomies, which are more economical in terms of the amount of liver parenchyma removed. According to the anatomical segmentation of the liver, all the individual or associated segmentectomies can be theoretically described. In fact, the number of segmental liver resections really performed is more limited [2]:

1. Single segmentectomies
   Segmentectomy 4: anterior partial segmentectomy 4 (resection of the quadrate lobe) and complete segmentectomy 4
   Segmentectomy 5
   Segmentectomy 7
   Segmentectomy 8
2. Bisegmentectomies
   Bisegmentectomy 6-7: the right posterior sectoriectomy
   Bisegmentectomy 4-5: removing the parenchyma from both sides of the gallbladder bed

Conclusion

The surgeon can choose among any techniques of hepatectomy with or without primary ligation of the vessels, radical or limited, classical hemihepatectomies or segmentectomies in order to adapt as precisely as possible the technique of liver resection to the disease to be treated: benign or malignant, small or large lesion, peripheral or central in the liver, in normal or cirrhotic liver. Sound knowledge of anatomy is necessary for anatomical surgery.

References

1. Bismuth H (1982) Surgical anatomy and anatomical surgery of the liver. World J Surg 6: 3-9
2. Bismuth H, Houssin D, Castaing D (1982) Major and minor segmentectomies "réglées" in liver surgery. World J Surg 6: 10-24
3. Couinaud C (1957) Le foie. Etudes anatomiques et chirurgicales. Masson, Paris
4. Goldsmith NA, Woodburne RT (1957) Surgical anatomy pertaining to liver resection. Surg Gynecol Obstet 195: 310
5. Castaing D, Kunstlinger F, Habib N, Bismuth H (1985) Intra-operative ultrasound study of the liver: methodology and anatomical results. Am J Surg (in press)

Concepts of Liver Resection for Primary and Secondary Tumors

L. H. Blumgart

Hepatobiliary Surgical Unit, Department of Surgery, Royal Postgraduate Medical School, Ducane Road, London W12 OHS, Great Britain

The amazing potential of the human liver to regenerate after hepatic resection allows removal of large portions of liver substance. The remnant, provided its blood supply, particularly portal blood supply and biliary drainage, is maintained, undergoes rapid regenerative hyperplasia and restoration of function. Detailed anatomical studies have defined the lobes and segments of the liver and provide the surgeon with the necessary planes for safe dissection.

The use of hepatic resectional procedures for diseases of the liver has become more common and it has become recognised that, for the successful performance of major hepatic resection, special skills and support services are required.

Technique of Hepatic Resection

The standard techniques for hepatic resection have been widely described [1-4] and will not be covered in detail. However it is important, as will be emphasised below, to define, particularly in the case of tumours, the limits of resectability. There are now techniques available which allow hepatic resection even in the presence of tumour involvement of one or other branch of the portal vein and, indeed, tumours involving the portal vein bifurcation may be resected [5]. Portions of the retrohepatic inferior vena cava may also be excised. These innovations have extended the range of hepatic resections and have an important bearing on the management of some tumours of the liver (vide infra) and of hilar cholangiocarcinoma [5].

Primary Hepatic Malignancy

Hepatocellular cancer, while a major health hazard in Africa and Asia, is relatively uncommon in the Western World. Available evidence suggests that resection is probably the only treatment method that may lead to cure. Although most reports of a large experience of resection of primary liver cancer in Africa and Asia are discouraging [6-9] results reported for the treatment of Western patients are considerably better [6, 10-12]. Indeed, hepatic resection may be carried out with a mortality that averages some 13% [2], but mortality figures as low as 3% have been recorded by some [4, 10]. Survival in the Mayo Clinic series and in the collected series of Foster and Berman [6] was approximately 30% at 5 years in patients with non-cirrhotic livers.

Recent Results in Cancer Research. Vol 100

Most liver cancers remain confined to the liver for a relatively long period before metastases develop and indeed the history may be prolonged even in cirrhotic patients. When primary epithelial liver cancer is found in a non-cirrhotic patient, then resection is justified so long as there is no evidence of distant spead. The presence of multiple nodules, if confined to one lobe and histological type, or even invasion of the diaphragm or rupture into the peritoneal cavity does not exclude the possibility of cure. Similarly, age and sex have not been shown to correlate with immediate or prolonged survival [6]. Resection is probably not justified for tumours occurring in cirrhotic livers in Western patients, although segmental resections guided by intraoperative ultrasound may change the situation in the future. Unless there is clear evidence of bilateral involvement or distant metastases, laparotomy is indicated. It is very important that size alone or even multiple tumours within a resectable area of the liver are not regarded as contraindicating surgical resection. Preliminary angiography and, for very large tumours, inferior vena cavography are important and assist the surgeon. However, involvement, certainly of one branch of the portal vein, or extensive compression, or even involvement of the vena cava should not preclude attempted resection. Methods for excision of such large tumours offering repair of the portal vein or of the involved vena cava have been described.

It has become evident in our practice at the Royal Postgraduate Medical School that some of the largest and slowest growing tumours are of the fibrolamellar variant of hepatocellular cancer and may have a better than average prognosis. The presence of such a lesion may be suspected in a patient with hepatocellular cancer often with low or normal alpha-feto protein levels with a raised serum vitamin-B_{12}-binding capacity [13] and with an elevation of the plasma neurotensin [14]. We have resected five of seven such lesions, all very large and all compressing the vena cava and involving the portal venous structures. Plasma neurotensin was elevated in all, and fell after resection. There was no mortality and all patients are alive and well at periods up to 3 years.

Liver transplantation has been used in the management of primary liver cell cancer, and it is usually stated should be considered for patients found to be irresectable. However, it is the author's opinion that the definition of irresectability should be most carefully made and while preoperative investigations of the most elegant kind are extremely valuable, patients should not be deemed irresectable purely on the basis of size or vascular involvement.

Other Primary Malignancy

Hepatic resection is an appropriate method of therapy for a variety of other hepatic malignancies, particularly hepatoblastoma and hepatocellular cancer in children. Other malignant lesions which might require hepatic resection are cystadenocarcinoma and, rarely, angiosarcomata.

Cholangiocarcinoma

Cholangiocarcinoma at the confluence of the bile duct is irresectable in 80% or more of cases but in the remaining 20% may be managed by local excision and in some patients by means of partial hepatectomy encompassing the bifurcation of the bile ducts with subsequent reconstruction by means of hepaticojejunostomy to the remnant [5]. Precise preoperative evaluation will define most clearly irresectable lesions and leave selected cases for attempted cure [15]. Again, involvement of a branch of the portal vein is not necessarily a contraindication to partial hepatectomy. In a series of 94 patients recently reported the author has resected tumour in 18 cases, 6 by local resection and 12 by hepatic resection, 9 of these patients having portal venous involvement and 3 requiring portal venous reconstruction procedures. The results indicated no mortality (30-day hospital mortality) for local resection and a 16.5% mortality for partial hepatectomy, the overall mortality for resection being 11%. The 30-day mortality was entirely related to infection usually acquired during a period of preoperative percutaneous transhepatic drainage. Indeed, the mortality for those patients treated without prior surgical intervention or intubation was only 9% [5].

The results indicate surgical resection of hilar cholangiocarcinoma is associated with very good quality of life. The mean duration of survival following resection was 17 months, and 7 patients were still alive for periods of just over 5 years, with a mean survival of 22.2 months. Others have reported encouraging results for resection, (including hepatic resection) for hilar cholangiocarcinoma [16-18]. Certainly resection offers potential cure and removal of the tumour with restoration of continuity of the gastrointestinal tract and this is associated with excellent palliation.

Metastatic Liver Tumours

Results for excision of secondary tumours arising from primary sites in the stomach, pancreas and breast are poor. Hepatic resection for secondary liver deposits arising from Wilms' tumour from hypernephroma, and particularly from the colon, is however advisable in selected cases [6].

There is evidence that liver secondary deposits from colorectal cancer are found in over 20% of patients at the time of initial presentation and many studies show that there are no 5-year survivors after diagnosis, most patients being dead within 2 years of presentation. Solitary liver deposits have a better prognosis than those with more widespread lesions and occasional survivors for 5 years are found [19]. However, all die from their tumour. In contrast, the mortality for hepatic resection from metastatic lesions in experienced hands has been recorded as low as 4% [11]. Five-year survival figures as high as 40% and a 28% survival at 10 years have been reported where the lesion is solitary [20]. Foster and Berman [6] in a collected series suggest that the 5-year survival figures should be approximately 20%.

In 34 major hepatic resections reported from the Mayo Clinic, Adson and Van Heerden [21] conclude that the risks of surgery are justified by lengthened survival and certainly good palliation in many patients.

In general, metastatic liver cancer arising from the colon should be excised if preoperative and operative assessment indicate no extrahepatic metastatic disease and if the lesions are located within a resectable area of liver tissue and preferably if the lesion is solitary. The primary lesion of course is important although there is no hard evidence that patients with Dukes' C_1 lesions fare any worse that those without nodal involvement [6]. Patients with locally invasive cancer and many involved nodes have a poor prognosis and should probably not be submitted to subsequent hepatic resection. Better results appear to be obtained for small rather than large lesions [20]. Rarely, resection may be indicated for the removal of a painful abdominal mass or for the control of haemorrhage.

At the Royal Postgraduate Medical School, Hammersmith Hospital, over the past 5 years 19 patients within hepatic metastases have been submitted to resection. There was only one hospital death within 30 days in a patient who underwent combined hepatic and pancreatic resection for symptomatic gastrinoma and 10 patients remain alive at periods from 1 month to 2.5 years.

Hepatic resection may also be indicated for metastatic lesions arising from other primary sites, and in particular resection for solitary carcinoid tumours may give excellent results in terms of palliation and with prolonged survival. Resection of solitary metastases from other endocrine lesions may occasionally be of value [22].

Personal Experience

The author has had a personal experience of 134 consecutive liver resections. Of these, 33 have been for liver injury or major vascular injury associated with the liver and of these patients 10 died, the majority of the deaths occurring in patients with liver necrosis and referred late. Eight patients have had resection for benign tumour, 14 for hepatocellular cancer, 22 for cholangiocarcinoma or gall bladder cancer and 34 for secondary liver tumours. There have been 23 other resections for a variety of benign conditions, including high bile duct strictures, cysts and intrahepatic stones.

Results for the resection of solid liver cancers at Hammersmith Hospital over the past 5 years are of some interest. There has been hepatic resection carried out for hepatoma in eight patients, five of whom have had very large fibrolamellar tumours involving portal vessels or the vena cava. There were no deaths in this group, all eight patients being alive at 1 month to 5 years, with a mean follow-up of 22 months. Two other primary liver tumours were resected; one patient with an apparently primary carcinoid of the liver and associated moderate cirrhosis died, the other patient with a large cystic mesenchymal lesion is alive at 21 months.

Seventeen patients with secondary deposits from colorectal cancer have also been approached with no operative deaths, 11 patients being alive with a mean follow-up of 18.2 months and 6 having died at a mean time of 15.6 months postresection. Five other patients with secondary deposits have been operated upon, one of whom died in the perioperative period; two others died at 17 months. The remaining patient submitted to hepatic resection for an apparently large solitary secondary from a breast carcinoma is alive, symptom-free, and apparently without recurrence at 16 months.

References

1. Bismuth H (1982) Surgical anatomy and anatomical surgery of the liver. World J Surg 6: 3-9
2. Longmire WP Jr, Tompkins RK (eds) (1981) Manual of liver surgery. Springer, New York
3. Blumgart LH (1983) Hepatic resection. In: Dudley H, Pories W, Carter D (eds) Operative surgery. Alimentary tract and abdominal wall, part 2. Butterworths, London, pp 477-499
4. Starzl TE, Bell RH, Bennt RW, Putman CW (1975) Hepatic trisegmentectomy and other liver resections. Surg Gynecol Obstet 141: 429-437
5. Blumgart LH, Benjamin IS, Hadjis NS, Beazley R (1984) Surgical approaches to cholangiocarcinoma at confluence of hepatic ducts. Lancet 1: 66-70
6. Foster JH, Berman MM (1977) Solid liver tumors. Major problems in clinical surgery, vol 22. Saunders, Philadelphia, pp 29-56
7. Ong GB, Chan PKW (1976) Primary carcinoma of the liver. Surg Gynecol Obstet 143: 31-38
8. Balasegaram M, Joishy SK (1981) Hepatic resection: pillars of success built on the foundation of 15 years of experience. Am J Surg 141: 360
9. Ong GB, Leong CH (1969) Surgical treatment of primary liver cancer. J R Coll Surg Edinb 14: 42-55

10. Adson MA, Sheedy PF (1974) Resection of primary hepatic malignant lesions. Arch Surg 108: 599-604
11. Fortner JG, Kim DK, MacLean BJ, Barret MK, Iwatsuki S, Turnbull AD, Howlands WS, Beattie EJ Jr (1978) Major hepatic resection for neoplasia: personal experience in 108 patients. Ann Surg 188: 363-370
12. Longmire WP Jr (1974) Hepatic resection. In: Zollinger RM (ed), Advances in surgery, vol 8. Year Book, Chicago, pp 29-61
13. Paradinas FJ, Melia WM, Wilkinson ML, Portmann B, Johnson PJ, Murray-Lyon IM, Williams R (1982) High serum vitamin B_{12} binding capacity as a marker of the fibrolamellar variant of hepatocellular carcinoma. Br Med J 285: 840-842
14. Collier NA, Weinbren K, Bloom SR, Lee YC, Hodgson HJF, Blumgart LH (1984) Neurotensin secretion by fibrolamellar carcinoma of the liver. Lancet 1: 538-540
15. Voyles CR, Bowley NJ, Allison DJ, Benjamin IS, Blumgart LH (1983) Carcinoma of the proximal extrahepatic biliary tree. Radiologic assessment and therapeutic alternatives. Ann Surg 197: 188-194
16. Skoog V, Thoren L (1982) Carcinoma of the junction of the main hepatic ducts. Acta Chir Scand 148: 411-414
17. Launois B, Campion JP, Brissot O, Gosselin M (1979) Carcinoma of the hepatic hilus. Surgical management and the case for resection. Ann Surg 190: 151-157
18. Evander A, Fredlund P, Hoevels J, Ihse I, Bengmark S (1980) Evaluation of aggressive surgery for carcinoma of the extrahepatic bile ducts. Ann Surg 191: 23-39
19. Wood CB, Gillis CR, Blumgart LH (1976) A retrospective study of the natural history of patients with liver metastases from colorectal cancer. Clin Oncol 2: 285-288
20. Wilson SM, Adson MA (1976) Surgical treatment of hepatic metastases from colorectal cancers. Arch Surg III: 330-333
21. Adson MA, Van Heerden JA (1980) Major hepatic resection for metastatic colorectal cancer. Ann Surg 191: 576-580
22. Nagorney DM, Bloom SR, Polak JM, Blumgart LH (1983) Resolution of recurrent Verner Morrison syndrome by resection of metastatic vipoma. Surgery 93: 348-353

Surgical Treatment of Primary Liver Cell Carcinoma in China

Z. D. Wu, S. S. Xia, and F. Z. Qiu

Second Department of Surgery, Wuhan Medical College, Wuhan, China

Primary liver cell carcinoma (PLC) is a frequent disease in China. Its incidence is five to ten times higher than in European and American countries. Annual mortality from PLC is 10.07/100000 of the population, which is about 100000 PLC deaths per year. PLC is more frequent in males, the male to female ratio being between 3 to 1 and 5 to 1, and the peak incidence of the disease is between 40 and 50 years of age.

Treatment of PLC is an urgent and very important task for Chinese hepatic surgeons. They have been tackling the problem for the past 30 years.

Hepatic surgery, hepatic resection for the treatment of PLC, started to develop in China in the early fifties. In the sixties, due to improved knowledge of liver anatomy and physiology and improvements in anesthesia and surgical technique in the treatment of PLC, much progress was made. The standard was raised in the seventies on the basis of better methods for early diagnosis and early treatment and many new techniques. The rate of resection increased from 20% to 40%; the operative lethality fell from 20%-30% down to 10%, in some instances to 0%. Furthermore, the number of patients with liver resections with a 5-year survival time rose to about 20%.

In China, at least eight reports, each of which presents more than 100 hepatic resections due to PLC, have been published. The long-lasting experiences have shown that besides the development of surgical technique, early diagnosis and early treatment are the key to successful surgical treatment of PLC [1].

Early Diagnosis of Primary Liver Cell Carcinoma

In the early diagnosis of PLC, the determination of AFP (alpha-fetoprotein) in the serum is known to play an important role. Since 1971 mass screening in more than 5 million inhabitants of our country with measurements of the serum AFP values have been carried out. During this trial more than 1000 cases of PLC, 400 of which were so-called subclinical cases with no signs and symptoms, were found.

Sufficient experience in mass screening and in clinical practice has proven the value of serum AFP measurements: (1) PLC can be detected using a less-sensitive method of AFP determination, so-called countercurrent immunoelectrophoresis (CIEP) at an average of 3.1 months prior to clinical signs and symptoms; or it can be detected with a more sensitive method, so-called radiorocket electrophoresis autography (RREA) or radioimmunoassay (RIA) even at an average of 8 months prior to a clinical manifestation of the dis-

Recent Results in Cancer Research. Vol 100

Table 1. Postoperative survival rate after liver resection for primary liver cell cancer (PLC)

	Number of resections	Survival rate (%)			*p*
		1 year	2 years	3 years	
Mass-screening group	66	64.2	39.3	28.9	<0.01
Consultation group	220	14.8	7.4	5.5	<0.01

ease. (2) The percentage of the so-called subclinical cases was 44.7% in the mass-screening group, but only 0.4% in that group that consulted a physician because of physical complaints. (3) In the mass-screening group, in 72.7% of hepatic resections a so-called small PLC was found, which means a single tumor mass with a diameter of less than 5 cm. (4) The rate of resection in patients of the mass-screening group was three times higher than that which was found in patients of the so-called consultation group. (5) The postoperative survival time of resected patients from the mass-screening group was considerably longer (Table 1).

As a consequence of the above-mentioned experiences our surgeons considered the possibility of diagnosing PLC only by measuring the serum AFP value as the only criterion. The following was found: in patients who were not pregnant and did not have active liver disease or embryonal tumors of the reproductive system, the diagnosis of PLC could be made if the serum AFP value exceeded 500 ng/ml for more than 4 weeks or if the CIEP stayed positive for the same time (according to a report of the Chinese conference for prevention and treatment of PLC, 1977), or with a serum AFP value above 200 ng/ml for more than 8 weeks if a normal serum glutamic pyruvic transaminase (SGPT) value was found simultaneously (according to Tang Zhouyou [2]), even if the patients had no symptoms of PLC.

During the diagnostic procedure of localizing the PLC, scintigraphy, sonography, computed tomography, and angiography, especially celiacography are of decisive importance. Sonography is simple and harmless and may be repeated; it is of excellent value in diagnosing tumors with a diameter of more than 2 cm. In addition to the determination of the serum AFP value, sonography is the most frequently used examination method for early diagnosis of subclinical PLC. Recently some reports were published in China concerning the use of angiography for the diagnosis of PLC [3, 4]. The rate of detection is 95%. The smallest PLC found by celiacography had a diameter of only 0.5 cm.

Hepatic Resection for the Treatment of Primary Liver Cell Carcinoma

Early reports concerning hepatic resection for the treatment of PLC originated in Changchun. During the resection procedure, the hepatic vessels and bile ducts are dealt with not intrahepatically but extrahepatically at the liver hilus. For this reason, Xia and Qiu [5] at our university carried out detailed examinations of the anatomy of the liver hilus, which were described extensively in 1962 using 100 total liver preparations. This research was very helpful for correct vascular and ductular surgery during liver resection. Wang Chengen has proposed ligating the liver vessel and bile ducts of the segment at the liver hilus prior to isolation and mobilization of the liver in order to prevent spread of tumor cells during operative manipulation. Wu Mengchao [6] has recommended the blood-saving liver resection with intermittent clamping of the hepatoduodenal ligament. Each clamping lasts 10–15 min; then a free interval of 3–5 min follows. During one liver resection usually one to two clamping procedures are sufficient. Wu Mengchao [6] has reported extensively 144 liver resections carried out with this technique and described no complications. This technique has advantages: it is simple, time saving, almost without bleeding, and easy to control.

Since the early 1980s three authors have reported good experiences with extensive hemihepatectomy. Yu Yeqin [7] carried out this procedure in three cases during vascular isolation and hypothermic liver perfusion, Wu Mengchao [8] and Si Chengrang [9] in three cases with total hepatic vascular isolation under normothermic conditions, and in one case with total hepatic vascular isolation under whole body hypothermia. Yu Yeqin [7] used the Nd-Yag laser, which was guided through an arm-like device, for hepatic resection and tumor vaporization; and later on successfully carried out hepatic resection with the Nd-Yag laser guided through a flexible fiber-optic system [10].

The total number of liver resections in China to date is more than 1400 cases, taking into account only large series with at least 100 cases. According to the literature, the operative mortality is between 2.8% and 14.7%, on average about 10% (Table 2) [11–15].

Surgical Treatment of the Unresectable Primary Liver Cell Carcinoma

Not until 1978 was a report published, in Shanghai, concerning the use of cryotherapy [16] using liquid nitrogen in the treatment of PLC in 28 cases. The 1-, 2-, and 3-year survival rates were 58.3%, 18.2%, and 12.5% respectively. One patient survived following cryotherapy 4 years and 2 months without tumor and died from pneumonia.

Favorable palliative results were often seen following ligation of the hepatic artery [17, 18]. In the majority of patients their overall condition and the symptoms improved. In 80% of patients the serum AFP level dropped; occasionally it even became negative. In addition, in some patients even the tumor mass was reduced. One hundred and twenty-two cases with ligation of the hepatic artery were collected in three series. The longest survival time was 48 months. Nearly 30% of the patients lived longer than 1 year (Table 3).

The ligation of the hepatic artery, in combination with systematic chemotherapy or infusion chemotherapy, and embolization of the hepatic artery have also been used by Chinese surgeons in the treatment of PLC [19].

Table 2. Lethality of liver resection in China (only reports with more than 100 resections included)

Year of publication	Authors	Number of resections	Operative lethality (%)
1974	Shanghai cooperative group for PLC (see [1])	258	14.7
1981	Tang Zhouyou [11]	153	12.7
1981	Wu Mengchao et al. [6]	246	6.9
1982	Huang Xingyao et al. [12]	181	2.8
1982	Li Guocai et al. [13]	114	11.4
1982	Zheng Zhaoyao [14]	128	4.6
1983	Shen Kangnian et al. [15]	195	8.2

Table 3. Results of hepatic artery ligation for treatment of PLC

Authors	Number of cases	Relief of symptoms (%)	Reduction of tumor size (%)	Survival at 1 year (%)	Survival (months)	
					Median	Maximum
Chang Xiaohua [17]	68	84.8 (56/66)	3.0 (2/ 66)	21.8 (12/55)	8.3 ± 6.25	33
Zhou Nanqiao [19][a]	40	50.0 (20/40)	25.0 (10/ 40)	40.0 (16/40)	12.5	48
Cai Zhongren [18]	14				8.5	
Total	122	71.7 (76/106)	11.3 (12/106)	29.5 (28/95)		

[a] Survival rate at 2 years: 20% (8/40)

Table 4. Results of resection for recurrence or metastases of PLC

Second operation	Number of cases	Interval between first and second operation (months)	+	Length of survival after second operation (months)	
Resection of liver recurrence [21-23]	9	10.5	+	7.5 (16.8[b])	
		83	+	13	
		34.5	+	10.5	
		19	+	18	
		4	+	53	
		14	+	18	
		21	+	15	
		30	+	11	
		47	+	5	
Hepatic artery ligation	2	9	+	13	14.0[b]
		10	+	15	
Laparotomy only	3	35	+	6	10.3[b]
		38	+	23	
		36	+	2	
Resection of peritoneal metastases	2	29	+	9	10.0[b]
		2.5	+	11[a]	
Cryotherapy	1	48	+	9	9.0[b]
Resection of lung metastases	4	33	+	24	18.0[b]
		30	+	24	
		44	+	17	
		49	+	7	
Total	21				
Conservative treatment	12				4.6[b]

[a] Still alive

[b] Mean

Table 5. Cause of death in eight male patients after allogeneic orthotopic liver transplantation for PLC

Case	Age	Date of transplant.	Survival time (days)	Main cause of death
1	47	30.12.1977	6	Acute hepatic and renal failure
2	36	01.02.1978	93	Infection by Candida albicans
3	29	08.10.1978	264	Generalized metastases
4	36	18.05.1979	22	Acute rejection crisis
5	29	12.06.1979	93	Hemorrhage caused by arrosion of the hepatic artery by subhepatic abscess
6	38	26.12.1979	7	Acute hepatic and renal failure
7	30	25.01.1980	12	Hemorrhage caused by rupture of hepatic artery (by localized Candida albicans infection)
8	37	13.11.1980	199	Hepatitis and generalized candidiasis

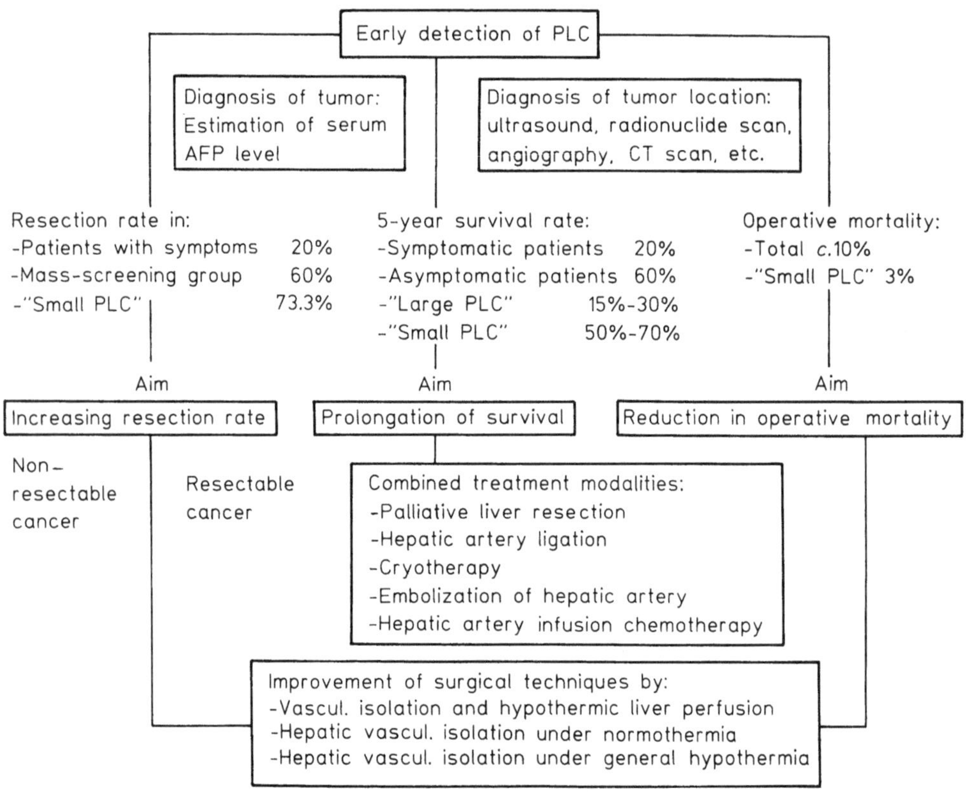

Fig. 1. Scheme for improvement of therapy results

Occasionally a positive result can be obtained in unresectable PLC by using so-called treatment in stages [20]. If the tumor mass following the above-mentioned combined treatment is reduced in size, occasionally PLC becomes resectable during repeated laparotomy. For example, one patient was suffering from an unresectable PLC. After chemotherapy for 9 months the tumor mass was reduced to 60%; after this, liver resection was carried out. Because of pulmonary metastases, 2½ years later pulmonary resection was also carried out. This patient survived the first operation for 7 years.

Hepatic Resection in Recurrent Primary Liver Cell Carcinoma

There is a tendency at present for hepatic resection to be used for the treatment of recurrent PLC. In three series nine patients were described [21-23]. The survival time following resection of the recurrent PLC was an average of 16.8 months, and 50% of the patients survived for more than 1 year. It is a fact that in recurrent PLC the result of surgical treatment is much better than that of chemotherapy if tumor resection is possible. The 1-year survival rate in both methods is 50% and 4.6% respectively (Table 4).

Hepatic Transplantation for the Treatment of PLC

Experimental research in China on hepatic transplantation commenced in 1958. Since 1973 at the Wuhan Medical College we systematically carried out 130 orthotopic hepatic transplantations in canines. In 1977 the clinical application of hepatic transplantation was achieved first in Shanghai and Wuhan [24]; so far a total of 57 cases have been transplanted, 52 of which had PLC. In our university we have carried out ten hepatic transplantations, eight cases with PLC [25]. One patient from our series survived 264 days, which is the longest survival time after hepatic transplantation in China, and he died from metastatic tumor disease. The results of hepatic transplantation in our hands are still not very good. A large number of patients have died from recurrence or metastases, because almost all of our patients suffered from late PLC. Table 5 shows the causes of death in liver recipients of our series.

Concluding Remarks

Until now radical hepatic resection is still the best method for the treatment of PLC. In order constantly to improve the results of the treatment, the following three objectives should be pursued: an increase of the resection rate of PLC, a decrease of the operative mortality, and an increase of survival time. As can be seen in Fig. 1, early diagnosis is the key for an improved treatment of PLC.

References

1. Tang Zhouyou (1981) Primary liver cancer, 1st ed. Shanghai Scientific Technical Publishing House, Shanghai
2. Tang Zhouyou (1982) Die Probleme der chirurgischen Behandlung des Leberkarzinoms in China. Chin J Surg 20 (2): 65

3. Wang Shouzhong et al. (1981) A study on selective angiography in 80 cases of primary hepatocellular carcinoma. Tumor 1 (4): 23
4. Lin Gui et al. (1982) Value of selective angiography in diagnosis of primary hepatocellular carcinoma. Chin J Surg 20 (2): 71
5. Xia Suisheng, Qui Fazu, et al. (1982) Chirurgische Anatomie des Leberhilus. Acta Acad Med Wuhan 2 (1): 25
6. Wu Mengchao et al. (1981) Experiences in surgical treatment of primary liver cancer. Tumor 1 (4): 20
7. Yu Yeqin et al. (1980) Bloodless hepatectomy. Chin J Surg 18 (2): 146
8. Wu Mengchao et al. (1981) Normothermic total hepatic vascular exclusion for hepatectomy. Chin J Surg 19 (1): 36
9. Si Chengrang (1983) Hypothermic hepatic vascular exclusion for extensive hepatectomy. Pract. Surg 3 (5): 253
10. Wu Zaide et al. (1982) Die experimentelle Forschung und klinische Verwendung des Nd-YAG Laser. Praktisch Laser 2 (2): 12
11. Tang Zhouyou (1981) Factors affecting survival after resection of primary liver cancer (with analysis of 153 cases). Nation Med J Chin 61 (2): 93
12. Huang Xingyao et al. (1982) Results of surgical treatment of carcinoma of liver: report of 181 cases. Chin J Surg 20 (2): 68
13. Li Guocai et al. (1982) Klinische Untersuchung der chirurgischen Behandlung des primären Leberkarzinoms bei 536 Fällen. Cancer 1: 9
14. Zheng Zhaoyao (1982) Surgical treatment of primary liver cancer (analysis of 128 cases). Shanghai Med 5 (2): 82
15. Shen Kangnian et al. (1983) Analyse des Resultates der Leberresektion zur Behandlung des primären Leberkarzinoms bei 195 Fällen. Cancer 2 (2): 81
16. Zhou Xinda et al. (1979) Cryosurgery for liver cancer: experimental and clinical study. Chin J Surg 17 (6): 480
17. Chang Xiaohua et al. (1981) Ligatur der A. hepatica zur Behandlung des Leberkarzinoms (Erfahrung bei 68 Fällen). Shanghai Med 4 (9): 1
18. Cai Zhongren (1981) Erfahrung über die Ligatur der A. hepatica zur Behandlung des Leberkarzinoms. New Med 3: 135
19. Zhou Nanquiao (1983) Treatment of unresectable hepatocellular carcinoma by hepatic artery ligation with and without chemotherapeutic perfusion: A follow-up study of 40 cases. Acta Acad Med Primae Shanghai 11 (3): 195
20. Yu Yeqin et al. (1983) Treatment of huge primary liver cancer in stages. Chin J Surg 21 (2): 92
21. Chen Han et al. (1979) Relaparotomie bei Patienten mit primärem Leberkarzinom. Shanghai Med 2: 794
22. Yu Yeqin (1980) Bewertung von Relaparotomie zur Behandlung des primären Leberkarzinoms. Jiangsu Med 11: 4
23. Shen Kangnian (1982) Bewertung der Reoperation bei Patienten mit primärem Leberkarzinom. Chin J Surg 20 (2): 128
24. Wu Zaide et al. (1979) Orthotope homologe Lebertransplantation (Klinische Erfahrung bei 3 Fällen). Acta Acad Med Wuhan: 17-8
25. Xia Suisheng et al. (1981) Erfahrungen über die orthotope Lebertransplantation. Acta Acad Med Wuhan 1 (1): 1

Surgical Therapy of Primary Liver Tumors

M. Trede and M. Raute

Chirurgische Klinik, Fakultät für klinische Medizin Mannheim, Universität Heidelberg,
6800 Mannheim, FRG

Figure 1 shows the angiogram of a 40-year-old technician in whom a small liver tumor was discovered in the right lobe during laparoscopy elsewhere. He had refused any treatment at the time and now presented to us 6 years later with a huge painful, palpable - and visible (!) - liver tumor.

Figure 2 shows the tumor, which had penetrated into the diaphragm and given rise to a solitary, well-encapsulated metastasis in the hepatoduodenal ligament.

In view of the patient's age, excellent condition, and long history we decided to attempt a cure by extended right hemihepatectomy and excision of the metastasis along with the common bile duct. The specimen showed a hepatocellular carcinoma weighing over 2 kg (Fig. 3).

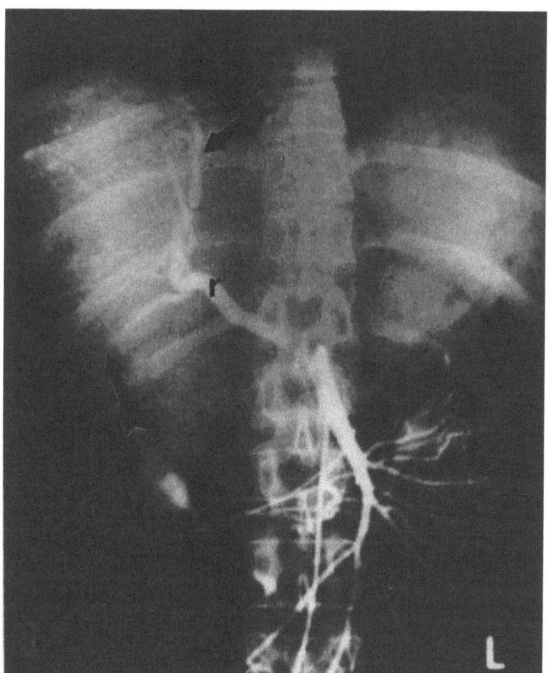

Fig. 1. Patient K. B., male, 46 years old. Mesenteric arteriography shows a hepatoma in the right lobe supplied largely by an aberrant right hepatic artery *(r)*

Recent Results in Cancer Research. Vol 100

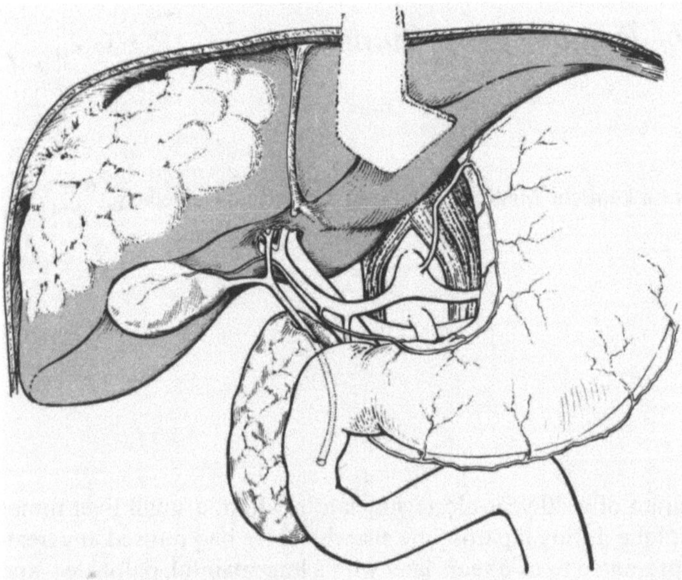

Fig. 2. Patient K. B., male, 46 years old. Schematic drawing showing the hepatoma occupying the right hepatic lobe and the medial segment of the left lobe. Large metastasis impinging on the common bile duct and pancreatic head

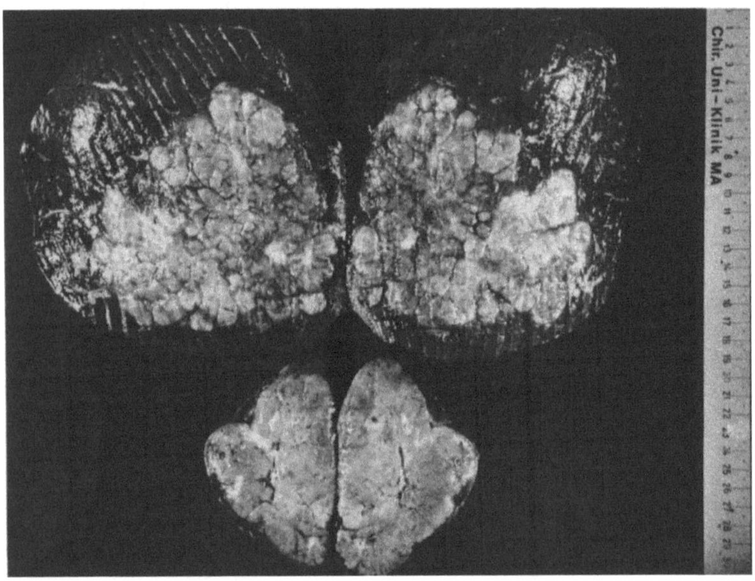

Fig. 3. Patient K. B., male, 46 years old. Operative specimen including the primary hepatocellular carcinoma and metastasis

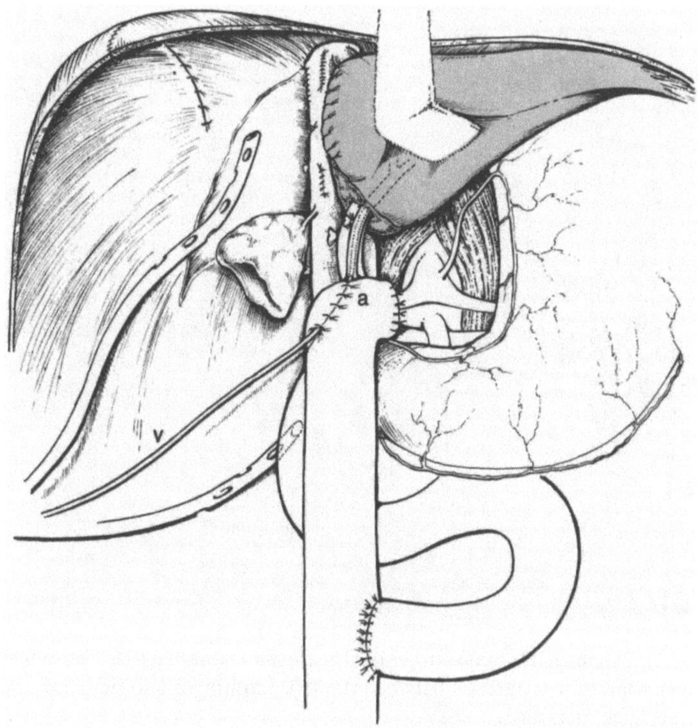

Fig. 4. Patient K. B., male, 46 years old. Operative sketch following extended right hemihepatectomy, leaving the two left lateral segments and a left hepaticojejunal anastomosis *(a)* drained by a silastic tube *(v)*

After reconstruction of the tenuous left bile duct draining the remaining second and third segments by means of a Roux-en-Y loop, the patient recovered uneventfully (Fig. 4). Histologic evidence of carcinomatous lymphangiosis of the diaphragm led to a course of betatron irradiation.

Nine months later a routine CT scan showed up a completely "silent" metastasis hidden between the left diaphragm and pericardium (Fig. 5). It too was removed uneventfully. He then enjoyed another symptom-free 1½ years but finally this man did succumb to his disease: 9 years after his carcinoma was first discovered and 3 years after its removal.

This case history illustrates some of the points I will briefly touch on in this paper:

1. The incidence of primary liver tumors
2. Some diagnostic problems from the surgeon's point of view
3. Technical aspects of hepatic resection
4. The results, including mortality, the chances of survival, and the complications

But first I would like to pay brief tribute to two surgical pioneers: C. Langenbuch, credited with the first major liver resection in 1888 [17], and Walter Wendel, who performed the first anatomic right hepatic lobectomy successfully in 1911 [30]. While we may wonder if Langenbuch's operation was really necessary - after all he only removed a congenital anomaly (a *Schnürlappen* of the left lobe) - there can be no doubt that Wendel's anatomic hemihepatectomy prolonged his patient's life for 9 years. She then died of a recurrence of her malignant hepatoma [31].

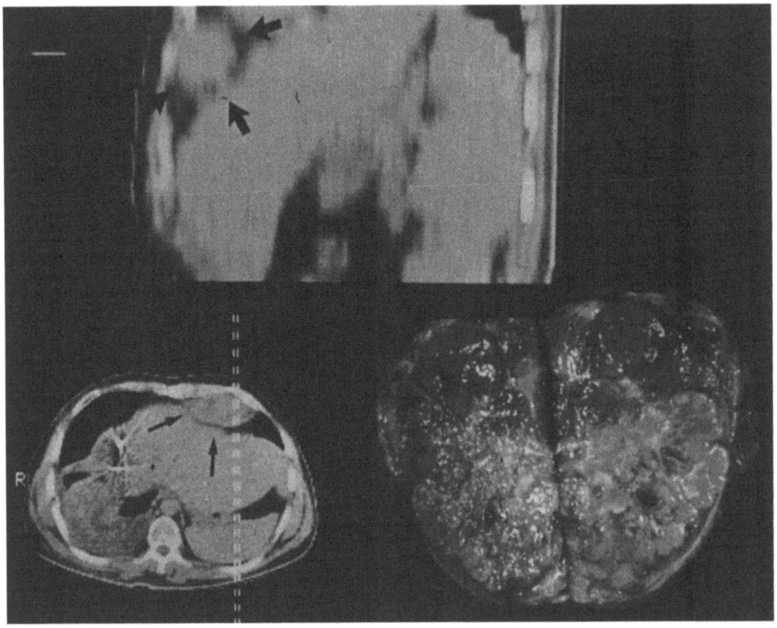

Fig. 5. Patient K. B., male, 46 years old. *Top and bottom left:* CT scan 9 months post-operatively; *arrows* point to a metastasis between the left diaphragm and pericardium. *Bottom right:* Completely enucleated metastasis

Incidence of Primary Liver Tumors

Primary liver malignancies are rare in Europe and the Western world, a fact I am painfully aware of, having to follow Prof. Wu's impressive presentation from China, where of course these tumors are common.

There is some comfort in the fact that Foster and Berman needed to visit 98 centers throughout the United States to collect 127 cases of resected primary liver tumors in adults for their famous survey of solid liver tumors [9]. And even the Lahey Clinic, renowned for its expertise in hepatobiliary surgery, could present only 48 hepatic resections in 26 years and only 18 of these were for primary liver malignancies [5]. There are indeed few clinics who see more than one or two of these cases per year.

In the Surgical Clinic in Mannheim out of 113 major hepatic resections (not including wedge resections or biopsies) performed over a 12-year period (1.10.72–30.6.84), 62 were carried out for metastases and 37 for benign hepatic tumors. There were only ten major resections performed for primary liver tumor:

Primary	liver tumors	10	
Secondary	liver tumors	62	
Benign	liver tumors	37	
Hydatid	liver disease	2	(out of 29)
Trauma		2	
		113	

Considering our special interest in gastrointestinal surgery at Mannheim, Table 1. puts these figures into perspective: We saw a total of 23 primary liver tumors, 10 of which were

Table 1. Total number of resections, resection rate, and operative (hospital) mortality for four different gastrointestinal tumors. Surgical Clinic, Mannheim, 1.10. 72-30.6. 84

Carcinoma	Number	Resection rate	Operative mortality
Colorectal	2123	1655 (78%)	115 (5.4%)
Gastric	1208	794 (66%)	[a] (8.7%)
Pancreatic	501	118 (23%)	3 (2.5%)
Hepatic	23	10 (43%)	1 (10%)

[a] For total gastrectomy

operable, with a mortality of one. Over the same 12-year period, for every primary liver malignancy we resected 12 carcinomas of the pancreas and 80 gastric and 160 colorectal cancers.

There were more women than men in this group; the average age was 54 years. In view of the fact that this is a wine-drinking part of the country and that we see many sequelae of cirrhosis (e.g., bleeding esophageal varices), it is perhaps surprising that only 7 of our 23 cases showed evidence of hepatic cirrhosis. And each one of these was inoperable.

Patients with primary liver tumors	23 patients
m/f 13/10	
Average age	54 years
Cirrhosis present in	7 patients
Resectability	10 patients
Hepatocellular Ca.	7 patients
Cholangiocellular Ca.	3 patients
Operative + hospital mortality	1 patient.

Symptoms, Signs, and Preoperative Diagnosis

According to Longmire, primary hepatic tumors can be grouped into five clinical types [18]:

Asymptomatic hepatomegaly
Upper abdominal pain
Fever
Acute abdomen (rupture)
Occult tumor (autopsy)

Half of our patients presented with an asymptomatic mass in the right upper quadrant. The other half complained of vague upper abdominal pain. We have seen pyrexia that ceased promptly with removal of the tumor as well as an acute abdomen on account of rupture - but both events occurred in our small experience only in benign lesions.

Jaundice occurs late and with the exception of some cholangiocarcinomas (e.g., Klatskin tumors) it is usually associated with inoperability.

With regard to *diagnostic procedures,* the surgeon is interested in the answers to four questions concerning the tumor: (1) where is it? (2) is it resectable? (3) will the remaining liver suffice for survival? and, finally (4), what is it?

1. Localization of the tumor is pinpointed first by the least expensive noninvasive method: ultrasound. The more elaborate CT is useful particularly with contrast enhancement. Whether or not NMR will really prove to be better remains to be seen.
   Hepatic scintiscans, while abandoned for preoperative diagnosis, remain useful in postoperative sequential examinations to demonstrate the passage of bile from the remaining liver segments into the gut. This reassures the surgeon in cases with prolonged postoperative jaundice.
2. The single most effective instrument for predicting the technical resectability of a liver tumor is angiography [32]. We ask our radiologists for celiac (and mesenteric) arteriography in every case and are so able to plan the extent of resection in advance.
   Furthermore, it is useful to be aware beforehand of any anatomic anomaly of the hepatic artery (seen in 20% of cases). That is why mesenteric arteriography is so useful - an aberrant right hepatic arising from the superior mesenteric artery is the commonest arterial anomaly found (see Fig. 1).
   We pay great attention to the portal venous phase of angiography. Infiltration of the portal bifurcation precludes any attempt at radical cure. But if only one branch of the portal vein is involved (Fig. 6) a curative hemihepatectomy may still be feasible. (Fig. 7).
   A transfemoral inferior cavogram is indicated only in selected cases with very large tumors. Mere compression of the IVC does not usually indicate inoperability. Infiltration of the IVC, however, was suggested in a 52-year-old woman by CT scan and confirmed by a constant caval defect (Fig. 8). This was caused by a metastasis and so a palliative resection of the severely symptomatic primary liver tumor was all that could be done.

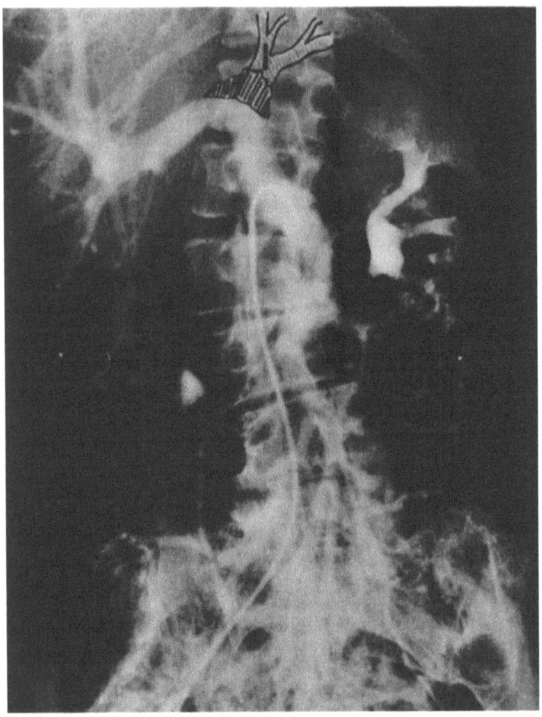

Fig. 6. Patient L. B., female, 55 years old. Portal venous phase of arteriography showing occlusion of the left branch of the portal vein *(1)* due to a cholangiocellular carcinoma (Klatskin tumor)

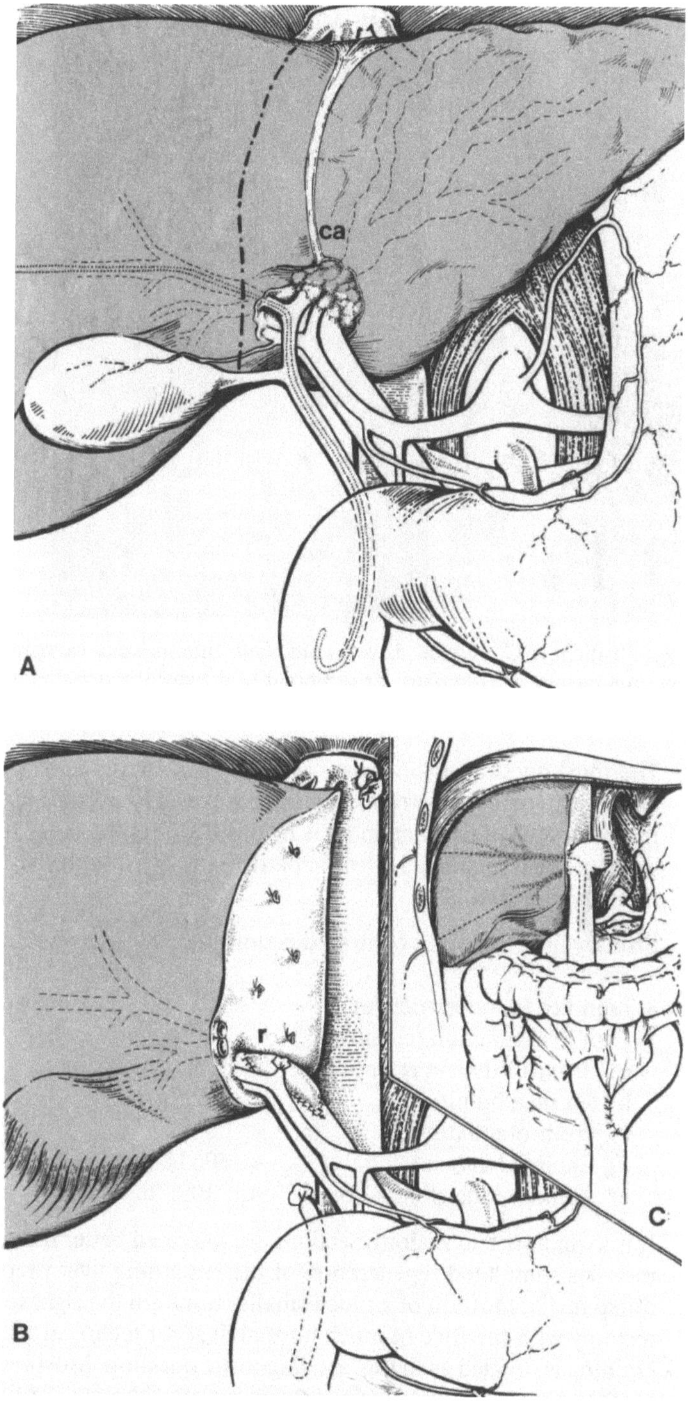

Fig. 7. A-C Patient L. B., female, 55 years old. **A** Sketch showing Klatskin tumor *(ca)* occluding the left hepatic duct and plane of resection for left hemihepatectomy *(s)*. **B** Operative site after left hemihepatectomy, resection of hepatic duct confluence and common bile duct and Goretex reconstruction of the right portal vein *(r)*. **C** Reconstruction of biliary drainage by right hepaticojejunostomy, splinted by two silastic tubes

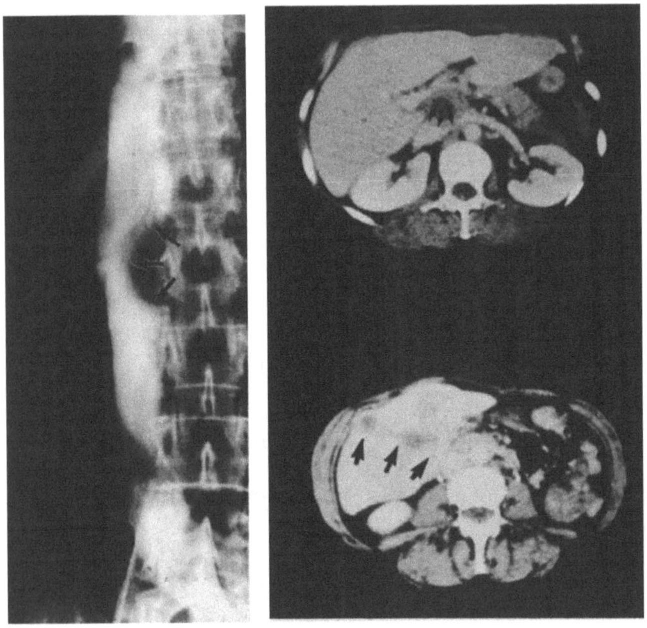

Fig. 8. Patient A. G., female, 52 years old. *Left:* Inferior vena cavogram showing a constant defect due to a metastasis. *Top right: Arrows* point to the caval impression at the level of entry of the left renal vein. *Bottom right:* Arrows point to the primary hepatocellular carcinoma in the right lobe

3. The third question is one that concerns radiologists and hepatologists - but the final answer can come only from the surgeon. We all know that up to 85% of the liver may be resected safely if the remainder is healthy [25]. It is not easy to predict the functional reserve of the remaining 15% of hepatic tissue quantitatively, but it is wise to follow certain guidelines [10, 20]:

   Primary liver tumours: contraindications to extensive resection
   1. Ascites
   2. Jaundice (nonobstructive)
   3. Poor liver function (cirrhosis):

a) Bromsulfthalein retention	>	35%
b) Serum albumin	<	2.5 g%
c) Prothrombin time	<	60%
d) Choline esterase	<	1500 U/liter
e) Aminopyrine elimination	<	10%/h

   It is axiomatic that major resections are tolerated better if the slow growth of a large tumor has stimulated regeneration of the remaining liver preoperatively. In contrast the dorsomedial location of a much smaller tumor in the right lobe may require hemihepatectomy with sacrifice of much normal liver for technical reasons.

4. Opinion is divided as to the last diagnostic question. Most internists and some surgeons prefer to have preoperative histologic proof of the type of tumor concerned. They recommend liver biopsy under laparoscopic control [3, 14]. We reserve this investigation - which after all carries some risk of bleeding, seeding of tumor, and equivocal findings - for cases with clinical suspicion of unresectability (e.g., cirrhotic patients) and avoid it whenever an operation is indicated anyway [2, 13, 28].

Resectability and Technical Aspects of Hepatic Resection

In the past 12 years we have performed 41 anatomic liver resections in Mannheim (Fig. 9). The resections for primary liver tumors are analyzed in Table 2. Ten patients were found to be inoperable (due to previously unrecognized metastatic spread to the other lobe or to lymph nodes outside the liver). A further three patients were shown to be inoperable by the diagnostic work-up. These meagre figures cannot of course be interpreted as a true resection rate of 43% (10 out of 23) since this group of patients was selected before being referred for surgery. The rate of resectability of primary liver carcinoma the world over is said to lie between 10% and 30% [14, 18].

Even among that very favorable group of 300 patients with tumors of less than 5 cm in diameter collected in Shanghai by means of an early detection program (α-fetoprotein test), the resection rate amounted to only 58% [23].

The extent of resection depends on the size and location of the tumor. If it is small and located peripherally - a segmental resection is perfectly adequate. And this may be all the patient will tolerate if the liver is cirrhotic. But as a rule we prefer the more extensive but far safer (and often quicker) procedures of right or left hemihepatectomy. Taking the former as a model I will now briefly look at some aspects of operative technique.

Both the incision and the exposure must in these cases be ample. We begin with a small right subcostal incision. But as soon as operability is assured, this is extended - for all right lobectomies - into the right thorax (in the bed of the eighth rib). Together with many others we feel that only a wide exposure with complete mobilization of the right lobe can make this operation reasonably safe [1, 28].

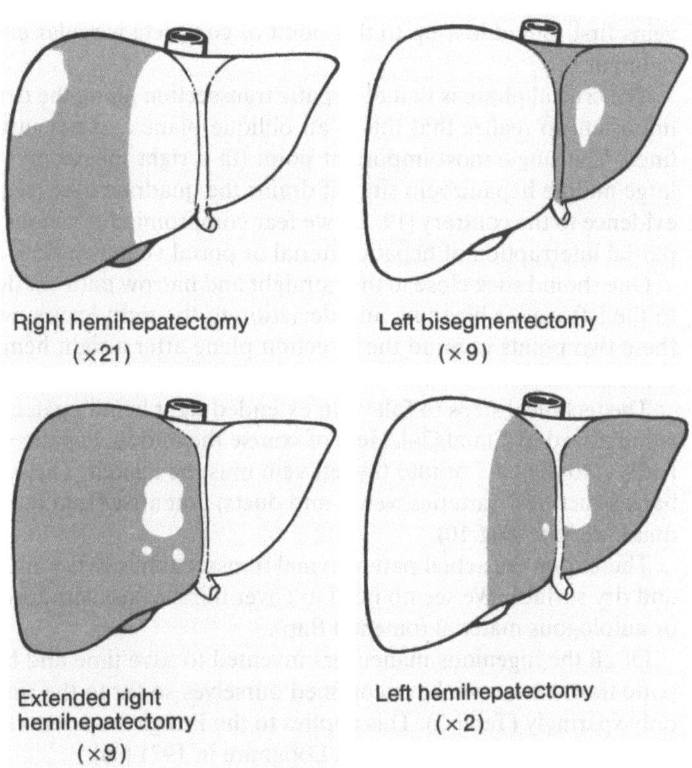

Fig. 9. Location of 41 anatomic liver resections performed in the Surgical University Clinic of Mannheim

Table 2. Treatment in 23 cases of primary liver cancer. Surgical University Clinic of Mannheim, 1.10.72–30.6.84

1. "Curative" resection	
Right hemihepatectomy	2
Extended right hemihepatectomy	4
Left hemihepatectomy	1
Atypical resections	3
Fifth segment	
Fourth segment + hepatic confluence	
	10
2. Laparotomy	
Showed inoperability	10
3. Conservative	
Inoperability shown preoperatively	3
Total	23

Opinion is divided about the next step. Some very experienced hepatic surgeons go right ahead with the parenchymal division of the liver under cover of inflow occlusion (Pringle maneuver), the biliary and vascular structures being tied and divided as they are encountered within the liver parenchyma [4, 7, 15]. Apparently normothermic occlusion can be extended to more than 1 h - the record with full recovery being 74 min [29].

In Mannheim we prefer to avoid this by dissecting the hilar structures and retrohepatic veins first. Blood loss up to this point of complete vascular exclusion of the right lobe is minimal.

The crucial phase is that of hepatic transsection along the demarcation plane - and it is important to realize that this is an oblique plane and not just a "gallbladder-vena cava line." The single most important point (in a right lobectomy) is to avoid damage to the large middle hepatic vein since it drains the quadrate lobe (segment IV). In spite of some evidence to the contrary [19, 21] we fear compromise of venous outflow as much as we do partial interruption of hepatic arterial or portal venous inflow.

One should stick close to the "straight and narrow path" of demarcation since deviation to the left causes bleeding and deviation to the right leaves necrotic tissue behind. With these two points in mind the resection plane after a right hemihepatectomy should look clean and dry.

The technical steps to follow in extended right hemihepatectomy have been beautifully summarized by Starzl [24]. Here of course the middle hepatic vein which drains either directly into the IVC or into the left vein must be ligated. The same applies to those "feedback structures" (arteries, veins, and ducts) that arise from the left branches to supply the quadrate lobe (Fig. 10).

Thereupon the actual parenchymal transsection is easier and it too should leave a clean and dry surface. We see no need to cover this surface with foreign (Gelfoam, Fibrin, etc.) or autologous material (omental flap).

Of all the ingenious maneuvers invented to save time and blood during the actual hepatic transsection we have confined ourselves so far to the simplest and have used these only sparingly (Table 3). This applies to the Pringle manoeuvre [22] and to the very useful clamp introduced by Storm and Longmire in 1971 [26].

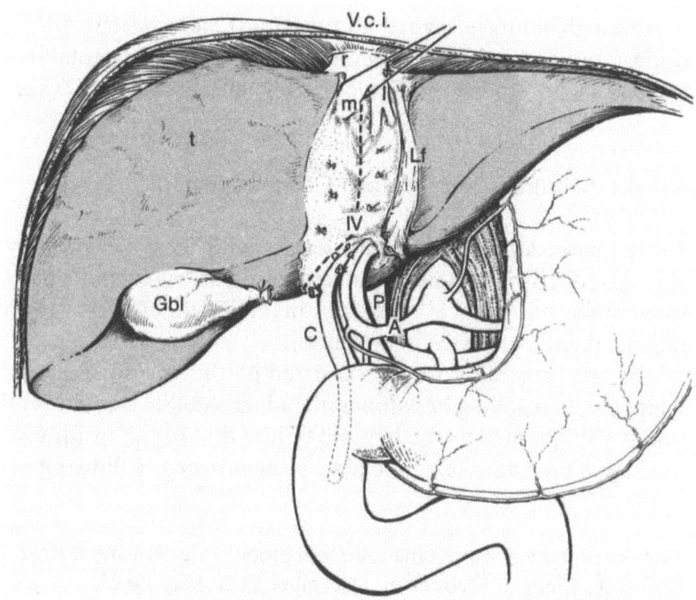

Fig. 10. Patient H.G., female, 44 years old. Operative sketch showing a large tumor *(t)* extending from the right hepatic lobe into the medial segment of the left lobe. *r,* right; *m,* middle; *l,* left hepatic vein; *Vci,* inferior vena cava; *Lf,* falciform ligament; *Gbl,* gallbladder; *C,* common bile duct; *P,* portal vein; *A,* common hepatic artery; *IV,* "feedback" vessels supplying the medial segment of the left hepatic lobe

Table 3. Methods intended to save time and blood during hepatic resection

Ⓐ ① Pringle Maneuver	Pringle [22] and
② Noncrushing clamp	Longmire [26]
	Storm 1971
③ Vascular isolation	Fortner et al. [8]
a) ± Hypothermic perfusion	Delva et al. [6]
b) ± Caval shunt	Testas et al. [27]
Ⓑ ① "Finger-fracture-dissection"	Lin [16]
② Crushing clamp	Lin et al. [17]
③ Laser	Durtschi [6a]
④ Ultrasonic surgical aspirator	Hodgson [12]
Ⓒ ① Autotransfusion	
② Preoperative hemodilution	Grundmann et al. [11]

As for the actual transsection, we prefer the "finger-fracture" technique. The crushing clamp is not adequately controllable nor is the laser beam, when it impinges on larger structures [18].

The new Ultrasonic Surgical Aspirator has earned applause from some surgeons [12]. To us it seemed rather a tedious, expensive instrument which still has to prove its superiority over the surgeon's finger.

Although we have owned an autotransfusion system since 1983, we have not had the opportunity to use it during hepatic resections. In fact, total blood loss for the last six anatomic resections performed in our clinic averaged 800 ml/case (Table 4).

Results: Mortality, Survival, and Complications

Table 5 summarizes our overall results with these ten primary liver tumors. There were four extended right hemihepatectomies, two right and one left hemihepatectomy, and three major but atypical resections involving the fifth and fourth segments (including the hepatic duct confluence in one case).

The one hospital mortality occurred on the seventh postoperative day in a 55-year-old woman with a 3000-g hepatoma including satellite tumors. At the end of a smooth operation nothing poited to the hepatic failure that began insidiously on the fourth postoperative day. Three days later she died of hemorrhage following rupture of the capsule of the

Table 4. Blood loss during the last six anatomic resections performed in a 6-month period. Surgical University Clinic of Mannheim, December 1983-May 1984

Patient	Age (years)	Procedure	Weight of specimen (g)	Intraoperative blood loss (ml)	Time for hepatic transsection (min)	Postoperative course
E. H.	57	Right hemihepatectomy	620	500	13	Alive 11 months
G. W.	49	Extended right hemihepatectomy	1350	250	14	Alive 9 months
L. B.	75	Right hemihepatectomy	760	400	9	Alive 9 months
P. H.	73	Left hemihepatectomy	1115	2700	-	Alive 6 months
E. H.	67	Extended right hemihepatectomy	1300	700	7	Alive 4 months
E. P.	71	Left bisegmentectomy	405	600	-	Alive 2 months

Table 5. Results of ten resections for primary liver tumors. Surgical University Clinic of Mannheim, 1. 10. 72-30. 6. 84

Procedure	*n*	Alive	Died
Extended right hemihepatectomy	4	1:8 years 1:9 months	1:7th postoperative day 1:32 months
Right hemihepatectomy	2	1:18 months	1:15 months
Left hemihepatectomy	1	-	1:28 months
Fourth and fifth segment resection	3	1:2 years (with "pump") 1:6 months	1:12 months
Total	10	5	5 (1 postoperative death)

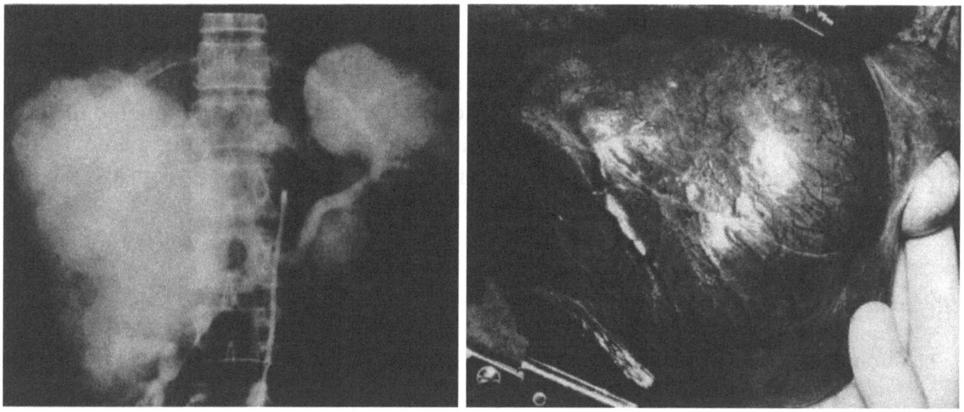

Fig. 11. Patient G.M., female, 45 years old. *Left:* Parenchymal phase of arteriography showing a large hepatocellular carcinoma reaching from the right lobe to the falciform ligament. *Right:* Operative photo showing the 3000-g tumor

remaining liver. It would seem that venous outflow obstruction was the cause but at autopsy no such obstacle could be found.

Of the remaining nine patients, four have since died of recurrent disease, having survived for an average of 22 months. This compares favorably with the life span of untreated (inoperable) cases [3].

The remaining five patients are still alive from 6 months to 8 years, although one of them, a 42-year-old lady, has had an Infusaid pump inplanted for treatment of satellite tumors. At the age of 4 years she had a carotid angiogram performed with Thorotrast (!).

There is an impressive list of specific postoperative complications following hepatic resection:

1. Hemorrhage from liver
   Due to coagulopathy from stress ulcer
2. Abscess - subphrenic
3. Pneumonia - right pleural effusion
4. Bile leak or
   bile duct obstruction
5. Hepatic insufficiency

Fortunately this group of ten patients was spared all but two of them. There were pleural effusions requiring aspiration in two patients and there was jaundice. Jaundice of a moderate and transient kind (< 5 mg%) is the rule following an extended right hemihepatectomy [24], which also applied to our four cases. But we have seen severe postoperative jaundice with values of 40 mg% and more requiring plasmapheresis for several weeks. And in no case was there any evidence of obstruction. In one patient (not part of this series) who had extended right hemihepatectomy performed for metastasis, bilirubin levels reached 25 mg%. The sequential technetium scan showed no excretion of bile from the remaining liver into the gut. And yet - the patient passed normally colored stools and the retrograde endoscopic examination proved that her remaining bile duct was patent. This particular patient had extended right hemihepatectomy performed for a 2.5-kg metastasis. She finally recovered and is alive and free of recurrence 3 years later. The explanation for her severe jaundice must lie in a transient hepatocellular insufficiency.

Our figures are small, but they happen to fit in nicely with the data collected by Longmire from nine centers of hepatic surgery: 684 patients out of a total of 2602 had major hepatic resection performed for primary liver cancer. The average operative mortality was 13.5%; the 3- and 5-year survival (though difficult to calculate exactly) amounted to about 35% and 10% [18]. Our longest survivor was also our first patient, who had an extended right hemihepatectomy for a 3000-g hepatocellular carcinoma almost 8 years ago. She remains alive, active, and free from recurrence (Fig. 11 a, b).

References

1. Adson MA (1983) Resection for primary liver tumor - 2nd advanced hepatobiliary course, Hammersmith Hospital, Nov. 1983
2. Adson MA, Weiland LH (1981) Resection of primary solid hepatic tumors. Am J Surg 141: 18
3. Bengmark S, Hafström L, Jeppsson B, Jönsson PE, Nagasue N, Persson B, Sundquist K, Szeleczky M, Tranberg K (1982) Neuester Stand der Leberchirurgie. Zentralbl Chirurgie 107: 689
4. Bismuth H, Houssin D, Castaing D (1982) Major and minor segmentectomies "réglées" in liver surgery. World J Surg 6: 10
5. Cady B, Bonneval M, Fender HR (1979) Elective hepatic resection. Am J Surg 137: 514
6. Delva E, Barberousse JP, Nordlinger B, Ollivier JM, Vacher B, Guilmet C, Huguet C (1984) Hemodynamic and biochemical monitoring during major liver resection with use of hepatic vascular exclusion. Surgery 95: 3, 309
6a. Durtschi MB, Stothert JC, Ashleman B, Auth DC, Lee MJ, Heimbach DM, Carrico CJ (1980) Laser scalpel for solid organ surgery. Am J Surg 139 (5): 665
7. Eßer G (1979) Zeit- und blutsparende Leberresektion. Chirurg 50: 136
8. Fortner JG, Shiu H, Kinne DW, Kim DK, Castro EB, Watson RC, Howland WS, Beattie EJ (1974) Major hepatic resection using vascular isolation and hypothermic perfusion. Ann Surg 180: 4, 644
9. Foster JH, Berman MM (1977) Solid liver tumors. Saunders, Philadelphia
10. Gill RA, Goodman MW, Golfus GR, Onstad GR, Bubrick MP (1983) Aminopyrine breath test predicts surgical risk for patients with liver disease. Ann Surg 198: 6, 701
11. Grundmann R, Strümper R, Kürten K, Pichlmaier H (1977) Möglichkeiten der Bluterspamis bei Leberresektion. Langenbecks Arch Chir 345: 653
12. Hodgson WJB, DelGuercio LRM (1984) Preliminary experience in liver surgery using the ultrasonic scalpel. Surgery 95: 2, 230
13. Iwatsuki S, Shaw BW, Starzl TE (1983) Experience with 150 liver resections. Ann Surg 197: 3, 247
14. Lee NW, Wong J, Ong GB (1982) The surgical management of primary carcinoma of the liver. World J Surg 6: 66
15. Lin T-Y (1974) A simplified technique for hepatic resection: the crush method. Ann Surg 180: 3, 285
16. Lin T-Y, Chen KM, Liu TK (1960) Total right hepatic lobectomy for primary hepatoma. Surgery 48: 1048
17. Langenbuch C (1888) Ein Fall von Resektion eines linksseitigen Schnürlappens der Leber, Heilung. Berl Klin Wochenschr 25: 37
18. Longmire WP, Tompkins RK (1981) Manual of liver surgery. Springer, New York
19. Mays ET (1977) Vascular occlusion. Surg Clin North Am 57: 2, 291
20. Ong GB, Lee NW (1975) Hepatic resection. Br J Surg 62: 421
21. Ou QJ, Hermann RE (1984) The role of hepatic veins in liver operations. Surgery 95: 4, 381
22. Pringle JH (1908) Notes on the arrest of hepatic hemorrhage due to trauma. Ann Surg 48: 541
23. Shanghai Coordinating Group (1979) Diagnosis and treatment of primary hepatocellular carcinoma in early stage. Chin Med J [Engl] 92: 801
24. Starzl TE, Bell RH, Beart RW, Putnam CW (1975) Hepatic trisegmentectomy and other liver resections. Surg Gynecol Obstet 141: 429

25. Stone HH (1977) Preoperative and postoperative care. Surg Clin North Am 57: 2, 409
26. Storm FK, Longmire WP (1971) A simplified clamp for hepatic resection. Surg Gynecol Obstet 133: 103
27. Testas P, Bénchiou J, Benhamou M, Chanzy M (1977) Vascular exclusion in surgery of the liver. Am J Surg 133: 692
28. Thompson HH, Tompkins RK, Longmire WP (1983) Major hepatic resection. Ann Surg 197: 4, 375
29. Waltuck JL, Crow RW, Humphrey LJ, Kauffman HM (1970) Avulsion injuries of the vena cava following blunt abdominal trauma. Ann Surg 171: 67
30. Wendel W (1911) Beiträge zur Chirurgie der Leber. Arch Klin Chir 95: 887
31. Wendel W (1920) Ueber Leberlappenresektion. Arch Klin Chir 114: 982
32. Williamson BWA, Blumgart LH, McKellar NJ (1980) Management of tumors of the liver. Combined use of arteriography and venography in the assessment of resectability, especially in hilar tumors. Am J Surg 139: 210

Typical and Atypical Resection Techniques of Hepatic Metastases

F. P. Gall, J. Scheele, and A. Altendorf

Chirurgische Klinik der Universität Erlangen-Nürnberg, Maximiliansplatz, 8520 Erlangen, FRG

This report deals exclusively with liver metastases from colorectal cancer, since our experience with hepatic metastases from other primary tumors is very limited.

Liver metastases are a major limiting factor in the curative surgical treatment of colorectal cancer. A rather high incidence of such metastases is well documented. Sixty-five percent of patients dying from colorectal cancer have been found to have liver metastases at autopsy [2]. In surgical reports the rate of overt metastases at laparotomy ranges from 13% to 20% [4, 6, 17, 19], but a much higher percentage of occult lesions must be present at the same time. Recent studies by Finlay et al. [6] and Mooney et al. [13] have demonstrated occult metastases in 29% and 30% of patients at the time of laparotomy.

In the past, diagnosis of liver metastases left the patient in a hopeless situation and it signaled the physican's retreat to purely palliative therapy. In recent years, however, interest in aggressive surgical treatment of colorectal cancer metastatic to the liver has increased, since, treated conservatively, the lesions have a dismal prognosis, owing to the non-existence of any effective systemic therapy.

Natural History

The documented prognosis of untreated liver metastases varies in different series, with a mean survival from time of diagnosis of 4.5-9 months (Table 1). However, most of these reports do not take into account the extent of the liver involvement, the presence of un-

Table 1. Mean survival in untreated colorectal liver metastases

	n	Months
Bengtsson et al. [4]	155	4.5
Fisherman and Petersen [7]	49	6.5
Jaffe et al. [11]	177	5.3
Nielsen et al. [15]	49	7.0
Pestana et al. [18]	353	9.0
Wanebo et al. [22]	197	7.6
Wood et al. [23]	113	6.6

Recent Results in Cancer Research. Vol 100

controlled primary or regional growth, and the presence or absence of extrahepatic metastases. These overall figures are therefore of little value, since patients not suitable for surgical resection are also included.

The outlook is somewhat different when reports with staged liver involvement are considered. In solitary metastases Wood reported a 5-year survival rate of 16%. His figures are in contrast to the retrospective study of 252 patients of the Mayo Clinic by Wagner [21], who found in unresected liver metastases a 3-year survival rate for solitary, unilateral multiple, and bilateral diffuse lesions of 21%, 6%, and 4% and a 5-year survival rate of 3%, 0%, and 2% respectively. His conclusion was that patients with untreated solitary liver metastases live longer than we have been led to think, but, what is even more important, that only 0-3% are still alive at 5 years. From their survey, Foster and Lundy [10] came to almost the same conclusions with respect to untreated solitary metastases, with a 5-year survival rate of less than 1%.

For a discussion of the present status of the surgical treatment of liver metastases we have analyzed our own experience with 390 patients operated on between 1969 and 1983. A curative liver resection for solitary or unilateral multiple metastases was possible in only 20% (80/390) of the patients. Since 1978 a hepatic artery infusion catheter was inserted in 33 patients with diffuse lesions to both lobes, while the remaining 277 patients had only liver biopsy.

Liver Resection

For hemihepatectomy the standard technique with preliminary ligation of the arterial and venous vessels and the bile duct at the porta hepatis and finger fracture dissection was used until 1982. Since then a new resectional technique with the ultrasonic scalpel in atypical and typical resection has been used in 36 patients with 1 death. Its use has also resulted in a marked reduction in intraoperative blood loss and postoperative complications. Routine coverage of the raw resectional surface with collagen sponge attached by fibrinogen glueing is, in our experience, superior to heavy through and through sutures.

Mortality

Out of 80 patients with liver resection 12 died postoperatively, a mortality rate of 15%. However, since 1978 we have been able to decrease this to 7.8% (4/51) (Table 2). Up until 1977 for synchronous operations the major fatal factor was anastomotic leakage of the colorectal resection in 3/24 patients, but this has been completely avoided in the additional 18 operations performed since then.

Table 2. Overall operative mortality in 80 liver resections for colorectal metastases. Surgical Clinic of Erlangen University, January 1969 - December 1983

	n	Synchronous	Metachronous	Mortality (%)
	80	7/42	5/38	15
1969-1977	29	7/24	1/ 5	27
1978-1983	51	0/18	4/33	7.8

Table 3. Liver metastases from colorectal carcinoma. Surgical Clinic of Erlangen University, 1969-1983

Postoperative mortality in curative liver resection				
Type of resection	1969-1977 †/n	(%)	1978-1983 †/n	(%)
Typical resection	2/ 6	33%	4/33	12%
Wedge resection	6/23	26%	0/18	-
Total	8/29	28%	4/51	8%

Table 4. Operative mortality in liver resection (%)

Limited resection		Major resection	
(excision, small wedge resection)		Adson and Van Heerden [1]	5.9
Foster and Lundy [10]	5	Bengmark et al. [3]	6.0
Wagner et al. [21]	0	Cady et al. [5]	10.0
Raute and Trede [19]	6	Foster and Lundy [10]	11.0
		Fortner et al. [8]	9.0
		Logan et al. [12]	5.3
		Morrow et al. [14]	20.0
		Nims [16]	12.0
		Raute and Trede [19]	11.0
		Starzl et al. [20]	3.3
		Wagner et al. [21]	4.0

Since 1978, depending upon the extent of the liver resection, our operative mortality for excision (Table 3) has been 0% and for hemihepatectomy including trisegmentectomy 12%. In the literature the mortality rate for limited resection, such as excision or small wedge resection, ranges from 0% to 6%, while major resections like hemihepatectomy and trisegmentectomy are associated with a mortality of 3.3%-20%, but recently this has been reduced to 5%-10% by many authors (Table 4).

Complications

Postoperative complications occurred in 21% of patients, as compared with 19%-28% in the literature [5, 8, 14]. Biliary drainage occurred in two patients but it ceased spontaneously after 14 days. In two patients with abscess formation, relaparotomy had to be performed. All other complications were successfully treated by conservative measures.

Late Results

For calculation of our late results 10/80 patients had to be excluded, because their liver resection had been performed within the past 12 months. Our overall 4-year survival rate, including postoperative mortality, in 70 patients with curative resection of liver metastases

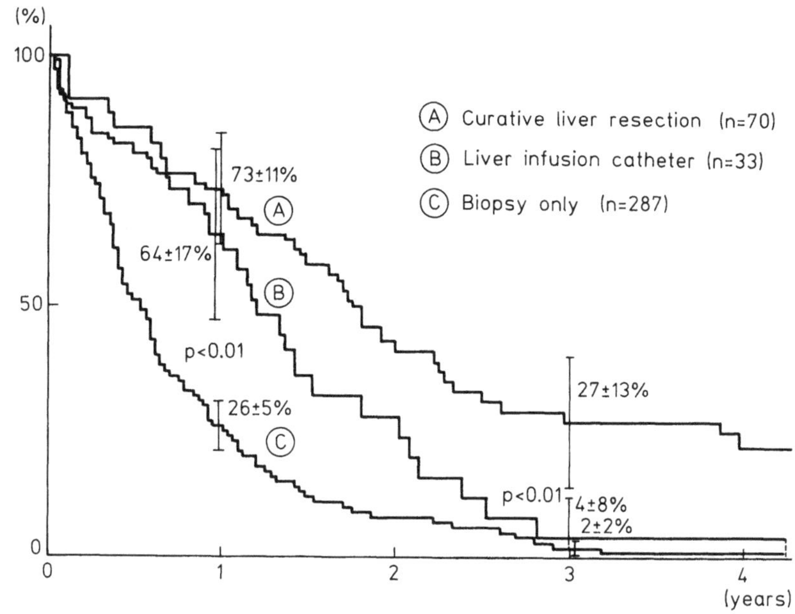

Fig. 1. Surgical treatment of liver metastases from colorectal carcinoma: modes of treatment in all patients. Surgical Clinic of Erlangen University, (Cumulative survival rates ±2SE, postoperative mortality included, 1969-1982/Dec. 31. 1983)

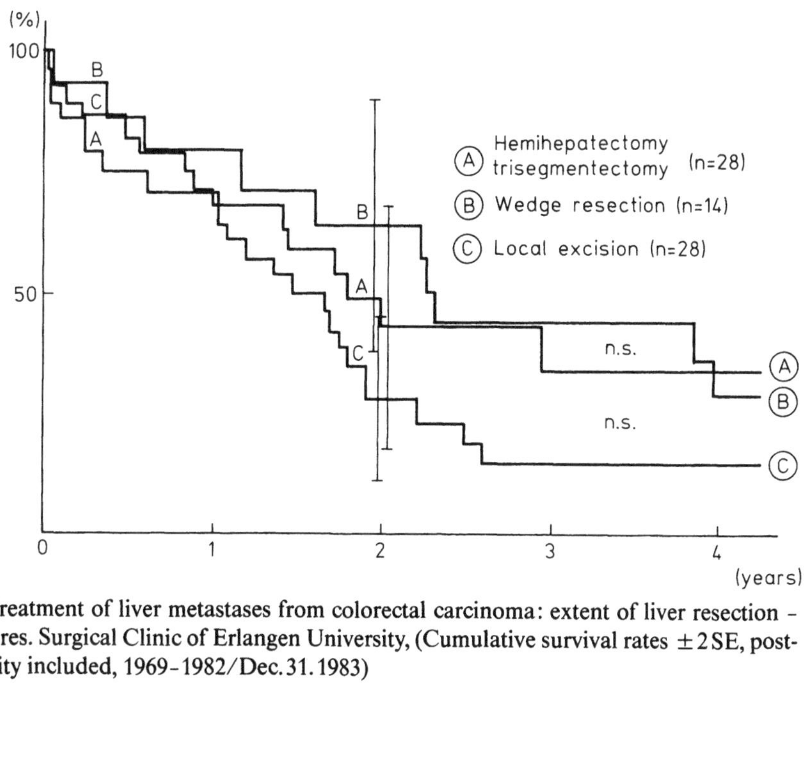

Fig. 2. Surgical treatment of liver metastases from colorectal carcinoma: extent of liver resection - curative procedures. Surgical Clinic of Erlangen University, (Cumulative survival rates ±2SE, postoperative mortality included, 1969-1982/Dec. 31. 1983)

from colorectal cancer was 24% (Fig. 1). This compares favourably with the 5-year survival rates of 20%-28% reported in the literature (Table 5).

The extent of the liver resection is of course dependent on the size of the metastases. An important question of interest is whether the different types of operative procedure all guarantee adequate radicality for a curative resection. On comparing excision, atypical resection, and hemihepatectomy (Fig. 2), we found no statistically significant difference in 2-year survival rates. In an earlier report by Foster and Lundy [10], results obtained with local excision were superior to lobectomy. If possible, therefore, a limited resection - local excision or wedge resection - with a margin of safety of at least 2 cm or more can be employed with no loss of radicality, to avoid a hemihepatectomy, which is associated with a much higher surgical risk, but no increase in effectivity.

The beneficial influence on survival of a long interval between resection of the primary tumor and the appearance of liver metastases has been overestimated in the past. In the analysis of our series the results of resection in synchronous and metachronous metastases

Table 5. Five-year survival of resected liver metastases from colorectal cancer

	n	%
Bengmark et al. [3]	39	20
Foster and Lundy [10]	231	23
Morrow et al. [14]	29	27
Wagner et al. [21]	141	25
Wanebo et al. [22]	27	28

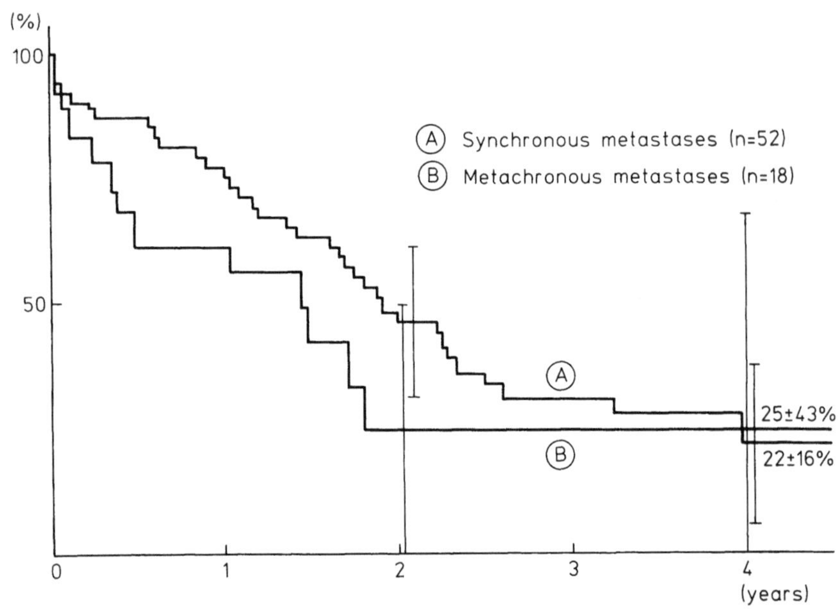

Fig. 3. Surgical treatment of liver metastases from colorectal carcinoma: time of diagnosis of metastases - curative procedures. Surgical Clinic of Erlangen University, (Cumulative survival rates ±2 SE, postoperative mortality included, 1969-1982/Dec. 31. 1983)

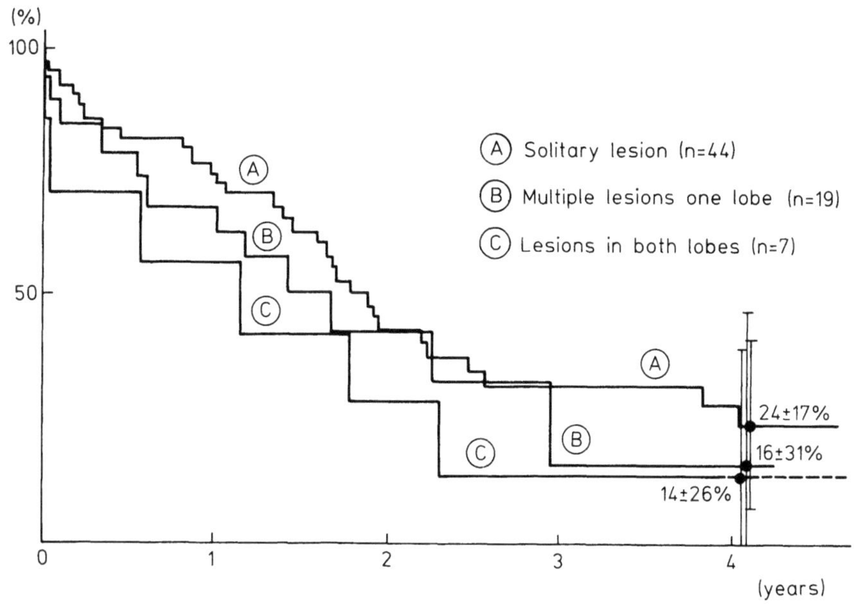

Fig. 4. Surgical treatment of liver metastases from colorectal carcinoma: extent of metastases - curative procedures. Surgical Clinic of Erlangen University, (Cumulative survival rates ±2 SE, post-operative mortality included, 1969-1982/Dec. 31. 1983)

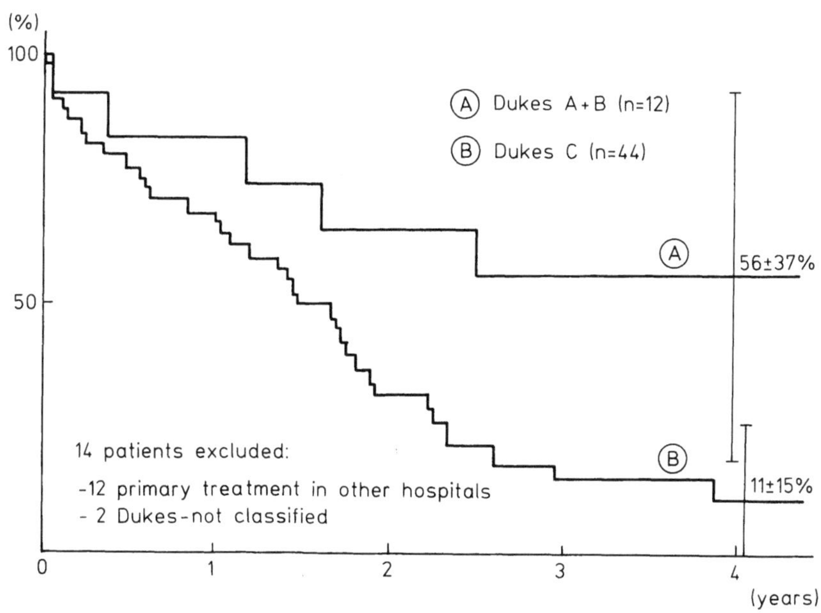

Fig. 5. Surgical treatment of liver metastases from colorectal carcinoma: Duke's classification of the primary tumor - curative procedures. Surgical Clinic of Erlangen University, (Cumulative survival rates ±2 SE, postoperative mortality included, 1969-1982/Dec. 31. 1983)

showed no statistically significant difference in survival rates at the end of the 3rd and 4th year (Fig. 3). Similar results for 5-year survival have recently been reported by Bengmark et al. and Foster [3, 9]. The generally accepted opinion that patients with metachronous lesions have a better survival chance is therefore no longer valid.

Controversy still exists as to the prognosis of solitary and multiple unilateral metastases. In their comprehensive study Foster and Lundy [10] reported a 5-year survival rate of 30% for solitary and 13% for multiple unilateral metastases. Even more unfavorable figures are reported by Bengmark and Hafström [2], Logan et al. [12], and Wilson and Adson [24], who observed that none of their patients submitted to resection for multiple unilateral metastases survived for 5 years.

In contrast to these reports our 2-year survival rates were 32% for solitary and 33% for multiple unilateral metastases, with expected 4-year survival rates of 24% and 16% respectively with no statistically significant difference (Fig. 4). Our own experience is supported by a recent analysis of the Mayo Clinic by Wagner et al. [21], who was unable to verify the previously reported prognostic difference between solitary and multiple metastases, published by Wilson and Adson [24], but now found equal 5-year survival rates for both lesions. Solitary metastases in each of the two lobes were removed by local excision in seven patients. This group is too small to obtain confirmation for this special indication on a statistical basis, but at present survival rate is almost identical with solitary or unilateral multiple lesions (Fig. 4).

A major determinant of the prognosis after resection of secondary liver lesions is the stage of the primary tumor. In Duke's A and B primary lesions the 4-year survival was 56% versus 11% in Duke's C lesions (Fig. 5). This difference was found to be almost statistically significant. A similar result has recently been reported also by Wagner et al. and Morrow et al. [21, 14].

With respect to the grade of malignancy of the colorectal carcinoma, no difference in survival after resection of liver metastases was found in our series.

In a small series of 14 patients the liver resection was classified as noncurative resection due to macroscopic or microscopic involvement of the resection line. The 1-, 2-, and 3-year survival rates were 57%, 7%, and 0% respectively. On comparing these results with the data on the natural history of untreated solitary or multiple unilateral metastases reported by Wagner et al. [21] it is evident that patients do not benefit from palliative resection of liver metastases.

During follow-up 50% (34/68) of patients who had a curative liver resection subsequently developed and died from liver, pulmonary, and bone metastases. Recurrent liver involvement was observed in 18/34 of these patients. This means that at the time of selection for liver resection about one-half of the patients had undetected diffuse metastases. A similar estimate was reported by Adson, which demonstrates that our present diagnostic facilities for reliable preoperative selection are far from optimal.

However, the following rules are generally accepted:
A synchronous liver resection should be performed when:

1. Extrahepatic metastases have been ruled out by the preoperative work-up.
2. Primary resection of the colorectal cancer has been classified as curative on macro- and microscopic findings.
3. The patient is in good condition and has tolerated the operation without difficulty.
4. A small solitary metastasis is present, which can be removed by an excision, small wedge resection, or lateral segmentectomy.

5. However, for large metastases requiring a hemihepatectomy the liver resection is postponed 14–21 days.

After curative resection of the primary colorectal cancer, about 30% of the patients will subsequently develop liver metastases. To detect these lesions as early as possible our regular follow-ups must include liver surveys with CT scans or ultrasonography at 6-month intervals.

A liver resection for metachronous metastases is advisable when:

1. A solitary or unilateral multiple lesions are present.
2. Complete removal seems possible.
3. The primary colorectal cancer has been removed by a prior curative resection.
4. Local or regional recurrence has been ruled out.
5. No extrahepatic metastases can be identified.

Contraindications

Cirrhosis of the liver, hepatic insufficiency or active hepatitis, as well as obstruction of the portal vein are considered contraindications for resection of liver metastases. In large symptomatic lesions a palliative resection or a debulking procedure before embarking on cytotoxic therapy may be indicated in rare cases on the request of the chemotherapist.

In closing, I would like to summarize:

Prior to laparotomy for colorectal cancer synchronous liver metastases should be identified.

Histological confirmation of liver metastases is mandatory to avoid unnecessary treatment of benign lesions.

A small solitary metastasis is removed by a local excision at the time of resection of the primary tumor. When in large or multiple unilateral metastases a major resection is required, the resection is postponed.

Operative mortality for excision or wedge resection is 0%–6%, while hemihepatectomy is still associated with a risk of 5%–10%.

Reported 5-year survival rates for curative resections vary from 20% to 28%. There is no significant difference in survival for solitary and multiple unilateral lesions nor for synchronous and metachronous lesions.

References

1. Adson MA, Van Heerden JA (1980) Major hepatic resection for metastatic colorectal cancer. Ann Surg 191: 576
2. Bengmark S, Hafström L (1978) The natural course for liver cancer. In: Ariel IM (ed) Progress in clinical cancer, Grune and Stratton, New York, pp 195–200
3. Bengmark S, Hafström L, Jeppsson B, Jönsson PE, Ryden S, Sundqvist K (1982) Metastatic disease in the liver from colorectal cancer. An appraisal of liver surgery. World J Surg 6: 61
4. Bengtsson G, Cansson G, Hafström L, Jonsson PE (1981) Natural history of patients with untreated liver metastases from colorectal cancer. Am J Surg 141: 586
5. Cady B, Bonneval M, Fender H (1979) Elective hepatic resection. Ann J Surg 137: 514
6. Finlay JG, Meek DR, Gray HW, Duncan JG, McArdle CS (1982) Incidence and detection of occult hepatic metastases in colorectal carcinoma. Br Med J 284: 803
7. Fisherman K, Petersen CF (1976) Survival among patients with liver metastases from cancer of the colon and rectum. Scand J Gastroenterol [Suppl] 37: 111

8. Fortner JG, McLean BJ, Kim DK, Howland WS, Turnbull AD, Goldiner P, Carlon G, Beattie EJ (1981) The seventies evolution in liver surgery for cancer. Cancer 47: 2162
9. Foster JH (1978) Survival after liver resection for secondary tumors. Am J Surg 135: 389
10. Foster JH, Lundy J (1981) Liver metastases. Curr Probl Surg 18: 157
11. Jaffe BM, Donegan WL, Watson F, Spratt JS Jr. (1968) Factors influencing survival in patients with untreated hepatic metastases. Surg Gynecol Obstet 127: 1
12. Logan SE, Meier SJ, Ramming KP, Morton DL, Longmire WP Jr. (1982) Hepatic resection of metastatic colorectal carcinoma. Arch Surg 117: 25
13. Mooney B, Critchley M, Grime S, Taylor J (1981) Portal vein scanning for early detection of liver metastases in colorectal cancer. Gut 25: 436
14. Morrow CE, Grage TB, Sutherland DER, Najarian JS (1982) Hepatic resection for secondary neoplasms. Surgery 92: 610
15. Nielsen J, Balsler J, Fenger HJ (1973) Carcinoma of the rectum with liver metastases. Prognosis and operative indications. Acta Chir Scand 139: 479
16. Nims, TA (1984) Resection of the liver for metastatic cancer. Surg Gynecol Obstet 158: 46
17. Oxley EM, Ellis H (1969) Prognosis of carcinoma of the large bowel in the presence of liver metastases. Br J Surg 56: 149
18. Pestana C, Reitemeier RY, Moertel CG (1964) Natural history of carcinoma of the colon and rectum. Ann J Surg 108: 826
19. Raute M, Trede M (1983) Metastasenchirurgie im Bereich der Abdominalorgane. Chirurg 54: 505
20. Starzl TE, Koep LJ, Weil III. R, Lilly JR, Putnam CW, Aldrete YA (1980) Right trisegmentectomy for hepatic neoplasms. Surg Gynecol Obstet 150: 208
21. Wagner JS, Adson MS, VanHeerden JA, Adson MH, Ilstrup DM (1984) The natural history of hepatic metastases from colorectal cancer. A comparison with resective treatment. Ann Surg 199, 502.
22. Wanebo HJ, Semoglou C, Attiyeh F, Stearns Jr. MJ (1978) Surgical management with primary operable colorectal cancer and synchronous liver metastases. Ann J Surg 135: 81
23. Wood CB, Gillis CR, Blumgart LH (1976) A retrospective study of the natural history of patients with liver metastases from colorectal cancer. Clin Oncol 2: 285
24. Wilson SM, Adson MA (1976) Surgical treatment of hepatic metastases from colorectal cancer. Arch Surg 111: 3330–334

Liver Transplantation for Liver Tumors

P. Neuhaus, C. E. Brölsch, B. Ringe, and R. Pichlmayr

Chirurgische Klinik, Städtisches Klinikum, Salzdahlumer Strasse 90, 3300 Braunschweig, FRG

Liver transplantation principally can be considered as a suitable form of treatment for any patient with progressive or end-stage liver disease, when no other standard therapy is available. The two main categories of indications are liver cirrhosis with severe complications from functional deterioration and primary malignancies of the liver.

When liver transplantation was first performed on humans by Starzl and Moore in 1963 [7], the widely accepted indication for several reasons was otherwise untreatable and unresectable malignancy - especially because a very short survival time of 2-6 months in patients with primary hepatic malignancy was well established, whereas the definition of end-stage liver disease and impending hepatic failure in cirrhotics was - and still is - very difficult.

Moreover, no other treatment modality for tumor patients like systemic or regional chemotherapy, hepatic artery ligation, and tumor embolization had been successful in terms of prolonged survival.

Recently Okuda [5] in a series of more than 150 untreated patients with primary hepatocellular carcinoma reported a mean survival time of 1.6 months and less than 15% lived for more than 6 months. He also showed that survival was better when only patients with small tumors without functional impairment of the liver were followed, and 35% of these patients lived for more than 1 year.

In comparison to the overall 1 year survival of less than 10% in his series *modern* forms of chemotherapy in different reports improved the 1-year survival to 30%-50%; results of surgical treatment with hepatic resection even show 40%-80% 1-year survival.

None of these figures must be taken as absolute values, since diagnostic tools like α-fetoprotein, ultrasound, and computed tomography have now made a much earlier diagnosis possible, since resection is feasible in only a few patients and since studies on the effect of chemotherapy do not usually have comparable control groups.

On the other hand, tumor patients do not carry the high surgical risk which in cirrhotic patients can be considerable and sometimes fatal. Tumor patients do not usually present with portal hypertension, and considerably less intraoperative bleeding can be expected.

Usually no other organ disease except of the liver is present in tumor patients, whereas cirrhotic patients often have developed impaired kidney function, pulmonary shunting, high cardiac output, and hypercirculatory syndrome and encephalopathy. Together with a poor general condition, metabolic derangement from bad liver function such as catabolism and muscle wasting, ascites, hypoalbuminemia, and clotting disorders as well as often prolonged treatment of infections, these produce severe intraoperative and postoperative problems in cirrhotic patients but not in tumor patients.

Recent Results in Cancer Research. Vol 100

Clinical Experience

From 1975 to 1984 liver transplantation was performed in 52 tumor patients and 81 patients with nonmalignant end-stage liver disease. Thirty-seven of these tumors were primary hepatic malignancies, 17 irresectable hepatocellular carcinomas in noncirrhotic livers, 15 hepatocellular carcinomas associated with cirrhosis, and 5 cholangiocellular carcinomas.

Nine patients had surgically untreatable adenocarcinomas of the biliary tract; six had metastatic disease, two of which were not correctly diagnosed before transplantation.

The first young patient presented with bleeding and coagulopathy from severe liver trauma, which had been unsuccessfully treated in another hospital. Because of impending hepatic failure, transplantation was performed and only after examination of the removed specimen was the diagnosis of a ruptured metastasis of the liver established. He was discharged from hospital before the exact diagnosis was made and died due to generalized metastasis 40 days after transplantation.

The second patient presented as having hepatocellular carcinoma, but turned out to have metastasis from melanoma; he died from postoperative septic problems.

Only one out of three patients with metastatic disease of colorectal carcinoma survived postoperatively for 11 months, but at operation tumor infiltration of the diaphragm had already been proven.

From the present results and also those of other groups it cannot be concluded therefore that liver transplantation in metastatic disease is totally unsuccessful. From the favorable results of liver resection for metastasis of colorectal carcinoma it could also be concluded that those patients, if carefully selected, could profit from liver transplantation. Adjuvant chemotherapy and eventually monoclonal antibodies against the residual micrometastasis could be helpful.

Another approach by Margreiter in his group included liver transplantation, total body irradiation, and high-dose cyclophosphamide followed by autologous bone marrow transplantation [4]. A young woman with metastasis from mammary carcinoma is now alive and without recurrence 2 years after this treatment.

The poor operative survival statistics in patients with metastatic disease do not apply to all tumor patients. Thirty-one of the 52 patients left hospital for some time, generally with very good palliation, although very few with the chance to be cured.

Another problem is the indication for liver transplantation in patients with biliary tract carcinomas, also referred to as Klatskin tumor or hepatic duct cell carcinoma. There was an argument between Starzl and Terblanche in 1979 about the best treatment of this slowly growing tumor, which can be successfully treated for some time by conventional palliative measures such as drainage by transhepatic tube or U-tube [8].

Most of the nine patients in our series who were transplanted had been treated in this way before. Only two died immediately after the operation; the others survived from 5 to 28 months. It is noteworthy that all of them except one had residual tumor or positive lymph nodes at operation, the growth of which has probably been accelerated by immunosuppression. But all patients were severely disabled by jaundice, repeated episodes of cholangitis, pain, and exclusion from social life. In this light transplantation may be justifiable, although to our knowledge no patient in the world with Klatskin tumor has so far survived for more than 6 years; most have died from metastatic disease after 1 or 2 years (Table 1).

Of the 37 patients who were transplanted for primary liver malignancies, 23 or 62% survived the operation. Survival times range from 3 months to more than 8 years; the 1-year

Table 1. Results of liver transplantation for carcinoma of the biliary tract. Medizinische Hochschule Hannover, 8.84, Klinik für Abdominal- und Transplantationschirurgie

	Age (years)	Survival (months)	Extrahepatic tumor left at operation	Metastases		Main cause of death
				Months post operation	Site	
N.H.	40	1	Recurrence of tumor 18 months after resection	-	-	Sepsis, liver failure
K.E.	55	9	> 12 months palliative drainage Positive lymph nodes, pancreas	0	Local	Chronic rejection
P.F.	30	28	-	22	Local, abdomen	Metastasis, chronic rejection, sepsis
M.M.	47	11	Positive lymph nodes, head of pancreas	0	Local, brain, bone	Metastasis
F.H.	56	14	Distal common bile duct	0	Local, brain, lung	Metastasis
K.J.	50	1	Distal common bile duct	0	Local	Rejection, sepsis
S.B.	28	5	Head of pancreas	0	Local, abdomen	Metastasis
O.U.	30	7	Head of pancreas	0	Local, abdomen	Metastasis
A.K.	40	2[a]	Head of pancreas duodenopancreatectomy	-	-	-

[a] Living

survival is around 30%, which is about the same as reported from other centers [1, 2, 3, 6, 7].

In most patients the methods available for detection of extrahepatic tumor spread have been used, but small lymph nodes, infiltration of the diaphragm, and small pulmonary metastases are still often not found before the operation. Diagnostic laparotomy and biopsy were suspected to promote tumor spread and therefore were only carried out in a few patients. In addition the risk of surgical infection and surgical difficulties at the time of transplantation were feared. When extrahepatic tumor was found at laparotomy for transplantation, the operation was continued despite the poor prognosis, because this was usually the only hope and chance of palliation for an individual patient, who after full explanation of his disease had given his consent to liver transplantation.

The results, as survival times, intraoperative assessment of extrahepatic tumor spread, clinical development of metastasis, and cause of death are listed in Tables 2 and 3.

The distinction between primary liver tumors with and without cirrhosis was made, because carcinomas in cirrhotic livers are usually smaller and are possibly found earlier in these patients, who are mostly under medical control, than in otherwise healthy subjects.

Table 2. Results of liver transplantation for hepatocellular carcinoma in patients who survived operation. Medizinische Hochschule Hannover, 8.84, Klinik für Abdominal- und Transplantationschirurgie

	Age (years)	Survival (months)	Extrahepatic tumor at operation	Metastases		Main cause of death
				Months post operation	Site	
D.I.[a]	41	> 8 years	-	30	Lung - removed	-
H.S.	14	25	Positive lymph nodes, diaphragm	12	Lung, local	Metastatic disease
M.F.	18	6	Positive lymph nodes	1	Lung	Metastatic disease + rejection
L.H.	48	5	-	5	-	Rejection
G.P.	39	8	Positive lymph nodes, diaphragm	5	Lung	Rejection, biliary complications
M.C.	14	11½	Positive lymph nodes	2	Lung	Metastatic disease + sepsis
U.J.[a]	55	>40	-	-	-	-
W.W.	56	4	Positive lymph nodes, diaphragm	3	Abdomen, lung, pleura	Metastatic disease, CMV
B.G.	52	3	Positive lymph nodes, diaphragm	3	Peritoneal carcinosis, lung, liver	Metastatic disease
D.A.	20	12	-	6	Abdomen	Metastatic disease
O.M.[a]	45	>16	-	6	Lung - resection	-
S.H.[a] Chol. cell. Ca.	57	22	-	22	Liver	-
B.M. Chol. cell. Ca.	48	6	-	3	Pleura, bone	Metastatic disease
R.M.[a] Hepatoblastoma	1	>33	-	-	-	-

[a] Patient living

Apparently almost half of these patients already had extrahepatic metastasis at the time of transplantation and there was no difference between both groups.

However five out of nine patients with hepatocellular carcinoma in cirrhosis had portal vein thrombosis containing tumor cells, which is of poor prognostic influence, even when no other extrahepatic metastases are found.

Since the overall survival curve in tumor patients probably would not justify any other effort in transplantation of these patients, the problem of pre- and intraoperative assessment of extrahepatic tumor spread needs to be evaluated.

Two possibilities exist, first to compare assessment of extrahepatic tumor spread at operation and at autopsy in patients who did not survive transplantation and secondly to compare survival times of patients with and without clinical signs of extrahepatic tumor spread at operation.

Table 3. Results of liver transplantation for hepatocellular carcinoma in cirrhotic patients who survived operation. Medizinische Hochschule Hannover, 8.84, Klinik für Abdominal- und Transplantationschirurgie

	Age (years)	Survival (months)	Extrahepatic tumor at operation	Metastases		Main cause of death
				Months post operation	Site	
S.H.	30	3	Positive lymph nodes, retroperitoneal space	1	Lung, abdomen, liver	Metastatic disease
T.B.	29	4	Diaphragm [b]	3	Lung	Metastatic disease
A.A.	42	30	Positive lymph nodes	28	Liver - resection	Sepsis after liver resection
W.K.	58	11	Omentum, diaphragm [b]	0	Bone (preoperative), liver, abdomen, lung	Metastatic disease
E.K.	46	8	- [b]	3	Thorax - liver	Sepsis, metastatic disease
U.R. [a]	50	> 20	-	-	-	-
V.U. [a]	42	> 9	-	8	Abdomen, liver	-
J.J. [a]	22	> 7	- [b]	-	-	-
D.S. [a]	42	> 7	- [b]	6	Bone	-

[a] Patient living
[b] Tumor cell thrombosis of portal vein

Table 4. Survival of patients with primary liver tumors after liver transplantation (months). Medizinische Hochschule Hannover, 8.84, Klinik für Abdominal- und Transplantationschirurgie

	Intraoperative assessment of tumor spread			
	N	Extrahepatic tumor, positive lymph nodes	N	"tumor-free"
Hepatocellular carcinoma	6	3, 4, 6, 8, 11½, 25 +	8	/ 5 [b], 6, 12 + \ > 16 > 22 > 33 > 40 > 116
Hepatocellular carcinoma in cirrhosis	4	3, 4 [a], 11 [a], 33 +	5	/ 8 [a] + \ > 20, > 9, > 7 [a], > 7 [a]

[a] Portal vein thrombosis with tumor cells
[b] Death due to rejection, no metastasis

Twenty-one patients died shortly after transplantation; 11 of these were judged to be macroscopically tumor-free; only in five of them could this assumption be confirmed at autopsy. Especially patients with hepatocellular carcinoma in noncirrhotic livers had undetected small metastasis in lymph nodes and elsewhere; none of them was tumor-free. Altogether only in 5 of these 21 patients who died was no extrahepatic tumor spread found. These patients could have been candidates for longer survival (Table 4).

Table 5. Tumor spread in patients who did not survive liver transplantation. Medizinische Hochschule Hannover, 8.84, Klinik für Abdominal- und Transplantationschirurgie

Diagnosis	N	Intraoperative/at autopsy		
		Tumor-free	Positive lymph nodes	Extrahepatic tumor
Hepatocellular carcinoma (HCC)	5	4/0 [a]	1/4	1/2
HCC + cirrhosis	6	4/3	2/3	2/2
Cholangiocellular carcinoma	3	2/1	0/2	1/2
Biliary carcinoma	2	1/1	1/1	1/1
Metastases	5	0/0	5/5	5/5

[a] One patient without autopsy

If survival times are compared between patients with and without signs of extrahepatic tumor spread at operation excluding operative mortality, significantly better results are found in the latter group. Whereas in the first group only 2 out of 10 patients survived for more than 12 months - and these 2 have also died - only 3 out of 13 patients, who were classified as tumor-free at the time of transplantation, have died from metastasis. Three more patients are alive with known metastasis after 16 months in the first group and 7 and 9 months in the second group. Together these 6 out of 13 patients account for this 50% of false-negative diagnoses "tumor-free" at operation, which could be shown in patients who did not survive the early phase after transplantation (Table 5).

Discussion

Altogether these results can be interpreted in different ways: possibly one conclusion could be that the overall 1-year survival rate of about 30% and the small number of long-term survivors and therefore eventually cured patients does not justify the high personal and financial input. Therefore liver transplantation should no longer be performed in tumor patients.

On the other hand, total liver replacement has obviously cured some patients, who otherwise certainly would have died, and has been a valuable palliation and prolongation of life for a considerable number of patients. Therefore it should be offered to such patients also in the future. Both standpoints can be supported with arguments, but with growing experience a more critical position will certainly evolve.

In the early phase of liver transplantation tumor recurrence was not expected to occur so soon after operation and with such regularity as it appears now. The overall results of total liver replacement were poor and physicians were often very reluctant to transfer patients with nonmalignant disease for transplantation until shortly before death.

Operative and postoperative problems in transplanted patients with cirrhosis were also much higher than in tumor patients and were aggravated by the adverse effects of immunosuppression with azathioprine, antilymphocyte globulin, and prednisolone. In this phase only three centers in the world performed liver transplantation continously. They carried the burden of disappointing results and slowly gained experience in surgical techniques, organ procurement and preservation, pre- and postoperative treatment of the transplant patient, and immunosuppression. Operative survival was estimated as successful.

When tumor recurrence killed most of the successfully transplanted patients end-stage cirrhosis more and more became the predominant indication for liver replacement. Tumor patients were carefully evaluated preoperatively with isotope scanning and computed tomography for metastasis. A high percentage of these patients had to be taken off the list of transplant candidates. Many more patients were faced with the choice of dying in a few months or of having liver transplantation. The lack of alternative treatment modalities led us to perform liver transplantation in these patients also when extrahepatic lymph nodes and metastases were found at the time of operation.

Our experience presented here supports to some extent this concept of palliative transplantation and many patients and their families have expressed the feeling that even a short period of life after transplantation has been very valuable for them.

A new chapter in liver transplantation was begun by Calne [2] and Starzl [7] with the introduction of the new immunosuppressant cyclosporin A in 1978. Rapidly improving results with the use of cyclosporin A and rising numbers of transplantations per year made liver transplantation a widely accepted alternative treatment for end-stage benign liver disease in adults and also in children with biliary atresia, where up to 80% 1-year survival has been achieved by our own group. Selection of patients therefore was carried out more and more in favor of the different forms of cirrhosis.

A careful analysis of our own as well as Calne's [2] and Starzl et al.'s [7] experience with liver transplantation in tumor patients, however, shows that there is a chance of long-term survival and even cure if extrahepatic tumor spread is excluded as much as possible pre- and intraoperatively. Moreover, it is possible that with adjuvant therapeutic modalities such as continuous infusion chemotherapy and monoclonal antibodies and through the use of bone marrow replacement after irradiation and chemotherapy, as Margreiter et al. [4] have shown, not only primary hepatic malignancies, but also metastases can be effectively treated with liver transplantation.

A side effect of the efforts at transplantation has been a steadily rising number of patients with liver tumors who were referred for liver transplantation because their tumors were thought to be unresectable by other surgeons. In Starzl's and also in our own experience a considerable percentage of these patients could be treated by extended or subtotal hepatectomy.

Of course the results of conservative surgical treatment, when possible, are better than the results of transplantation. But it still seems justified to keep an optimistic view on the prospect of liver replacement for irresectable malignancies.

References

1. Brölsch C, Neuhaus EP, Burdelski M, Wonigeit K, Lang W, Schmidt FW, Pichlmayr R (1984) Aktueller Stand der Lebertransplantation. Diagnostik 17: 12-16
2. Calne RY (1982) Liver transplantation for liver cancer. World J Surg 6: 76-80
3. Iwatsuki S, Klintmalm GB, Starzl TE (1982) Total hepatectomy and liver replacement (orthotopic liver transplantation) for primary hepatic malignancy. World J Surg 6: 81-85
4. Margreiter R, Huber C, Niederwieser D, Gratwohl A, Frommhold H, Schönitzer D (1985) Combined bone marrow and liver transplantation with total body irradiation and high dose cyclophosphamide in the treatment of metastatic liver disease. Transplant Proc 17 (1): 296-297

5. Okuda K (1983) Primary hepatocellular carcinoma, prognosis in 600 patients. NIH Consensus Development Conference, Liver transplantation. NIH, Bethesda, Maryland
6. Pichlmayr R, Brölsch C, Wonigeit K, Neuhaus P, Sigismund S, Schmidt FW, Burdelski M (1984) Experience with liver transplantation in Hannover. Hepatology 4: 56S-60S
7. Starzl TE, Iwatsuki S, van Thiel DH, Gartner JC, Zitelli BJ, Malatack JJ, Schade RR, Shaw BW, Hakala TR, Rosenthal JT, Porter KA (1982) Evolution of liver transplantation. Hepatology 2: 614-636
8. Terblanche J, Koep LJ, Starzl TE (1979) Liver transplantation. Med Clin North Am 63: 507

Requirements and Results of Liver Perfusion

K. Schwemmle and K. Aigner

Abteilung für Allgemeinchirurgie, Zentrum für Chirurgie der Justus-Liebig-Universität, Klinikstrasse 29, 6300 Giessen, FRG

Among the various treatment modalities for liver metastases such as resection, intraarterial infusion, isolated perfusion, or chemoembolization, isolated perfusion enables chemotherapeutic agents to be added to the perfusion circuit in dosages higher than could be tolerated by systemic administration. The upper limit of dosage is only the local toxicity. Because hepatic metastases are mainly vascularized by the hepatic artery, intraarterial infusion of cytotoxic agents provides a much higher concentration of the drug in these tumors than can be achieved by systemic chemotherapy.

To develop a method for intraarterial treatment with maximal doses of chemotherapeutic drugs, we started with isolated perfusion of the liver in animal experiments according to previously published methods [4-6]. Optimal surgical techniques and drug toxicity were studied in dogs. After these studies in animals had proved that the method was practicable and safe, in November 1981 we performed an isolated hepatic perfusion in two patients suffering from disseminated hepatic metastases of colorectal cancer [1]. After

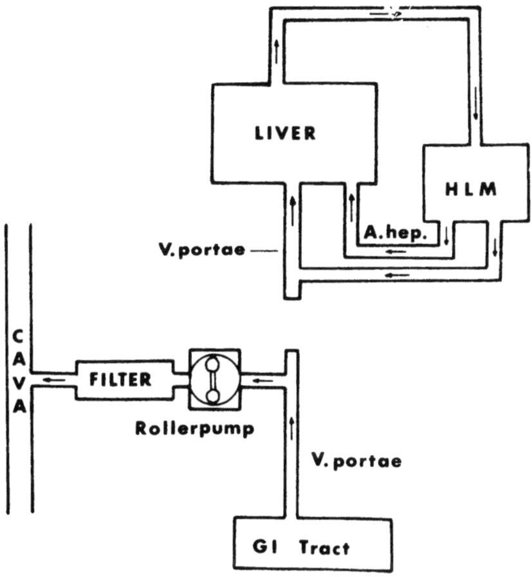

Fig. 1. Portocaval shunting and liver circulation during hepatic perfusion. *HLM*, heart-lung machine

Recent Results in Cancer Research. Vol 100

these two patients had survived 5 months without complications, another 38 patients were submitted to isolated hyperthermic perfusion of the liver with chemotherapeutics [2].

In the isolated perfusion circuit both the hepatic artery and portal vein are perfused and the hepatic venous return is collected via a single venous line. During isolated perfusion a portocaval shunt is established in which ammonium is filtered out of the portal blood (Fig. 1). Recently, we have omitted the filtration unit.

During the operative procedure through an abdominal midline incision the liver, the hepatoduodenal ligament, and the inferior caval vein are exposed. Tourniquets are placed around the gastroduodenal artery and portal vein and around the caval vein below and above the renal veins as well as intrapericardially.

In order to collect the hepatic venous outflow a double-channel catheter is inserted into the caval vein from below the renal veins. This special catheter consists of a longer channel shunting the caval vein to maintain cardiac venous return and a second shorter channel for the isolated hepatic venous return. The portocaval shunt tube is inserted into the caval vein channel, whereas two lateral openings collect the venous return from the kidneys.

After the perfusion catheter is inserted into the caval vein the portal vein is cannulated in both directions. The peripheral catheter is connected to the portocaval filtration unit, consisting of a roller pump and a hemofiltrating system. At flow rates of approximately 300-400 ml portal venous blood has been filtered and with adequate volume substitution returned to the caval shunt tube. Thus blood levels of ammonium have been kept within normal ranges during the period of isolated hepatic perfusion. In case of leakage to the systemic circulation a part of the cytotoxic drugs as well has been filtered out in that portacaval shunt. As soon as the shunt is established, the common hepatic artery is clamped and perfusion is started via the central portal vein catheter in a partial circuit. Then the arterial catheter is inserted into the gastroduodenal artery and the liver is perfused via two arterial lines at a flow rate of 200-350 ml/min in the hepatic artery and 150 ml/min in the portal vein. Heating the perfusion circuit the temperature of the hepatic tissue is increased. The temperature, which should not exceed 40 °C, is measured with needle probes in the right and left liver lobes. In our first 31 isolated liver perfusions we only applied 5-fluorouracil (5-FU) in a dosage between 500 and 1000 mg. In the last eight patients a combination consisting of mitomycin C and 5-FU was used.

Few complications occurred after isolated liver perfusion. Three patients died a short time after the operation. One patient died 2 hours later from intreatable bleeding after an isolated hepatic perfusion combined with a hemihepatectomy. The tumor had already infiltrated the caval vein. In an other patient septicemia and respiratory distress occurred 6 days after the perfusion. The third patient died from renal failure 2 weeks after the perfusion. His autopsy showed a 90% regression of the tumor. Seventy percent of the hepatic tissue in this case had been involved in metastases. In the last 30 patients there were no fatal outcomes.

Figure 2 shows the actual survival of two groups of 12 patients treated either by only one isolated liver perfusion with 5-FU (left curve) or by isolated liver perfusion combined with subsequent hepatic artery infusions as a maintenance therapy. Both groups of 12 cases were mainly clinical stage III in the Lausanne classification with disseminated disease and extreme hepatomegaly. For clinical staging total liver volumes and tumor volumes were measured by CT scan and not only estimated by the surgeon during operations. The median liver volume of these patients was 4.1 liters and the median tumor volume was 1.8 liters.

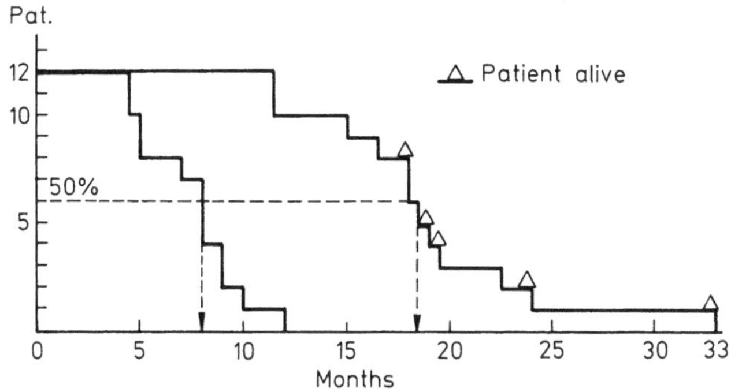

Fig. 2. Survival after isolated liver perfusion alone *(left curve)* and in combination with arterial infusion (mitomycin C and 5-FU, *right curve*)

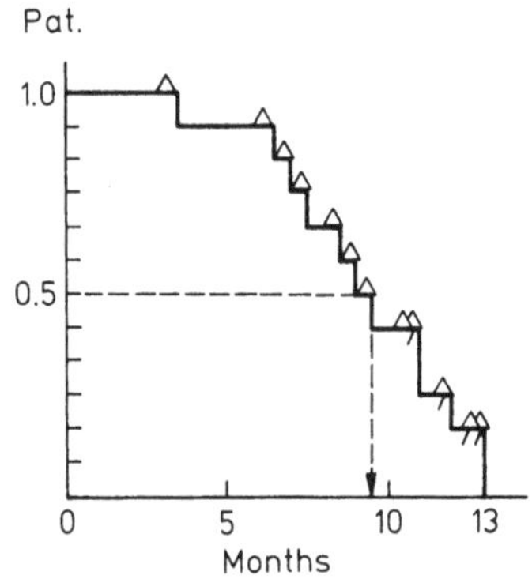

Fig. 3. Actual survival of the last group of 12 patients with liver metastases (Lausanne stage II). Perfusion with mitomycin C and 5-FU (eight patients) and 5-FU alone (four patients) in combination with subsequent hepatic artery infusion (all patients alive)

These two groups were formed in order to find out whether isolated liver perfusion combined with subsequent infusion was superior to isolated perfusion alone or not. Patients treated by isolated hepatic perfusion alone had a median survival of 8 months [3]. On the other hand patients with a combination treatment have been followed for a median of 18.5 months. The longest actual survival without progression of hepatic disease is 33 months. In the first group all patients ceased. The five patients still alive in the second group are indicated by vertical bars in fig. 2.

In spite of the increased survival time unfortunately in the combined group the patients developed extrahepatic metastases after the treatment. In ten cases (83%) metastases of the lung developed. Half of the patients developed peritoneal carcinosis or at least positive lymph nodes at the hepatoduodenal ligament and in three cases (25%) recurrences at the colorectal anastomoses or at the perineal scar developed.

A third group consisting of 12 patients in clinical stage II (Fig. 3) were perfused with 5-FU (4 cases) and with a combination consisting of 5-FU and mitomycin C. All patients had subsequent hepatic artery infusions with the same combination. Although in that group all patients are alive and median survival is 9.5 months, follow-up is still too short to draw any conclusions.

For hepatic artery infusions we use a so-called Implantofix permanent catheter with a subcutaneously placed port, which is inserted into the gastroduodenal artery. This catheter allows continuous access for intraarterial infusion chemotherapy after isolated perfusion and the tip of the catheter acting as a valve mechanism prevents reflux and clotting of blood.

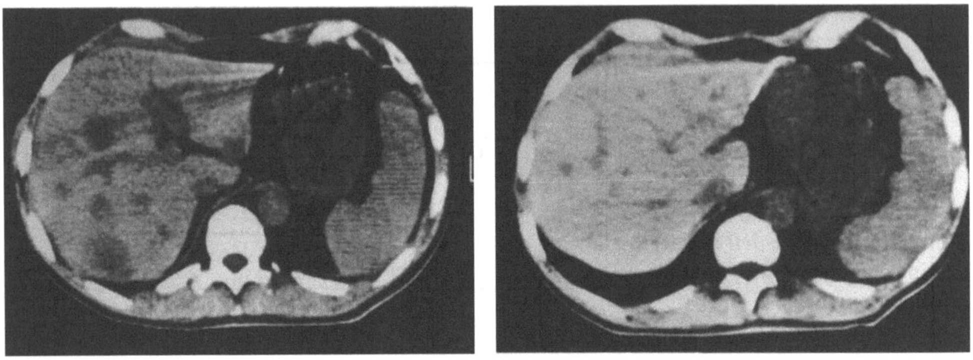

Fig. 4. Computed tomography scan before and after combined therapy (isolated perfusion and arterial infusion)

In CT scan usually only changes in tumor density are observed after isolated perfusion and it takes quite a few months until tumors diminish. The patient shown in Fig. 4 was treated by isolated perfusion and by hepatic artery short-time infusions. The CT scan taken 6 months after the initial treatment shows only a small amount of residual tumor in the liver parenchyma.

Estimation of total liver volume with CT scan usually shows a 20% decrease in total liver volume after isolated perfusion. After three additional courses of hepatic artery infusion a further decrease in total liver volume to 68% was seen. The estimation of tumor volume or tumor diameter by CT scan is much more difficult since edema or inflammatory changes can only hardly be differentiated from tumor tissue.

In most of our patients hepatic metastases had progressed to Lausanne stage III, which means an excessive hepatomegaly and elevation of the alkaline phosphatase. In these cases micrometastases to other organs such as lung and bones are usually assumed. It has been pointed out by Pettavel and Morgenthaler that the presence of concomitant metastases in other organs would not influence the length of survival of a patient with hepatic metastases [7]. However, in our stage III cases growth of hepatic lesions was surpassed by local recurrences or lung metastases several months after isolated perfusion, while the growth of their hepatic metastases remained stationary or suppressed. For this reason the most beneficial effect of isolated perfusion combined with three to six courses of intra-arterial short time infusions might be attained in patients suffering from only a few metastases in one or both liver lobes not resectable from technical reasons. Remaining micrometastases would represent a more susceptible target for regional chemotherapy. Although 60% of our patients had chemotherapy before perfusion and showed no response to systemic treatment, they did respond to high-dose locoregional treatment with the same drug and this is a strong additional argument for the benefit of isolated liver perfusion.

The requirements of isolated liver perfusion are summarized as follows:

1. Metastases of carcinoid or colorectal carcinomas
2. No evidence of tumor outside of the liver
3. Moderate enlargement of the liver: liver edge not more than 5 cm below the costal margin
4. If possible additional reduction of tumor volume (liver resection or enucleation of metastases)
5. Combination therapy with hepatic artery infusion

In conclusion we see the following advantages of liver perfusion:

1. We are able to use a high cytotoxic dosage which cannot be achieved by other methods, for example, intermittent or continuous intraarterial infusion.
2. The administration of the cytotoxic agents is performed via both the hepatic artery and the portal vein.
3. A combination with hyperthermia is given.

The most important disadvantage of this method is the fact that the perfusion cannot be repeated. However, it is possible at any time to continue the therapy with intraarterial infusions and/or with chemoembolization.

References

1. Aigner K, Walther H, Tonn JC, Krahl M, Wenzl A, Merker G, Schwemmle K (1982) Die isolierte Leberperfusion mit 5-Fluorouracil (5-FU) beim Menschen. Chirurg 53: 571
2. Aigner K, Schwemmle K (1983) Die isolierte Leberperfusion. In: Eigler FW, Gross E (eds) Ergebnisse der Chirurgischen Onkologie 6. Enke, Stuttgart
3. Aigner K, Walther H, Tonn JC, Link KH, Schoch P, Schwemmle K (1984) Die isolierte Leberperfusion bei fortgeschrittenen Metastasen kolorektaler Karzinome. Onkologie 7: 13
4. Ausman RK (1961) Development of a technic for isolated perfusion of the liver. NY State J Med 61: 3993
5. Boddie AW, Booker L, Mullins JD, Buckley CJ, McBride CM (1979) Hepatic hyperthermia by total isolation and regional perfusion in vivo. J Surg Res 26: 47
6. Kestens PJ, Farrely JA, McDermott WV (1962) A technique of isolation and perfusion of the canine liver. J Surg Res 2: 58
7. Pettavel J, Morgenthaler F (1969) Traitement chimiothérapique des métastases hépatiques en fonction de leur évolution spontanée. Schweiz Med Wochenschr 99: 588-590

Intraarterial Chemotherapy for Colorectal Liver Metastases and Hepatomas Using a Totally Implantable Drug Infusion Pump

C. M. Balch and M. M. Urist

M. D. Anderson Hospital & Tumor Institute, Division of Surgery, The University of Texas System Cancer Center, 6723 Bertner Dr., Box No. 112, Houston, TX 77030, USA

Introduction

Continuous regional chemotherapy for treating hepatic tumors is a rational pharmacological approach as palliative treatment in selected patients, such as those with hepatocellular carcinoma and metastatic colorectal carcinoma. Continuous regional chemotherapy has the following advantages: (1) it delivers a higher concentration of drug directly to the liver tumor since it avoids a dilutional effect that otherwise occurs with a systemic (intravenous) injection; (2) many antimetabolites have a more effective antineoplastic effect when administered by a chronic infusion rather than by pulse injection; (3) there is significant hepatic extraction of many drugs when injected directly into the hepatic circulation, particularly fluorodeoxyuridine (FUdR) and to a lesser extent 5-fluorouracil (5-FU), mitomycin C, and adriamycin; this further increases the concentration of the drug at the site of the liver neoplasm; and (4) continuous infusion (either intraarterially or intravenously) has a lower peak serum concentration, thus decreasing toxicity such as marrow depression with FUdR and 5-FU, or cardiotoxicity with adriamycin [15, 19, 22, 29]. There are some disadvantages to this approach as well. First, there is less systemic exposure of the drug so that metastases at extrahepatic sites are not treated to the same degree. Second, there can be significant local toxicity, especially chemical hepatitis, cholecystitis, and gastritis.

Intraarterial infusion for hepatic tumors has been utilized for several decades using externalized catheters and battery-driven pumps [1, 9, 26, 27, 28, 30, 31]. In the past, a broad application of this approach has been limited by frequent problems related to the externalized catheter, the necessity for repeated hospitalization, and the use of bulky external pump devices [14].

Furthermore, catheter complications were significant and included intraabdominal infections, thrombosis of the hepatic artery, and malfunction or migration of the catheter [8, 10, 25, 28]. These limitations, however, have now been surmounted with the availability of a totally implantable drug infusion pump (manufactured by the Infusaid Corporation, Norwood, Massachusetts, United States).

The Infusaid totally implantable pump system was first developed by Blackshear et al. at the University of Minnesota [6, 7]. It is a lightweight (180 g), small (9.5 cm in diameter), silent, and reliable device that is powered by charged freon and has a 50-ml chamber capacity. It delivers drugs at a fixed rate, ranging from 3 to 10 ml/day. Every 1-2 weeks the implanted pump is refilled and automatically recharged by a simple percutaneous injec-

Recent Results in Cancer Research. Vol 100

tion on an outpatient basis. The pump also has a sideport for direct access to the hepatic artery catheter for bolus injections or short-term infusions of drugs. Newer modifications of the Infusaid pump include the capability for simultaneous drug delivery through two catheters and altering pump flow rates with glycerol-saline solutions at different viscosities. More detailed descriptions about the technical features of this device have been published [3, 6, 7].

Indications

Numerous clinical investigations are being conducted throughout the world to evaluate the treatment efficacy of this approach. In general, only those cancers where primary carcinoma is confined to the liver should be considered for this regional chemotherapy approach. Most centers have restricted their evaluations to patients with metastatic colorectal carcinoma and metastatic carcinoid to the liver, while a few centers have evaluated hepatocellular carcinomas and other tumors as well. In general, patients with breast carcinoma, melanoma, or ovarian carcinoma are not considered as candidates, because their metastatic disease is often more widespread. Patients with carcinoma from the stomach and pancreas with hepatic metastases are generally not considered because their tumors are usually refractory to currently available chemotherapy. Patients with known extrahepatic metastases are also excluded because their treatment must utilize a systemic form of chemotherapy. Occasional exceptions to this are those patients whose extrahepatic disease can be surgically removed or treated successfully by irradiation therapy.

Pump Implantation Technique

Surgical technique of pump implantation and the perioperative management have been published [2, 3, 23]. Only the major points will be summarized here.

Preoperatively, potential candidates for pump implantation are assessed for: (1) surgical risk associated with underlying chronic disease or poor nutritional state; (2) adequate hepatic reserves (e.g., normal serum bilirubin and no ascites); (3) hepatic vasculature as delineated with a celiac axis and superior mesenteric arteriogram; and (4) evaluation for extrahepatic disease in the abdomen and lungs with radiological imaging techniques. A baseline level of carcinoembryonic antigen in the serum and an assessment of liver tumor size by sonography, computed tomography, or liver scintigram are also obtained. The patient's perioperative nutritional status is optimized and antibiotics are given.

The surgical technique consists of the catheter placement and the pump implantation. The hepatic artery catheter must be inserted so that the entire liver is perfused (including using two catheters if necessary). Approximately 85% of patients have a single hepatic artery supplying the liver. In this case, catheterization of the gastroduodenal artery is utilized (Fig. 1). The right gastric artery and any other branches of the hepatic artery distal to the gastroduodenal artery are ligated to prevent infusion of drug to the stomach and duodenum. Complete perfusion of the liver and absent perfusion to the intestinal tract is documented by injecting 2 ml of a 10% fluorescein solution through the catheter and exposing the upper abdominal contents with an ultraviolet (Wood's) light. In about 10%-15% of patients, there is a dual arterial blood supply with a replaced right hepatic artery arising from the superior mesenteric artery and a left hepatic artery from the celiac axis. In this situation, patients must have either a dual catheter pump or two separate

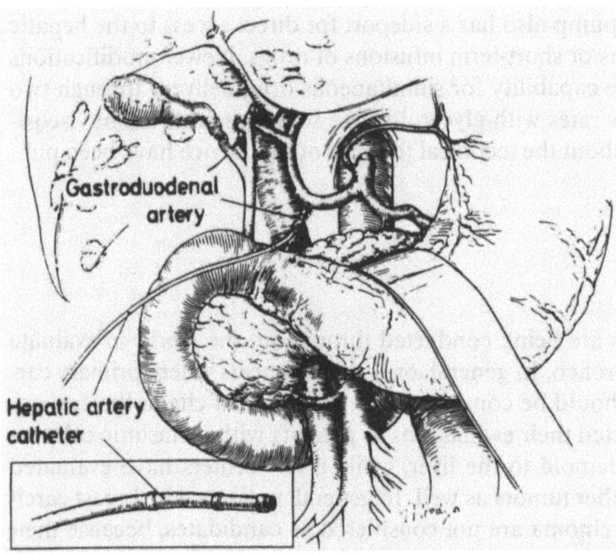

Fig. 1. Hepatic artery catheter placement in patients with standard arterial anatomy. The gastroduodenal artery is ligated and the catheter placed at the junction of the gastroduodenal artery and the hepatic artery. The right gastric artery has been ligated as well. A close-up of the beaded catheter is shown in the inset [23]

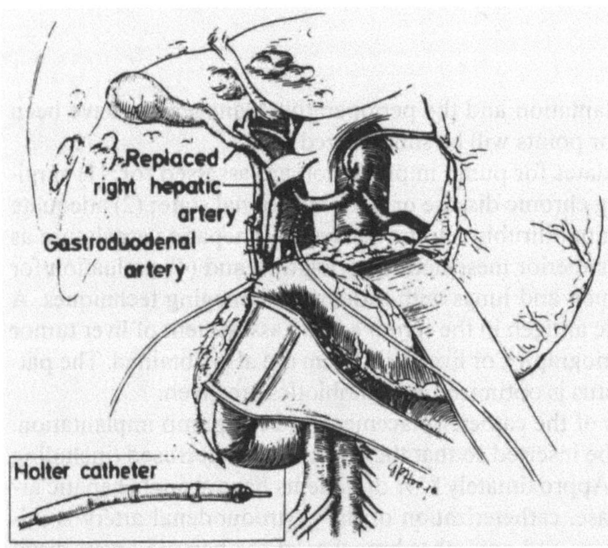

Fig. 2. Dual arterial blood supply to the liver, with a replaced right hepatic artery originating from the superior mesenteric artery and the left hepatic artery arising from the celiac axis. In this situation, it is necessary to place a catheter in each hepatic artery and use a dual catheter (arterial-arterial) Infusaid pump. A Holter catheter is used to cannulate the replaced right hepatic *(inset)* through an arteriotomy in the lateral wall of the replaced right hepatic artery. A 6-0 cardiovascular pursestring suture is placed around the arteriotomy, and the filiform tip is inserted. The catheter is then secured to the adventitia or surrounding tissues of the vessel. A second catheter is placed in the gastroduodenal artery in the usual position. The right gastric artery is ligated [23]

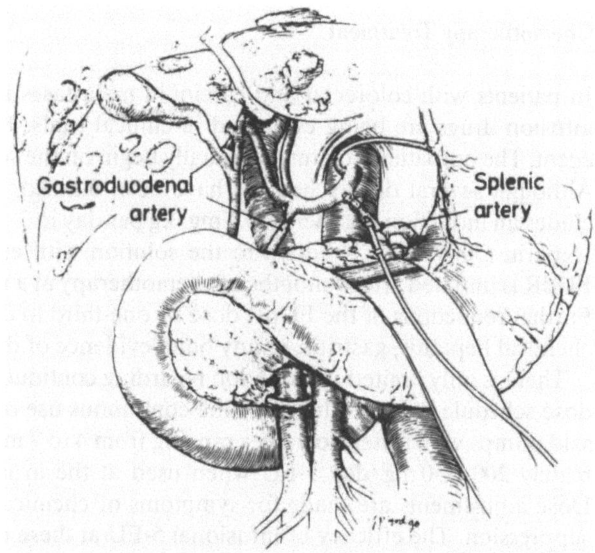

Fig. 3. Another anatomic variant requiring special catheter placement is a "trifurcation" of the hepatic branches with the gastroduodenal artery arising close to the junction of the right and left hepatic arteries. In some cases, the gastroduodenal artery actually branches from the right hepatic artery. In these instances, there would be preferential flow to the right hepatic artery if the catheter was placed in the gastroduodenal artery. To ensure equal distribution of drug to all areas of the liver, the most suitable placement is a retrograde cannulation of the splenic artery into the celiac axis. In this instance, the right and left gastric arteries and the gastroduodenal artery are ligated [23]

pumps implanted in order to perfuse the entire liver (Fig. 2). Occasionally, the gastroduodenal artery will come off the right hepatic artery or at the bifurcation of the right and left hepatic artery. In this circumstance, the best approach is to cannulate the celiac axis through the splenic artery and then ligate the left gastric artery, the gastroduodenal artery, and the right gastric artery to prevent drug infusion to the gastrointestinal tract (Fig. 3).

The Infusaid pump is implanted in a separate subcutaneous pocket of the lower abdominal wall. The hepatic artery catheter is spliced to the pump catheter over a small metal adapter. The catheter is then flushed with saline solution through the side port of the pump to ensure patency. Alternatively, the pump can be implanted in the subcutaneous pocket first and the catheter tunneled through the anterior abdominal wall. The catheter is then positioned in the gastroduodenal artery without having to splice two catheters together.

Several measures are used to minimize the risk of pump pocket infection. These include: (1) pre- and postoperative antibiotics (usually a cephalosporin), (2) shaving the abdominal wall immediately prior to surgery (rather than the night before), (3) irrigation of the pump pocket with an antibiotic solution (e.g., cloxacillin and polymyxin), (4) closure of the pump pocket incision with subcuticular sutures, and (5) occlusive plastic-film dressing over the pump pocket incision for 48 h. Using this approach, we have not had a single pump pocket infection in over 180 implantations.

Finally, a prophylactic cholecystectomy is performed to avoid symptoms of chemical cholecystitis. Previously, we have encountered both acute and chronic cholecystitis in a substantial number of patients that was induced by the FUdR chemotherapy. This potential complication, often associated with significant symptoms, can thus be prevented.

Chemotherapy Treatment

In patients with colorectal and carcinoid metastases to the liver, both FUdR and 5-FU infusion drugs are being evaluated in clinical trials. FUdR is the most commonly used agent. The outpatient treatments usually begin on the seventh or eighth postoperative day. Although several dose schedules have been utilized, our current regimen of FUdR includes an induction regimen at 0.3 mg/kg per day in 2-week cycles alternating with saline. Heparin (5000 units) is added to the solution with each refill. A maintenance dose of FUdR is initiated after 4 months of chemotherapy at a reduced dose of 0.2 mg/kg per day. Further reductions of the FUdR dose by one-third to one-half are made for symptoms of chemical hepatitis, gastritis, or any other evidence of drug toxicity.

There is only limited information regarding continuous 5-FU chemotherapy. One 5-FU dose schedule being evaluated is the continuous use of full-strength solution using Infusaid pumps with faster flow rates ranging from 4 to 7 ml/day. This would deliver approximately 200-350 mg/day 5-FU when used at the available concentration of 50 mg/ml. Dose adjustments are made for symptoms of chemical hepatitis, GI toxicity or marrow suppression. The efficacy of infusional 5-FU at these doses has not yet been proven, but preliminary results are encouraging.

Mitomycin C is often used as a supplement for patients with colorectal or carcinoid metastases. This is administered by a 1-h infusion through the side port of the pump at 10-15 mg/m^2 under any of the following conditions: (1) if the FUdR drug dose was reduced to one-half or less, (2) if there was any evidence of progression of disease in the liver, or (3) if there was any evidence of progression of disease in extrahepatic sites.

In patients who develop extrahepatic disease, intravenous (systemic) infusions of 5-FU (either 1 g/day each week or 20-30 mg/kg per day $\times$ 5 in 1-month cycles) can also be administered. This includes patients who subsequently develop multiple pulmonary metastases, abdominal carcinomatosis, or symptomatic metastases at other sites. Usually, reduced doses of FUdR regional chemotherapy are administered to the liver in alternating cycles with the 5-FU systemic chemotherapy to maintain a stable tumor response in the liver. In selected patients, extrahepatic metastases can be surgically excised (i.e., supraclavicular nodes, abdominal incision, adrenal gland). It is not uncommon for patients to develop nodal metastases along the hepatic artery or at the porta hepatis that may cause jaundice as a result of bile duct compression. These and metastases to the bone, brain, or distant lymph node sites can be treated with radiation therapy.

Regional Adriamycin chemotherapy is being evaluated for selected patients with hepatocellular carcinoma, especially those without evidence of diffuse disease arising in a cirrhotic liver. In this instance, the Infusaid pump is attached to a hepatic artery catheter to maintain catheter patency. Alternatively, an Infus-a-port can be attached to the hepatic artery and then flushed at regular intervals to maintain catheter patency [2]. The former approach is preferred, because there is some risk of thrombosis when the Infus-a-ports are used rather than a constant infusion of saline. Adriamycin is given with an externalized pump over a 2- to 4-day period, using an externalized bedside pump. We have generally used Adriamycin at a dose of 60 mg/m^2 as a constant 72-h infusion via the side port of the pump every 4-6 weeks. Patients are monitored for marrow suppression and for cardiac toxicity.

Results of Treatment

Colorectal Metastases to the Liver

The Surgical Oncology Unit at the University of Alabama in Birmingham, United States, has implanted Infusaid pumps in over 150 patients with colorectal metastases to the liver. This was a prospective phase II clinical trial evaluating continuous FUdR regional chemotherapy, supplemented with mitomycin C chemotherapy when necessary. The updated results of the first 110 consecutive patients will be summarized. Full details involving a statistical analysis of the first 81 patients have been published [4]. The results of these patients undergoing regional chemotherapy have been compared with a control population of 129 patients, whose clinical features were comparable to those undergoing pump implantation [4, 18]. The characteristics of the control patients and those treated with regional chemotherapy are shown in Table 1. The two patient groups were comparable with respect to age, sex, extent of liver metastases, and number of lobes involved.

There are several parameters used for measuring tumor response rates, such as measuring the serum levels of carcinoembryonic antigen (CEA) and the tumor dimensions by nuclear or radiological imaging techniques [21]. However, none of these parameters are sufficiently specific, reproducible, and accurate to report results. The most quantitative and reproducible end point is patient survival rates. It should be noted in passing that 88%

Table 1. Characteristics of patients

	Regional chemotherapy (110 patients)	Historical control patients (129 patients)
I. Clinical factors		
Median age (years)	57	61
Males	52%	62%
Primary tumor site		
Right colon	27%	27%
Transverse	3%	6%
Left colon	13%	9%
Rectosigmoid	57%	58%
II. Tumor features		
Lobe involvement		
Right only	31%	29%
Left only	5%	7%
Both lobes	64%	64%
Number of tumor nodules		
1	16%	20%
2-4	30%	14%
> 4	54%	66%
III. Liver function tests (at diagnosis of metastases)		
Alkaline phosphatase		
> 200 IU	75%	71%
Bilirubin < 1.0 mg%	85%	84%
CEA > 100 mg%	36%	48%

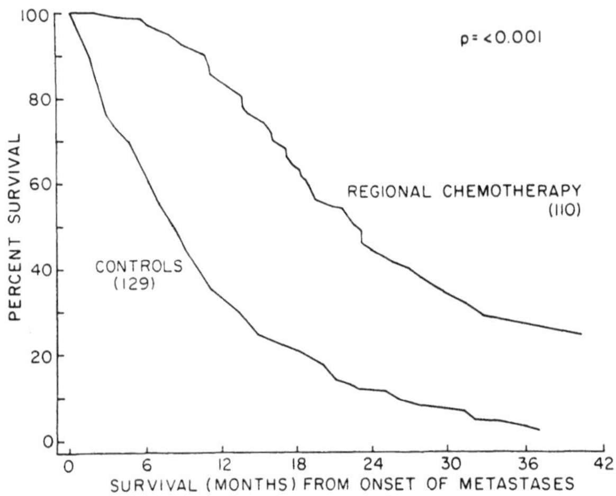

Fig. 4. Updated survival curves for 110 consecutive patients treated at the University of Alabama in Birmingham with regional chemotherapy using the Infusaid implantable pump. Those patients receiving regional chemotherapy had a significantly better survival than a historical control group of 129 patients with liver metastases not treated with regional chemotherapy ($P < 0.0001$). Characteristics of the two patient groups are listed in Table 1

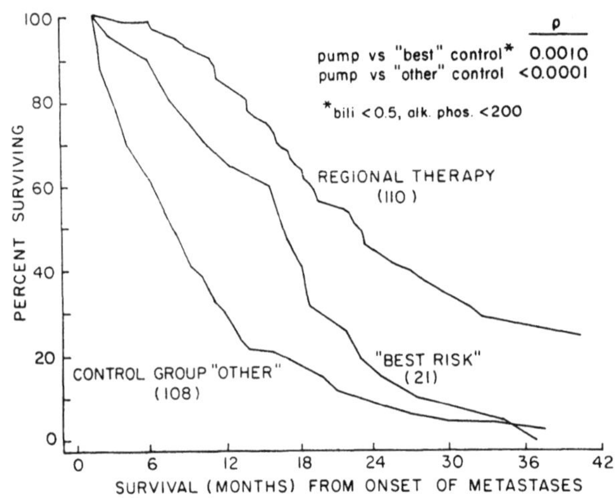

Fig. 5. The most favorable subgroup of patients from the control series was identified based upon a prognostic factors analysis [18]. The entire group of 110 pump patients (including nonresponders) had a significantly improved survival rate, compared with the "best risk" control subgroup, who had normal liver function studies, disease confined to one liver lobe, and the primary tumor resected ($P = 0.001$)

of our patients had a decrease in their preoperative CEA by one-third or more within 5 months of starting treatment. In fact, the average decrease of the CEA was 33% after 2 months of treatment and 80% after 5 months of treatment.

By four criteria, the regional chemotherapy patients had an improved survival rate compared with the control series. First, the 1-year survival and the median survival was better for the entire group of pump patients versus controls (84% versus 36%, 24 months versus 8 months, $P < 0.0001$) (Fig. 4). The survival for the regional chemotherapy patients was not influenced by the extent of tumor involvement, whether previous systemic 5-FU was given, or whether the patient had symptomatic disease [4]. Second, the entire group of regional chemotherapy patients (including nonresponders) had a greater 1-year survival compared with the most favorable subgroup of control patients with the following characteristics: normal liver function tests, no symptoms, and only one lobe involved (84% versus 66%, $P = 0.001$) (Fig. 5). Third, a subgroup of 68 pump patients, whose initial treatment for metastatic disease was regional chemotherapy (within 3 months of diagnosis) had a better

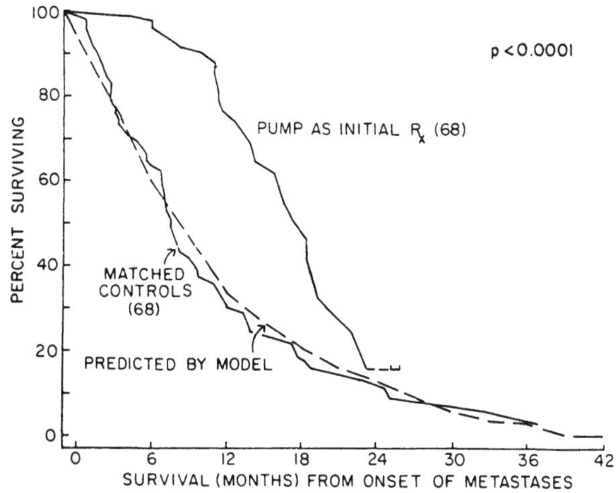

Fig. 6. A subgroup of 68 patients initially treated with regional chemotherapy was compared with an exactly matched group of 68 control patients selected by computer analysis (see Table 2). Patients receiving regional chemotherapy had an improved survival rate compared with the matched historical control ($P < 0.0001$). In addition, a mathematical formula was constructed to predict the outcome of the 68 control patients. Both the observed and predicted survival of the control series exactly coincided

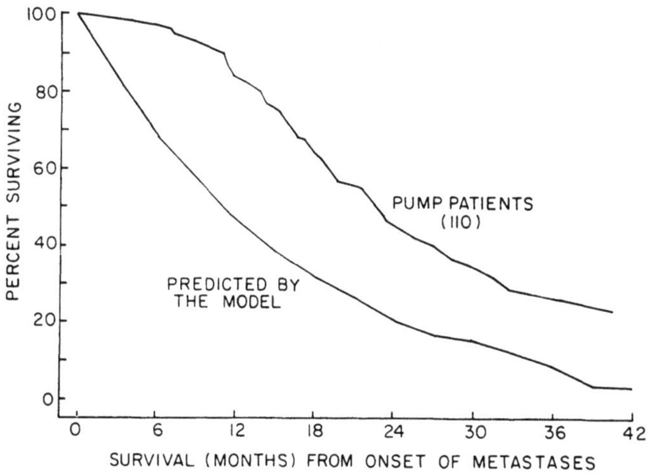

Fig. 7. A mathematical model based upon a prognostic factors analysis was constructed to predict the survival rate of the 110 pump patients. The observed survival rate for the pump patients was considerably better than that predicted by the mathematical model, presumably because of the regional chemotherapy

1-year survival than a computer-matched group of 68 control patients with the same prognostic factors (75% versus 33%, $P = < 0.0001$) (Fig. 6). This subgroup of patients was chosen because they were the most comparable with the controls, since the time of diagnosis and treatment was the same. The control patients were matched by computer with the prognostic factors of the pump patients (Table 2). Fourth, the actuarial survival for all 110 pump patients was significantly better than predicted by a mathematical model constructed to predict the patient's clinical course based upon the seven dominant prognostic variables identified in a multifactorial analysis (84% survival at 1 year versus 45% predicted survival) (Fig. 7). Presumably, this difference was due to the regional chemotherapy. The validity of the mathematical model was tested by comparing the predicted results for the 68 control patients based upon their prognostic factors with their observed results. The two curves were superimposable (Fig. 6).

Forty-eight patients (44%) have relapsed while receiving regional chemotherapy. The median time from pump implantation to first relapse was 6 months. Of these patients, only 23% showed evidence of tumor progression in the liver, despite intraarterial infusions of

Table 2. Comparison of pump patients treated at the time of initial diagnosis compared with a computer-matched control group

	Pump patients ($N=68$)	Controls ($N=68$)
Primary tumor resected	100%	100%
Alkaline phosphatase <200 IU	75%	77%
Bilirubin <1 mg%	60%	58%
Bilobar disease	77%	77%
1-3 metastatic nodes	48%	53%
Median age (years)	52	61
Males	52%	38%

Table 3. Relapses in 48 of 113 patients while receiving regional chemotherapy

Site	%
Lung	62
Abdominal nodes	32
Liver progression	23
Bone	12
Peritoneum	23
Pelvis	8
Brain	2
Other	18

Table 4. Status after 4 months of regional chemotherapy

	No S_x or Improved	Mild to Moderate S_x	Worse
Asymptomatic (⅔)	58%	36%	6%
Symptomatic (⅓)	52%	34%	13%

FUdR with or without mitomycin C. Most of these patients had progression of disease at other sites as well. The distribution of relapse sites and extrahepatic disease is shown in Table 3. The most common site was the lung, which occurred in 62% of the patients. The pulmonary metastases were treated with systemic chemotherapy, either in short-term infusions or in long-term continuous infusions using a catheter placed in a subclavian vein and connected to the drug infusion pump. The response rate was 33% in these patients. Metastases in the celiac, periportal, and retroperitoneal lymph nodes were the second most common site (32% of relapsed patients). These were generally treated by irradiation. Twelve percent of relapsed patients had bony metastases, while 8% had pelvic metastases, and one patient had brain metastases. These patients were generally treated with irradiation if they were symptomatic.

An independent observer evaluated each patient's life-style by personal interview to determine what changes had occurred prior to pump implantation and after 4 months of regional chemotherapy. The patients' symptoms of disease, drug toxicity, employability status, leisure time activity, and level of physical activity were ascertained. About one-third of the patients were symptomatic at the time of presentation (Table 4). After 4 months of treatment, 52% improved or became asymptomatic, 36% remained symptomatic (either because of the tumor or drug toxicity) but maintained a fairly normal level of physical activity, while 13% of the symptomatic patients became worse, usually because of tumor progression. Two-thirds of the patients were either asymptomatic or had only mild symptoms of their disease at the time of pump implantation. After 4 months of treatment, 58% remained asymptomatic; 36% had moderate symptoms (usually due to drug toxicity), but maintained a normal but slightly reduced level of physical activity, while 6% had significant symptoms interfering with their quality of life. Over 72% of employable patients returned to their work on either a part-time or a full-time basis. Many patients became symptomatic later in the course of treatment, usually due to disease progression or due to chronic symptoms of chemical hepatitis.

The implanted pump itself did not cause symptoms or interfere significantly with physical activites of any of the patients. A few had a physical awareness of the pump, especially when bending or stooping. No patient experienced pain or discomfort from the implanted device.

None of the patients had systemic toxicity while receiving FUdR alone, although some had marrow suppression, nausea, or diarrhea with regional mitomycin C infusions or with systemic chemotherapy. None had thrombosis of the hepatic artery, pump malfunction, catheter migration, pump pocket infection, or intraabdominal abscess. While most patients had chemical hepatitis, with elevations of serum liver chemistries, this was only clinically significant in half of them. About one-third of patients became jaundiced due to chemical hepatitis during the course of treatment. This risk increased proportionately with the duration and dose of the FUdR regional chemotherapy.

Hepatocellular Carcinoma

A consecutive series of 13 patients with histologically confirmed unresectable hepatomas were treated with regional adriamycin chemotherapy through a hepatic artery catheter. A Model 400 Infusaid pump was used to maintain catheter patency with saline between drug cycles. Three of 13 patients had chronic active hepatitis, four of 13 had hepatoma arising in a cirrhotic liver, and 4 of 13 had elevated alphafetoprotein levels. Patients received 60 mg/m^2 Adriamycin as a constant 72-h infusion via the side port of the pump every 4-6 weeks. There were no mechanical pump failures; one patient required early catheter replacement because of occlusion. Five of 13 patients developed cardiotoxicity and later received other drugs intraarterially. Only three patients developed total alopecia, and one patient required delay in treatment because of bone marrow toxicity. Six of 13 patients showed a decrease in tumor size by CT scan or ultrasound, while 6 of 13 had stable disease and one of 13 had progression on adriamycin therapy. Sixty-five percent of patients were alive at 1 year, while the median survival was 20 months. This compares to an expected median survival of only 6-10 months in most published series. This trial is continuing.

Experience at Other Institutions

Our experience is similar to that published by several other series using the Infusaid implantable drug infusion pump and the dose schedules of FUdR and mitomycin C described above. At the University of Michigan Medical Center the response rate was 83% for 93 treated patients, with a median duration of response of 13 months and a median survival of 25 months from the diagnosis of liver metastases [24]. Patients with extrahepatic disease treated with regional chemotherapy had a lower response rate (74%) and median survival (14 months). When calculated from the time of pump implantation, the median survival for patients with liver metastases only was 18 months, while those with liver plus other sites of metastases had a median survival of only 8 months (Fig. 8). Forty-five percent of these patients had failed prior systemic chemotherapy. In patients with metastatic colorectal cancer involving only the liver, regional chemotherapy provided excellent control of hepatic tumors, and none of the patients died solely as a result of uncontrolled tumor in the liver. In fact, progressive extrahepatic disease occurred in 75% of patients who relapsed, while their liver tumor remained stable. As in the Alabama series, the most common site of extrahepatic progression of disease was the lung or extrahepatic sites in the abdomen.

The University of California in San Diego Medical Center had a 67% response rate, with a median survival of 8 months in 18 patients treated with combined intraarterial regional chemotherapy and hepatic irradiation [5]. The ten patients with liver function tests less than twice normal had a median survival of about 25 months, while the 8 patients with liver function tests more than twice normal had a median survival of only 6 months ($P = 0.02$).

At the Massachusetts General Hospital, Cohen and colleagues have used a transaxillary hepatic artery in conjunction with the Infusaid implantable drug infusion pump. This approach permits the implantation of the catheter and the pump under local anesthesia or

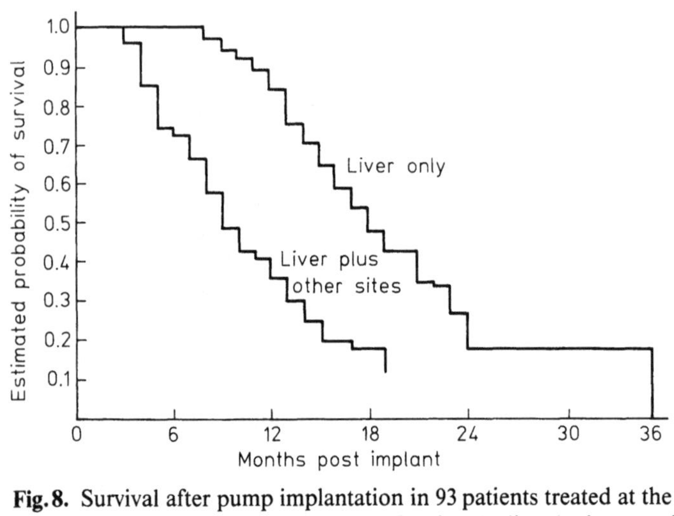

Fig. 8. Survival after pump implantation in 93 patients treated at the University of Michigan Medical Center. Patients with metastases confined to the liver had a more favorable outcome with regional chemotherapy compared with patients who had extrahepatic metastases at the time of pump implantation. The results are quite similar to those obtained at the University of Alabama in Birmingham as shown in Fig. 6 [24]

light general anesthesia [11, 12, 13]. The median survival for these patients was about 12 months after pump implantation, but many of these patients had more advanced disease (including some with incipient liver failure) compared with those in the Alabama and Michigan series. Complications were greater as well, including catheter migration and gastritis probably due to perfusion of FUdR through the right gastric artery.

At the University of Chicago, Levine and colleagues have implanted the Infusaid pump in 57 patients [20]. Their median survival from the onset of diagnosis was 23 months. They noted a 30% response using a 50% reduction in size by CT scanning, with a combination of dichloromethotrexate and FUdR. In their study, however, the FUdR was used at a dose one-half of that used in the Alabama and Michigan series. In addition, those patients with "stable" response by CT scanning had the same survival as those with a 50% reduction in size by CT scanning. In our opinion, CT scanning underestimates tumor size because some tumors may undergo necrosis and scarring rather than significant reduction in overall tumor mass. For this reason, survival is the more appropriate end point than measuring response rate by tumor imaging or CEA monitoring.

Weiss and associates from the Dana Farber-Harvard Group reported a partial response in only 30% of 17 patients with colon cancer assessed by computed tomography [32]. In this study, however, the substantial number of the patients did not have complete perfusion of the liver, indicating inadequate regional chemotherapy. Moreover, survival from the time of pump implantation was significantly better than a small control series of patients who did not undergo pump implantation, when calculated from the time of surgical evaluation.

Summary and Future Directions

Regional intraarterial chemotherapy for treating liver tumors is not a curative approach, but appears to achieve significant palliation in many patients, both in terms of quality and quantity of life. These results are somewhat better than those previously published using externalized arterial catheters and portable pumps. These earlier trials using externalized catheters have significant technical limitations, including vascular thrombosis, that limited their long-term usage. The major difference using the implantable drug delivery system is that long-term chemotherapy can now be given on a continuous basis with little or no risk of thrombosis, catheter migration, or infection.

The results described above demonstrate some significant limitations of regional chemotherapy. FUdR is efficiently extracted by the liver, so that extrahepatic sites are undertreated. Thus, while liver metastases could be controlled in most patients, the major cause of death was tumor progression in extrahepatic sites, particularly lung metastases and abdominal carcinomatosis.

Another approach for treating liver metastases is continuous systemic infusional chemotherapy with FUdR or 5-FU. Clinical trials to evaluate this are now in progress. Preliminary results from a randomized prospective trial involving 45 patients with liver metastases from colorectal carcinoma indicate no difference in survival rates or response rates in patients receiving continuous intraarterial versus intravenous chemotherapy [16, 17]. However, the data results are too early to make any definitive conclusions.

It should be emphasized that the clinical investigations published to date are nonrandomized prospective (phase II) clinical trials. Despite the fact that the results are encouraging, they must be confirmed by a randomized control series. The Hepatic Tumor Study Group has initiated a multi-institutional randomized prospective trial comparing regional

FUdR chemotherapy versus systemic 5-FU chemotherapy versus combined regional and systemic chemotherapy. A number of other clinical trials are ongoing, both in the United States and in Europe.

With respect to hepatocellular carcinoma, a pilot experience with 15 patients demonstrated that a 72-h Adriamycin infusion through a hepatic artery catheter is associated with a high response rate and prolongs survival compared with historical controls. The Infusaid pump was used to maintain catheter patency. Patients with diffuse hepatocellular carcinoma arising in a cirrhotic liver were specifically excluded from this study. Further experience with this approach is necessary to confirm these results.

Virtually all investigators using the Infusaid pump have found it to be a reliable, safe drug delivery device that represents a remarkable technological achievement as a drug delivery system. However, much work remains in learning how to use this device in an optimal fashion for cancer chemotherapy, how to use optimal dose schedules of various antimetabolites, and how to ascertain the optimal routes of administration (intraarterial, intravenous, or combined). It seems likely that current clinical trials now in progress and future investigations will allow a more rational and more effective use of this implantable drug delivery system.

Acknowledgments. This work was supported by PHS grants CA-33988 and RR-00032-24 awarded by the National Cancer Institute, DHHS. Dr. Balch is an American Cancer Society Professor of Clinical Oncology and Dr. Urist holds a Junior Faculty Fellowship from the American Cancer Society.

References

1. Ansfield FJ, Ramirez G, Davis HL, Jr, Wirtanen GW, Johnson RO, Bryan GT, Manalo FB, Borden EC, Davis TE, Esmaili M (1975) Further clinical studies with intrahepatic arterial infusion with 5-fluorouracil. Cancer 36: 2413
2. Balch CM, Urist MM (1983) Vollständig implantierbare Infusionspumpe. Eine neue Behandlungsmöglichkeit für ausgewählte Patienten mit Lebertumoren. Dtsch Med Wochenschr 108: 1008
3. Balch CM, Urist MD, McGregor ML (1983 a) Continuous regional chemotherapy for metastatic colorectal cancer using a totally implantable infusion pump: a feasibility study in 50 patients. Am J Surg 145: 285
4. Balch CM, Urist MM, Soong S-J, McGregor ML (1983 b) A prospective phase II clinical trial of continuous FUDR regional chemotherapy for colorectal metastases to the liver using a totally implantable drug infusion pump. Ann Surg 198: 567
5. Barone RM, Byfield JE, Goldfarb PB, Frankel S, Ginn C, Greer S (1982) Intra-arterial chemotherapy using an implantable infusion pump and liver irradiation for the treatment of hepatic metastases. Cancer 50: 850
6. Blackshear PJ (1979) Implantable drug-delivery systems. Sci Am 241: 66
7. Blackshear PJ, Dorman FD, Blackshear PL Jr, Varco RL, Buchwald H (1972) The design and initial testing of an implantable infusion pump. Surg Gynecol Obstet 134: 51
8. Cady B (1973) Hepatic arterial patency and complications after catheterization for infusion chemotherapy. Ann Surg 178: 156
9. Cady B, Oberfield RA (1974) Regional infusion chemotherapy of hepatic metastases from carcinoma of the colon. Am J Surg 127: 220
10. Clouse ME, Ahmed R, Ryan RB, Oberfield RA, McCaffrey JA (1977) Complications of long-term transbrachial hepatic arterial infusion chemotherapy. AJR 129: 799
11. Cohen AM (1984) Massachusetts General Hospital Infusaid pump experience. Presented at thirteenth annual cancer course: infusional cancer chemotherapy. Techniques and clinical trials in systemic and regional chemotherapy. Harvard Medical School, March 1-3

12. Cohen AM, Greenfield A, Wood WC, Waltman A, Novelline R, Athanasoulis C, Schaeffer NJ (1983a) Treatment of hepatic metastases by transaxillary hepatic artery chemotherapy using an implanted drug pump. Cancer 51: 2013
13. Cohen AM, Kaufman SD, Wood WC, Greenfield AJ (1983b) Regional hepatic chemotherapy using an implantable drug infusion pump. Am J Surg 145: 529
14. Dorr RT, Trinca CE, Griffith K, Dombrowsky PL, Salmon SE (1979) Limitations of a portable infusion pump in ambulatory patients receiving continuous infusions of anticancer drugs. Cancer Treat Rep 63: 211
15. Ensminger WD, Rosowsky A, Raso V, Levin DC, Glode M, Come S, Steele G, Frei E III (1978) A clinical-pharmacological evaluation of hepatic arterial infusions of 5-fluoro-2'-deoxyuridine and 5-fluorouracil. Cancer Res 38: 3784
16. Kemeny N (1983) The systemic chemotherapy of hepatic metastases. Semin Oncol 10: 148
17. Kemeny N (1984) A randomized study of intrahepatic vs systemic infusion of fluorodeoxyuridine in patients with liver metastases from colorectal carcinoma. Presented at thirteenth annual cancer course: infusional cancer chemotherapy. Techniques and clinical trials in systemic and regional chemotherapy. Harvard Medical School, March 1-3
18. Lahr CJ, Soong S-J, Cloud G, Smith JW, Urist MM, Balch CM (1983) A multifactorial analysis of prognostic factors in patients with liver metastases from colorectal carcinoma. J Clin Oncol 1: 720
19. Legha SS, Benjamin RS, Mackay B, Ewer M, Wallace S, Valdivieso M, Rasmussen SL, Blumenschein GR, Freireich EJ (1982) Reduction of doxorubicin cardiotoxicity by prolonged continuous intravenous infusion. Ann Int Med 96: 133
20. Levin B (1984) Therapy of metastatic colorectal cancer with hepatic artery infusion chemotherapy using a subcutaneous implanted pump: University of Chicago experience. Presented at thirteenth annual cancer course: infusional cancer chemotherapy. Techniques and clinical trials in systemic and regional chemotherapy, Harvard Medical School, March 1-3
21. Lokich JJ (1983) Determination of response in treatment of hepatic neoplasia. Semin Oncol 10: 228
22. Lokich JJ (1984) Hepatic artery chemotherapy: the relative importance of direct organ distribution vs. the constant-infusion schedule. American J Clin Oncol 7: 125
23. Niederhuber JE, Ensminger WD (1983) Surgical considerations in the management of hepatic neoplasia. Semin Oncol 10: 135-147
24. Niederhuber JE, Ensminger WD, Gyves J, Thrall J, Walker S, Cozzi E (1984) Regional chemotherapy of colorectal cancer metastatic to the liver. Cancer 53: 1336-1343
25. Oberfield RA, McCaffrey JA, Polio J, Clouse ME, Hamilton T (1979) Prolonged and continuous percutaneous intra-arterial hepatic infusion chemotherapy in advanced metastatic liver adenocarcinoma from colorectal primary. Cancer 44: 414
26. Patt YZ, Mavligit GM, Chuang VP, Wallace S, Johnston S, Benjamin RS, Valdivieso M, Hersh EM (1980) Percutaneous hepatic arterial infusion (HAI) of mitomycin C and floxuridine (FUDR): an effective treatment for metastatic colorectal carcinoma in the liver. Cancer 46: 261
27. Petrek JA, Minton JP (1979) Treatment of hepatic metastases by percutaneous hepatic arterial infusion. Cancer 43: 2182
28. Reed ML, Vaitkevicius VK, Al-Sarraf M, Vaughn CB, Singhakowinta A, Sexon-Porte M, Izbicki R, Baker L, Straatsma GW (1981) The practicality of chronic hepatic artery infusion therapy of primary and metastatic hepatic malignancies: ten year results of 124 patients in a prospective protocol. Cancer 47: 402
29. Seifert P, Baker LH, Reed ML, Vaitkevicius VK (1975) Comparison of continuously infused 5-fluorouracil with bolus injection in treatment of patients with colorectal adenocarcinoma. Cancer 36: 123
30. Sullivan RD, Norcross JW, Watkins E, Jr (1964) Chemotherapy of metastatic liver cancer by prolonged hepatic-artery infusion. N Engl J Med 270: 321
31. Watkins E Jr, Khazei AM, Nahra KS (1970) Surgical basis for arterial infusion chemotherapy of disseminated carcinoma of the liver. Surg Gynecol Obstet 130: 581
32. Wiess GR, Garnick MB, Osteen RT, Steele GD, Jr, Wilson RE, Schade D, Kaplan WD, Boxt LM, Kandarpa K, Mayer RJ, Frei ET III (1983) Long-term hepatic arterial infusion of 5-fluorodeoxyuridine for liver metastases using an implantable infusion pump. J Clin Oncol 1: 337

Vascular Access to Liver Tumors

Vascular Patterns of Liver Tumors and Their Consequences for Different Therapeutic Approaches

N. B. Ackerman and W. B. Hodgson

Department of Surgery, Metropolitan Hospital Center New York,
New York and Valhalla, NY, USA

In the therapeutic management of both primary and metastatic liver tumors vascularity assumes a major importance. The circulation of these tumors constitutes a pathway for the delivery of antitumor agents. In addition, the possibility of diminishing or eliminating oxygenation and blood flow to these tumors depends on knowledge of the vascularity. The vascularity of the liver tumors is more complicated than that of most other tumors because of the presence of both arterial and portal circulations. Both systems may play a role in the perfusion of tumors and arterioportal and arteriovenous shunting may further complicate the picture. Reestablishment of tumor circulation through collateral vessels and internal shunting soon after arterial occlusion is another major aspect of this subject.

The extent of vascularity, in both animal and human liver tumors, has a range varying from virtual avascularity to extreme hypervascularity. Changes occur as the tumors develop and grow. In addition, there is some evidence that tumor vessels may respond differently to chemical and physical changes than vessels of the host liver tissue.

Histological Types of Liver Tumors

The liver is a fertile soil for the development of malignant tumors. Primary cancers including hepatocellular and cholangiocarcinoma tumors vary significantly in regard to size, extent of involvement within the liver and degree of cellularity and stroma. Metastatic tumors are even more variable. The liver is the most frequent site for metastatic disease of tumors within the peritoneal cavity. In addition to adenocarcinomas, which are most common, other tumors include squamous cell carcinomas, carcinoids, sarcomas, lymphomas, melanomas, and functioning tumors from the glandular structures. The relationship of vascularity of liver tumors to the histological appearance has not been extensively studied.

Angiographic Variations of Liver Tumors

Vascularity of liver tumors may encompass a wide range of patterns in both experimental animals and patients. In patients, there have been several attempts to classify these patterns as to degree of vascularity. Suzuki and colleagues [23] performed microangiograms on patient specimens and classified their results. Grade 1 tumors were tumors that were almost avascular, grade 2 tumors were hypovascular, grade 3 tumors were more vascular

Recent Results in Cancer Research. Vol 100

than the surrounding areas of the liver, and grade 4 tumors were exceptionally vascular. Angiograms of grade 1 tumors showed only displacement and stretching of existing arteries. Thirteen percent of cancers were in this group. Grade 2 tumors included 23% of patients. Angiograms showed narrowing and irregular contours, and although some tumor vessels were seen, a tumor stain was not apparent during the capillary and venous stages. The grade 3 cancers included 39% of patients, and angiograms demonstrated an increased vascularity with irregular, tortuous vessels. There were 12% of patients at the grade 4 level. Angiograms of these patients showed extreme hypervascularity, with a chaotic arrangement of vessels with an intense tumor stain. The correlation between primary sites of the metastatic tumors and the angiographic grades was not clear cut.

Other investigators have tried to correlate the degree of vascularity with primary site of the metastatic tumor. Bragg [12] noted that renal cell carcinomas, leiomyosarcomas, carcinoids, and islet cell and papillary cell tumors of the pancreas tended to be more vascular than other tumors. Adenocarcinomas from the stomach, pancreas, and breast, and tumors from the lung, adrenal glands, and melanomas were usually avascular. This is, however, a generalization and other factors such as size and cellularity may be more significant.

Vascular Patterns in Experimental Tumors

Hepatic angiograms have been performed in experimental animals with implanted intrahepatic tumors. Assa [10] performed angiograms on rabbits with VX2 tumors implanted in the liver. Arterial vascularity differed widely, but in all animals portal venography demonstrated an absence of portal circulation in the tumors. Hypervascularity was seen when the implanted tissues were harvested from tumors growing in the donor animals for not more than 14 days. Relatively avascular tumors occurred when donor animals had tumors growing for at least 21 days. There were histological differences in the tumors from these two groups of donors.

Studies by Kido [18] graphically demonstrated the changes in vascularity with growth. These angiographic studies were performed on rats with implanted intrahepatic Walker carcinosarcoma tumors. During the first few days after implantation specific tumor vascularity was not apparent. The first vascular changes involved dilatation and tortuosity of vessels, and small encircling vessels became apparent. Over the next few days with increasing tumor growth new vessel formation occurred with continued encircling of the surface of the tumor. Connections between these encircling vessels became prominent. With further growth, the irregular pattern of vascularity on the tumor surface continued, but partial to complete avascularity was noted within the tumors.

Considerable work has been carried out in the investigations of vascular patterns of experimental tumors using pigmented silicone rubber (Microfil) injected into arterial and portal circulations. The tumors in these studies were Walker carcinosarcomas implanted in the liver of rats. In these studies of Ackerman [1] tumors measuring less than 1 mm in diameter had not developed any new vessel formation. With growth beyond this point, single, newly formed vessels began to encircle the tumors. The vessels were derived from either arteriolar or portal circulation in a completely random fashion. With further growth more vessels developed and in some specimens both arteriolar and portal vessels were involved, with mixing of the two circulations. As tumors continued to grow, reaching a size of between 5 and 7 mm in diameter, the encircling plexus became more extensive and better developed. As this occurred, the arterial circulation became predominant and in most specimens no portal circulation was seen (Fig. 1). In some of these specimens a very minor

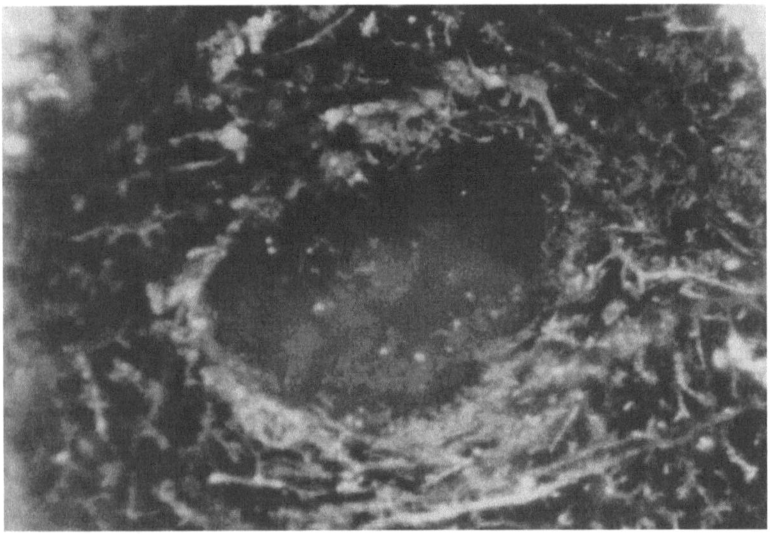

Fig. 1. Walker carcinosarcoma implanted in the liver of rat. Studied by perfused Microfil. The encircling plexus of vessels is derived from arterial circulation

portal component to the tumor circulation could be identified, usually in one small segment of the encircling plexus [22]. In general, portal vessels were compressed or displaced as the tumors grew. The tumor vessels were characterized as irregular in diameter, tortuous, and convoluted. With tumors of this size, central portions were generally avascular or at the most there were a few small vessels derived from the arterial circulation penetrating into the central portion.

In these studies, with further growth to massive size, a chaotic vascular picture became apparent [1]. In these tumors, which were as large as 33 × 33 mm in size, vascularity was usually markedly decreased. However, either arterial or portal circulations contributed to the vascularity of the tumors and it was often mixed. Vascularity surrounding the tumors varied from sparse to very dense. Central areas tended to be relatively avascular.

Effects of Drugs and Physical Conditions on Vascularity

There have been some attempts to change the circulatory pattern of liver tumors in patients with the use of vasoactive drugs. Most of these studies have been in conjunction with attempts to improve visualization of the tumors during angiography. Epinephrine has been used in some of these studies. As noted by Kahn et al. [17], epinephrine produced an intense vasoconstriction of the liver for about 15 s, followed by a gradual hyperemia with an increased diameter of arteries, an increase in blood flow, and a greater opacification of the veins. While the vessels leading to the tumors appeared to be less responsive, relatively vascular tumors were diagnosed more easily because of the increased blood flow. Avascular tumors were less responsive.

Experience with tolazoline (Priscoline) in patients with liver tumors was reported by Goldstein and associates [14]. Hepatic arterial blood flow increased with Priscoline and in some patients increased vascularity and staining of the metastatic liver tumors became ap-

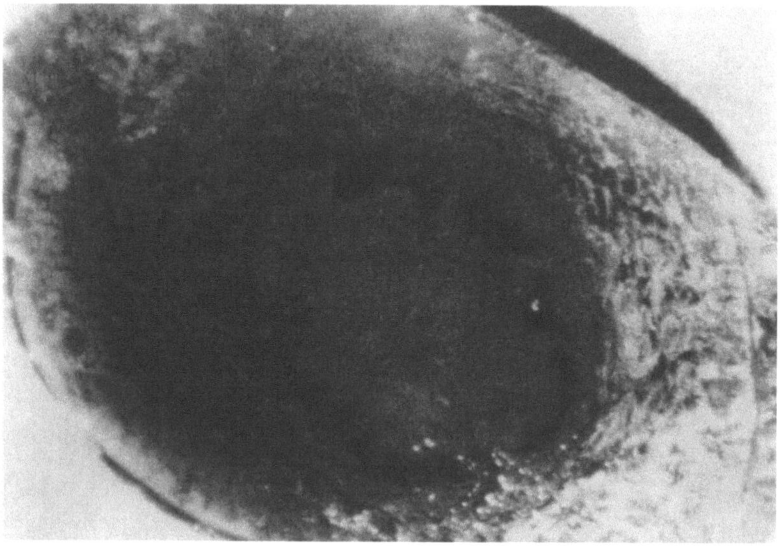

Fig. 2. Increased arterial vascularity of the encircling plexus as well as within the central area of a Walker tumor after administration of epinephrine

parent. A hypervascular effect in the encircling plexus around the metastatic tumors was often identified, resulting in an improved diagnosis of these tumors.

Considerable work has been accomplished observing the effects of certain vasoactive drugs on the perfusion of tumors in rats. Tumors studied were intrahepatic implants of Walker Sarcoma. As reported by Ackerman and Hechmer [3], epinephrine administered intraarterially immediately before Microfil injection resulted in increased perfusion of vessels in the encircling plexus as well as a very intense increase in vascularity within the central areas of the tumors (Fig. 2). Without epinephrine, these central regions appeared avascular. Epinephrine injected within the portal system produced a similar effect. This increased vascularity was noted both in moderate-sized tumors averaging 5-7 mm in diameter as well as in massive-sized tumors averaging 14 × 18 mm in size. The vessels in the central areas of the tumors were small and irregular, and measured 6-8 μm in diameter. In some specimens a structureless area was seen, possibly representing a vascular lake or cellular necrosis.

The effect produced by epinephrine is not totally understood. This effect was blocked by administration of phenoxybenzamine but not by propranolol [6]. Possible mechanisms involved may include changes in arterioportal shunting around the tumor with increased internal flow or acute production of decreased interstitial pressure within the tumors. Other experimental studies with epinephrine have been more variable [15, 16]. Some investigators have had similar experience while others have not identified this increase in vascularity. Variations in experimental design may account for these differences.

Norepinephrine has generally produced a decrease in tumor vascularity and perfusion [24]. In studies with Microfil by Ackerman et al. [8], central vascularity of the tumors was decreased (Fig. 3). However, some investigators have reported an increase in vascularity with norepinephrine using different experimental techniques [15].

There have been studies with other vasoactive drugs and Microfil, but the changes in tumor vascularity were less impressive that that seen with epinephrine [8]. Some increases in

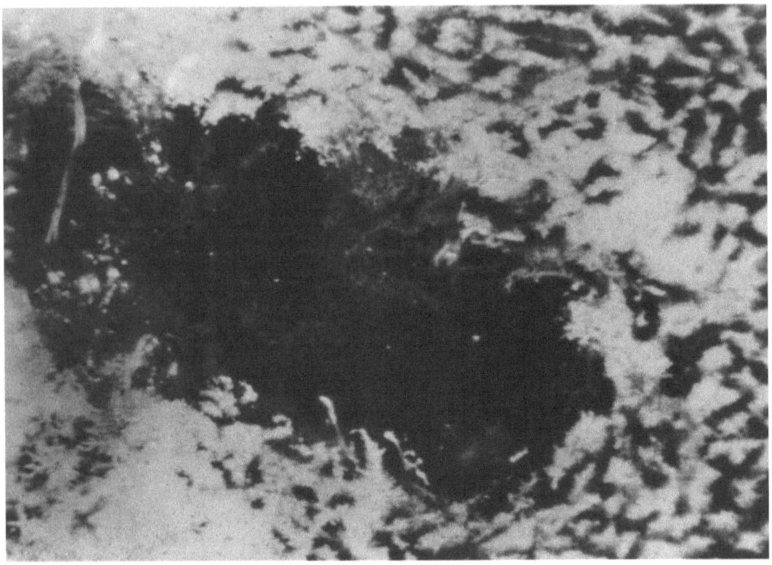

Fig. 3. Decreased vascularity of a Walker sarcoma after administration of norepinephrine

vascularity were seen with glucagon, bradykinin, and vasopressin. Decreased perfusion within the tumors was seen with histamine, lidocaine, angiotensin, and acetylcholine. The possibility of improving the delivery of chemotherapeutic agents to the liver tumors with the use of an appropriate vasoactive drug such as epinephrine warrants further research in this field.

The effects of extremes of temperature on tumor vascular perfusion have also been studied by Ackerman and Makohon [4]. The vascular perfusion of experimental tumors decreased when tumors were cooled to 5 °C. However, when these tumors were frozen with liquid nitrogen and then allowed to thaw, significant acute increases in tumor vascularity were seen both in the encircling vessels as well as within the tumors. However, it would be expected that, in time, blood flow to tumors exposed either to extreme heat or to freezing would decrease as increased permeability, viscosity, and thrombosis occurred.

The permeability of tumor vessels probably plays an important role in the uptake of antitumor agents. The neovascular circulation formed as the tumor grows apparently is more permeable than vessels in host tissues [2]. These tumor vessels lack a definite smooth muscle layer and have only an endothelial lining. In some of these vessels the endothelial lining is defective. There are fenestrations present in the walls of the vessels and increases in permeability may be related to these structural changes. There is also some evidence of permeability-promoting factors produced by the tumors. The tumor vessels are not responsive to chemical agents which are known to produce increased permeability in other vessels. As reported by Ackerman et al. [7], administration of histamine, bradykinin, or serotonin to experimental animals with intrahepatic Walker tumors produced increased permeability in the normal liver vessels but no increase within the tumor. It has been speculated that the fenestrations may be maximally opened in these vessels and may not respond further. Antiinflammatory drugs including antagonists to histamine and serotonin have decreased tumor permeability, and similar results were seen with steroids and nonsteroidial antiinflammatory drugs including indomethacin, phenylbutazone, ibuprofen, and naproxan [5].

Permeability of the tumor vessels has been increased by changes in physical conditions. Reactive hyperemia produced by temporary arterial occlusion produced a relatively short-lasting increase in tumor vessel permeability, seen at 5 min after releasing the occlusion but not at 30 min or 6 h [7]. More impressive changes were produced by freezing the tumors with liquid nitrogen and permitting thawing, as reported by Ackerman and Makohon [4]. This effect occurred rapidly and persisted as long as 24 h. This is probably due to direct damage produced in the endothelial lining. Extreme hyperthermia produced similar results. Interestingly, temperatures increased to 40 °C had no effect on vascular permeability, but at 43 °C major increases in permeability occurred in studies by Lefor et al. [21]. This is of particular interest since 40 °C is not an effective dose therapeutically, but 43 °C is within the therapeutic range. This increase in permeability with development of vascular stasis and decreased blood flow to tumors may play a role in the therapeutic effect of hyperthermia.

When vascular perfusion of tumors is improved by the use of certain chemical and physical changes, it becomes apparent that these tumors often have a well-developed vascular structure within the central internal areas. It is not known why these vessels are not ordinarily perfused. One possibility is related to high interstitial pressures within the tumors. That these pressures may be elevated is not unreasonable considering the increased vascular permeability of tumor vessels, the absence of lymphatic vessels within the tumors, and the pseudoencapsulation around the tumors. Studies on the measurement of tumor interstitial pressure are currently underway. Preliminary results measuring pressures within metastatic liver tumors of patients have demonstrated pressures more than 7.5 times higher than in the surrounding normal liver tissue. It is conceivable that if interstitial pressures could be reduced, perfusion of the tumors could be enhanced.

Relationships of Vascularity to Chemotherapy, Embolism, and Vessel Ligation

Nonexcisional approaches to liver tumors have generally involved administration of chemotherapeutic agents into the blood stream or interruption of the vessels feeding the tumors. Obviously these techniques are dependent upon a satisfactory blood supply leading to the tumor. The use of hepatic artery infusion to deliver chemotherapeutic agents more directly to liver tumors has been in practice for many years. There has been some recent interest in using the portal system or the obliterated umbilical vein for the same purpose. Attempts have been made to decrease perfusion of these tumors by hepatic artery ligation or dearterialization. A combination of hepatic artery ligation with simultaneous infusion of chemotherapeutic agents distal to the ligation has also been employed. Other techniques used to decrease arterial blood supply to the tumors have involved the use of embolization techniques with a variety of embolic substances. The study by Kim and associates [19] clearly demonstrated the importance of a good vascular supply to liver tumors in terms of improved survival time. Patients were treated by a combination of hepatic artery ligation and distal hepatic artery infusion chemotherapy. The results indicated that survival time was greater in patients with more vascular tumors, both primary or metastatic. For example, patients with highly vascular metastases from colon carcinomas had an average survival time of 17 months compared with 7.2 months survival time in those with less vascular tumors. This is the only study, thus far, that suggests this relationship.

As a consequence of vascular interruption procedures and infusion therapy changes in the patterns of vascularity often occurred. Blood flow studies by Gelin et al. [13] at the time of operation when the hepatic artery was acutely ligated demonstrated a decreased flow to 66% of control levels in the normal liver, and a decrease in flow to 8% of control levels in the liver tumors. Portal perfusion of liver tumors increased during this time. Hemorrhage and gas formation can be identified in some of these tumors on angiographic and dynamic CT scans after vascular embolization. Unfortunately, collateral arterial flow to the liver developed rapidly and may account for the limited success of this therapeutic technique. Studies by Bengmark and Rosengren [11] and by Koehler et al. [20] identified collateral flow developing as early as 4 days in the former study and as early as 4 h after ligation in the latter study. Collaterals developed from pancreaticoduodenal, phrenicoabdominal, intercostal, and gastroduodenal arteries as well as from the proximal part of the main hepatic artery.

Similar results were seen in studies on experimental animals with implanted Walker tumors in the liver. Collateral flow was identified from peritoneal adhesions to the liver. Studies by Ackerman et al. [9] with Microfil injected intraportally after acute hepatic artery ligation demonstrated filling of the encircling plexus of the tumors via the portal vein in half the animals studied. The portal system may be able to assume a role in the nourishment of these tumors after hepatic artery interruption. In spite of the fact that most primary and metastatic tumors have a predominately arterial circulation, it is difficult to dearterialize these tumors completely because of the adaptation in terms of collateral formation and shunting. However, these procedures when applied in appropriate cases have provided significant palliation and prolongation of life.

References

1. Ackerman NB (1974) The blood supply of experimental liver metastases. IV. Changes in vascularity with increasing tumor growth. Surgery 75: 589-596
2. Ackerman NB, Hechmer PA (1978) Studies on the capillary permeability of experimental liver metastases. Surg Gynecol Obstet 146: 884-888
3. Ackerman NB, Hechmer PA (1980) The blood supply of experimental liver metastases. V. Increased tumor perfusion with epinephrine. Am J Surg 140: 625-631
4. Ackerman NB, Makohon S (1981) The effects of cooling, freezing and thawing on vascular permeability and perfusion in experimental liver metastases. Surg Gynecol Obstet 152: 262-267
5. Ackerman NB, Makohon S (1982) The effects of steroidal and non-steroidal anti-inflammatory agents on vascular permeability in intrahepatic tumors. Int J Microcirc 1: 254
6. Ackerman NB, Makohon S (1984) The blood supply of experimental liver metastases. VII. Further studies on increased tumor vascularity caused by epinephrine. Microcirc Endothel Lymph 1: 547-568
7. Ackerman NB, Hechmer PA, Makohon S (1980) Failure of histamine type mediators to enhance vascular permeability in experimental liver metastases. Surg Gynecol Obstet 151: 647-651
8. Ackerman NB, Hechmer PA, Makohon S (1982) The blood supply of experimental liver metastases. VI. Comparison of the effects of epinephrine and other catecholamines on tumor vascularity. Microcirculation 2: 111-125
9. Ackerman NB, Lien WM, Silverman NA (1972) The blood supply of experimental liver metastases. III. The effects of acute ligation of the hepatic artery or portal vein. Surgery 71: 636-641
10. Assa J (1970) Differential patterns of vasculature to liver tumors. Br J Cancer 24: 360-363
11. Bengmark S, Rosengren K (1980) Angiographic study of the collateral circulation to the liver after ligation of the hepatic artery in man. Am J Surg 119: 620-624
12. Bragg DG (1976) Angiography of hepatic neoplasm: a review. Int J Radiat Oncol Biol Phys 1: 965-971
13. Gelin LE, Lewis DH, Nilsson L (1968) Liver blood flow in man during abdominal surgery. II. The effect of hepatic artery occlusion on the blood flow through metastatic tumor nodules. Acta Hepatosplen 15: 21-24

14. Goldstein HM, Thaggard A, Wallace S, Neiman HL (1976) Priscoline-augmented hepatic angiography. Radiology 119: 275-279
15. Hafström L, Nobin A, Persson B, Sundqvist K (1980) Effects of catecholamines on cardiovascular response and blood flow distribution to normal tissue and liver tumors in rats. Cancer Res 40: 481-485
16. Iwaki A, Nagasue N, Kobayashi M, Inokuchi K (1978) Intra-arterial chemotherapy with concomitant use of vasoconstrictors for liver cancer. Cancer Treat Rep 62: 145-146
17. Kahn PC, Frates WJ, Paul RE Jr (1967) The epinephrine effect in angiography of gastrointestinal tract tumors. Radiology 88: 686-690
18. Kido C (1970) Hepatic angiography of experimental transplantable tumor. Invest Radiol 5: 341-347
19. Kim DK, Watson RC, Pahnke LD, Fortner JG (1977) Tumor vascularity as a prognostic factor for hepatic tumors. Ann Surg 185: 31-34
20. Koehler RE, Korobkin M, Lewis F (1975) Arteriographic demonstration of collateral arterial supply to the liver after hepatic artery ligation. Radiology 117: 49-54
21. Lefor AT, Makohon S, Ackerman NB (1985) The effects of hyperthermia on vascular permeability in experimental liver metastasis. J Surg Oncol 28: 297-300
22. Lien WM, Ackerman NB (1970) The blood supply of experimental liver metastases. II. A microcirculatory study of the normal and tumor vessels of the liver with the use of perfused silicone rubber. Surgery 68: 334-340
23. Suzuki T, Sarumaru S, Kawabe K, Honjo I (1972) Study of vascularity of tumors of the liver. Surg Gynecol Obstet 134: 27-34
24. Young SW, Hollenberg NK, Kazam E, Berkowitz DM, Hainen R, Sandor T, Abrams HL (1979) Resting host and tumor perfusion as determinants of tumors vascular responses to norepinephrine. Cancer Res 39: 1898-1903

Changes of Vascular Pattern of Tumors and Surrounding Tissue During Different Phases of Metastatic Growth

R. Bassermann

Pathologie, Ganghofer Strasse 12, 8950 Kaufbeuren, FRG

The vascular systems of metastases exhibit changes with increasing growth. These changes in the vascular systems depend on certain factors in the surrounding tissue, i. e., in the parent tissue of the metastases, and on the specific characteristics of the malignant tumor. These various factors are as follows:

1. Histological type of metastasis
2. Histological degree of differentiation
3. Rate of growth
4. Induction of stroma
5. Incidence of necrosis
6. Location of the organ
7. Preexisting vascular structures or, as the case may be, relationship to the vascular system in the host organ

The growth of malignant tumors - and this applies to metastases as well, of course - is inconceivable without their own vascular system, i. e., without neoangiogenesis in the tumor. There is no doubt that in practice every growing tumor sooner or later produces angiogenetic stimuli which lead to neoangiogenesis [9]. The process of angiogenesis in metastases does not begin immediately after the invasion of the first tumor cells into the host organ [2]. This may constitute a difference from angiogenesis in primary tumors, which mostly develop out of preneoplasia and which, already in that form, exhibit characteristic changes in the vascular system [10].

The prerequisite is rather a certain tumor cell mass or tumor size: the endothelial proliferation within and around the tumor in micrometastasis is relatively slight as long as the tumor cells are orientated to the available vascular structures of the host organ and are nourished by them.

Folkman characterizes this stage, in which no angiogenetic activity of the endothelium is yet identifiable, as the stage of diffusion, i. e., an avascular tumor stage [8]. In this phase of growth the micrometastasis is supplied through the acquired and local capillary network. At this stage, one can observe in micrometastases of the liver how the tumor cells, which have penetrated into the trabeculae, compress the sinusoids down to narrow vestigial luminae, in which nevertheless erythrocytes can still be identified (Fig. 1 a, b).

In the lung, tumor cells in the micrometastases seem to line the alveolar walls; the alveolar capillaries here are also compressed by the pressure of growth of the tumor. Basically

Recent Results in Cancer Research. Vol 100

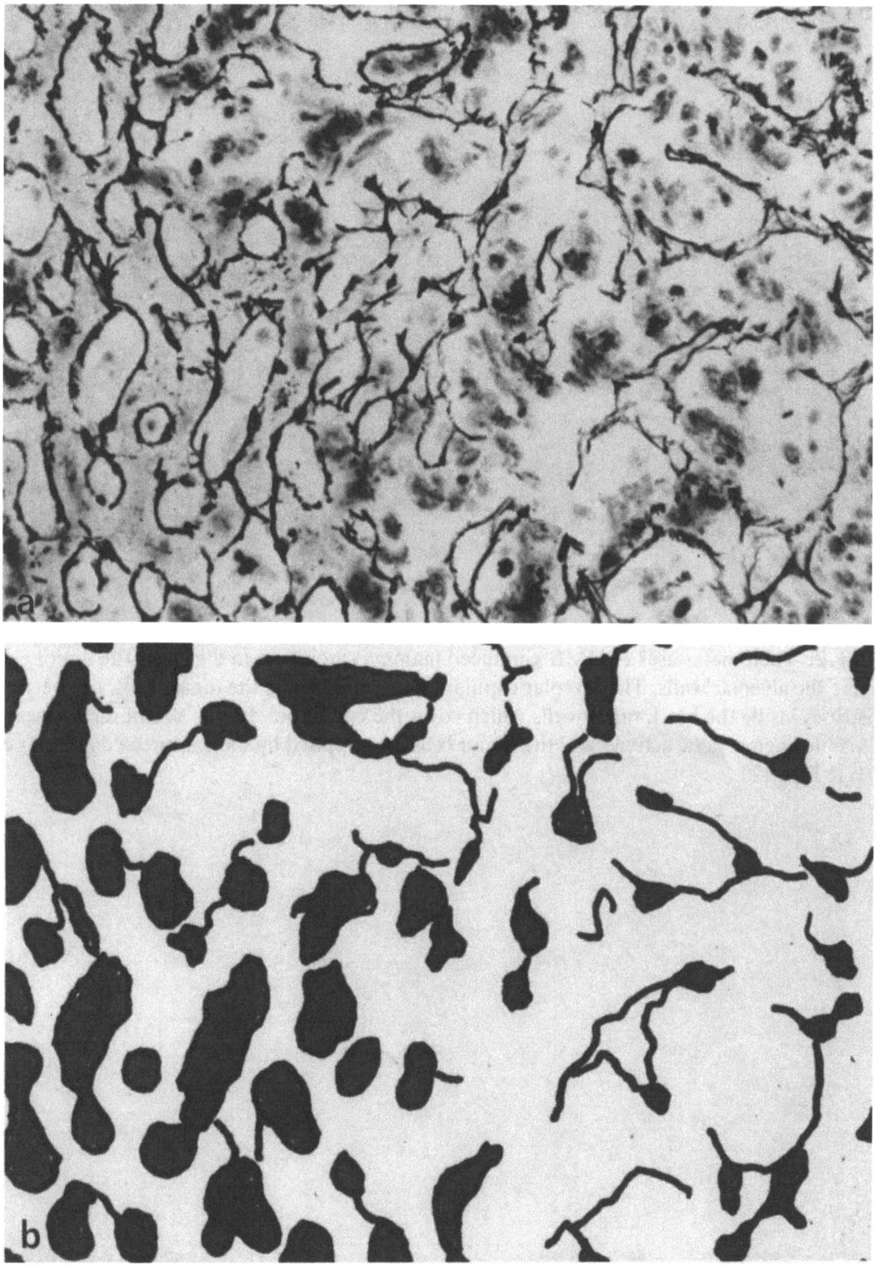

Fig. 1. a Vascular system of micrometastases of a small cell bronchial carcinoma. *On the right* the vascular area of the sinusoids is compressed by the infiltration of the tumor cells into the trabeculae. The micrometastases are supplied by the acquired and compressed sinusoid vessel system and there is no visible neoangiogenesis. Approximately *in the middle* is the beginning of the normal liver parenchyma *on the left*. Gomorri, × 520. **b** Schematized representation of the histological picture of **a**. The vascular area in the region of the metastases is greatly compressed compared with the normal liver parenchyma on the left (vascular system in *black*)

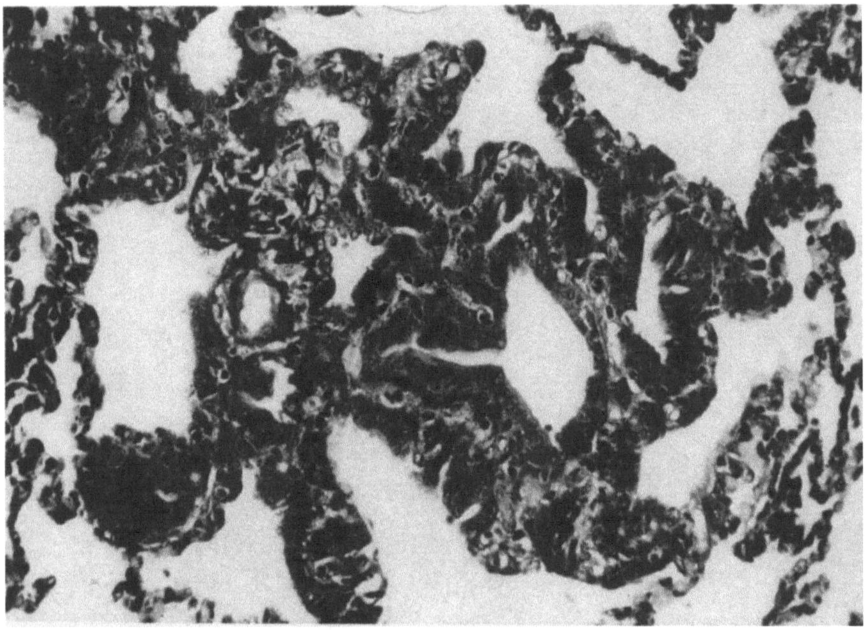

Fig. 2. Micrometastases of DMBA-induced mamma carcinoma in the lung. The tumor cells seem to line the alveolar walls. The alveolar capillaries, compressed by the tumor cells, can be seen as small stripes inside the black tumor cells which cover the capillaries. In this size of metastases there is no visible angiogenetic activity and the tumor cells are supplied by the compressed alveolar capillaries. H & E × 420

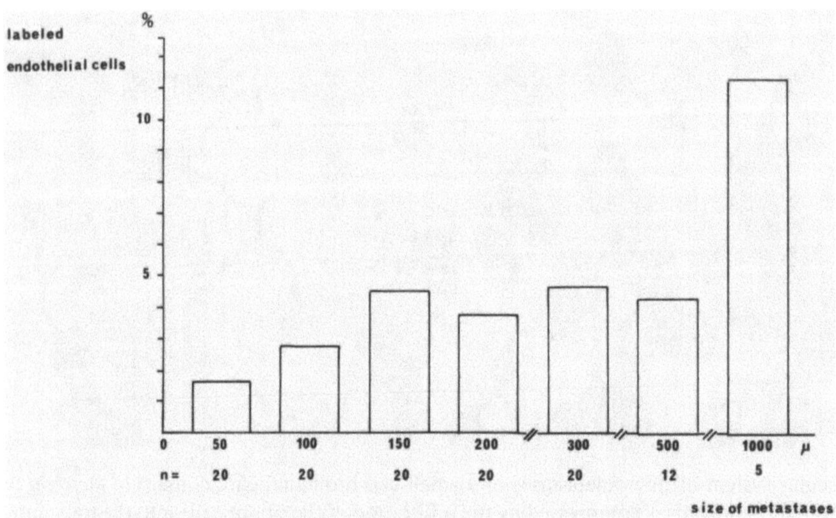

Fig. 3. Endothelial proliferation depending on the size of metastases in lung metastases of DMBA-induced mammary carcinoma of the rat after labeling with ^{3}H-thymidine. Up to the size of 500 μm there is only a small amount of proliferating endothelium in and around the metastases and the amount hardly exceeds the normal degree of endothelial regeneration in the lung. Between 500 and 1000 μm diameter a spontaneous and marked increase of endothelial proliferation appears in the metastases and their surroundings

similar phenomena are exhibited here as in the micrometastases of the liver (Fig. 2). In this phase of tumor growth there is no discernable neoangiogenesis.

When the original vascular system no longer suffices for the blood supply of the micrometastases, because it has been destroyed, or because the diffusion distance has become too great, a spontaneous and marked growth spurt appears in the endothelium of the metastases and their surroundings (Fig. 3).

The order of magnitude at which one can see such growth, in the case of lung metastases of dimethylbenzanthracene (DMBA)-induced mammary carcinomas in the rat, is approximately 500 μm. At this metastasis size one finds a clear growth spurt in the endothelium as compared with smaller metastases, as can be seen from Fig. 3. Up to the size of 500 μm, there is only a small amount of proliferating endothelium in and around the metastases, and the amount hardly exceeds the normal degree of endothelial regeneration in the lung. This can be seen as indicating:

1. That the amount of angiogenetic stimulus secreted by the carcinoma cells is, in the case of micrometastases up to a certain size, insufficient to induce effective proliferation of the endothelium.
2. Alternatively, that the growing metastasis does not yet require any angiogenesis and that only when it has reached a critical size or a critical diffusion distance does the endothelium begin to react to the angiogenetic stimulus and proliferate.

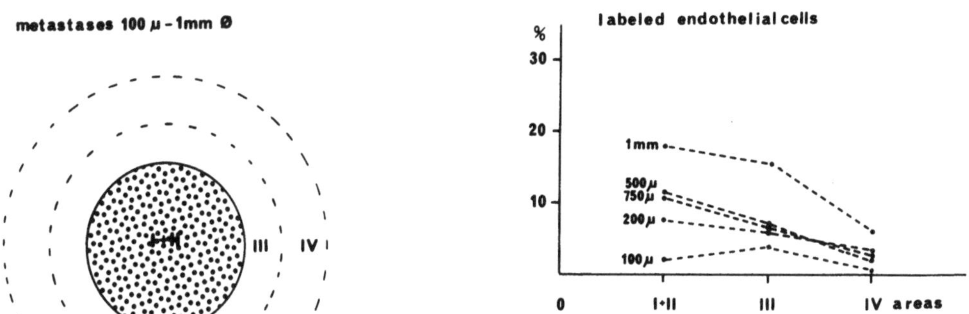

	I+II	III	IV
100 μ P :	2.1	3.9	0.3
200 μ P :	7.2	6.8	2.0
500 μ P :	11.5	6.2	3.5
750 μ P :	10.9	6.6	3.0
1 mm P :	18.0	15.3	6.0

a b

Fig. 4. a Measuring endothelial proliferation in liver metastases of Walker carcinosarcoma of the rat after radioactive labeling with ^{3}H-thymidine. The metastases are divided (on the histological sections) into different zones of equal size and at intervals of approximately 250 μm. The labeled endothelium was counted. Up to a size of 1 mm of a metastasis it was not possible to divide the metastases into two different zones and they were combined (zones 1 and 2, *dotted circle*). The third zone is the normal liver parenchyma immediately bordering the metastases; the fourth zone is called the peripherically outer liver zone. **b** In metastases of up to 1 mm in size a continual increase in endothelial proliferation can be observed, both within the micrometastases (zones 1 and 2) and also in their immediate surrounding zone. The greatest proliferative activity in the endothelium is found in the metastases themselves and to a lesser extent in the immediately surrounding liver tissue

With further growth of the metastases increasing proliferation of the endothelium occurs in the metastases and their surroundings, which emanates from the local and acquired vasculature. This can be clearly demonstrated by distributing ^{3}H-thymidine on histological section of experimentally induced liver metastases of Walker carcinosarcoma 256 in different zones of equal size and at intervals of approximately 250 µm, and then counting the ^{3}H-thymidine-labeled endothelia cells (Figs. 4a, b, 5a, b) [3].

At a metastasis size up to 1 mm, the greatest proliferative activity in the endothelium is found in the metastases themselves and also in the immediate vicinity and to a lesser extent at a distance of roughly 250 µm from the edge of the metastases.

In metastases of approximately 1 mm upward (Fig. 5a, b), the endothelial proliferation inside the metastases in the central sections continually decreases. The maximum endothelial proliferation activity is shifted in these metastases to the border area of the tumors or to the immediately surrounding liver tissue. This activity of endothelial proliferation leads finally to a newly formed vessel system of the metastases and, according to Folkman [9], to the stage of active perfusion of the tumor (Fig. 6). Denekamp and Hobson [6] and Gunduz [11] have been able to show that in the central sections of malignomas, during growth, even the proliferative activity of the tumor cells decreases. It now appears that the growth activity of the endothelium in the central sections also constantly declines. The maximum proliferation in tumor cells and in the endothelium (and also the new construction of vessels) is shifted to the periphery of the metastases. This is an important starting point for a therapeutic concept, and this does not only apply to liver metastases.

The cause of this is to be sought in the disturbance of the microcirculation in the metastases or the malignant tumors. It is well known that in malignant tumors disturbances in the microcirculation occur at a very early stage and in most cases this leads to a collapse of the vascular system, i.e., in most cases to central necrosis. The cause of this disturbance in the microcirculation is principally to be sought in the special nature of the newly formed vascular system of the metastases [7, 17].

Other factors which lead to a disturbance of the microcirculation are also directly or indirectly connected with the structure of the newly formed vascular system, factors such as the slowing down of the blood flow in the capillaries, the increase in transcapillary filtration, and the lack of lymph drainage in the early stage of tumor growth. This means that the neoangiogenesis in metastases ultimately leads to an ineffective vascular system, although it is possible for the vascular density in malignant tumors to be sufficient for their blood supply, as Denekamp has been able to show.

Apart from what has already been mentioned, it is especially the histological tumor type which influences the vascular pattern during further growth in metastases [14]. The more differentiated the histological appearance of the metastasis, the more specific is the appearance of its vascular system, i.e., every tumor forms its own characteristic vascular bed. Otherwise it is very difficult to reach a conclusion as to the histological tumor type from the vascular pattern of the metastases or primary tumor (Figs. 6–8). In summing up, one can but confirm the statement by Lewis [12] in 1927 that it is not the induced vascular system that shapes the tumor but that each histological tumor type develops its specific vascular system. He conducted investigations on five different experimental tumors. But the histological tumor type determines not only the vascular pattern of metastases, but clearly also its vascular density. Thus radiologists already know that metastases of squamous cell carcinomas show a lower vascular density than do those of adenocarcinomas. Highly differentiated carcinomas almost show as high a density of vasculature as poorly differentiated carcinomas (Figs. 6, 8).

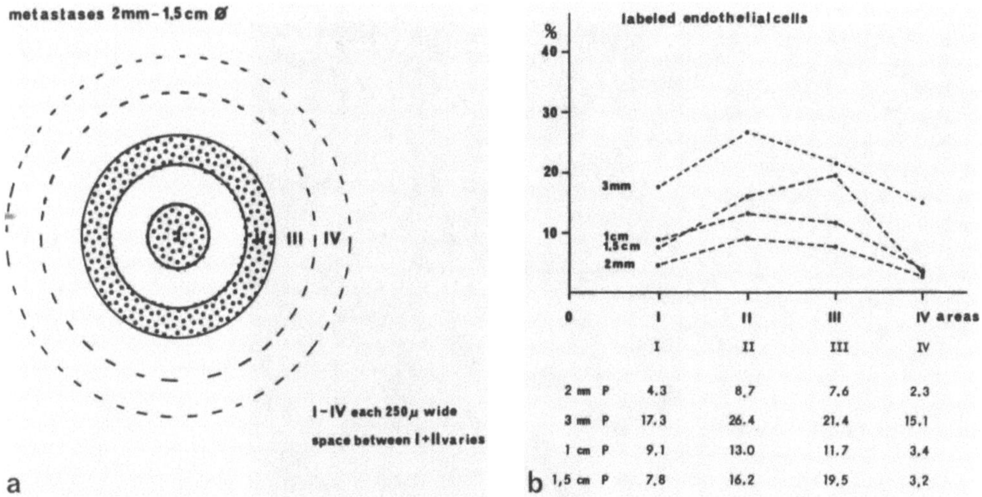

Fig. 5. a In the cases of metastases which are larger than 1 mm it was possible to divide them into an inner (zone 1) and an outer zone (zone 2) of 250 μm in width respectively, whereby the distance between zones 1 and 2 constantly changed with increasing size. **b** Here can be shown that in metastases of approximately 1 mm upward the endothelial proliferation inside the metastases in the central sections (zone 1) continually decreases. The maximum endothelial proliferation activity is shifted to the border area of the metastases (zone 2) and to the immediately surrounding liver tissue (zone 3)

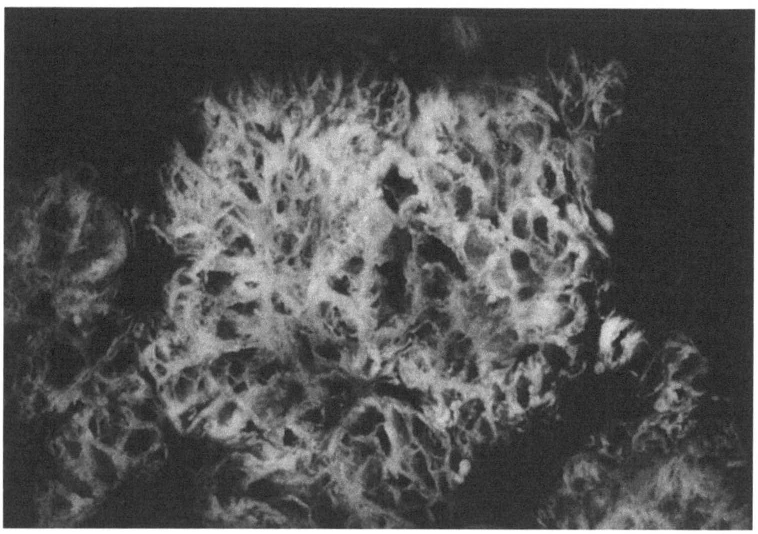

Fig. 6. Contrast photograph of the very characteristic vessel system of a liver metastases of a well-differentiated adenocarcinoma of the stomach. The newly formed vessels extend around the large gland complexes and the mucus. A. hepatica contrasted with $BaSO_4$ (Micropaque, Nicholas)

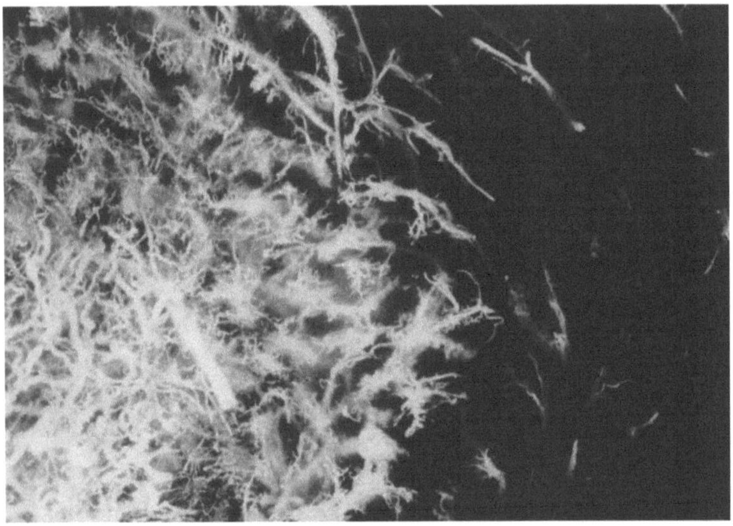

Fig. 7. Contrast photograph of the vessel system of a moderately differentiated adenocarcinoma of the breast. The tumor vessels became part of the metastases in regular stages extending from the portal areas. There is a very dense, but rather regular, tumor vessel system but in contrast to Fig. 3 the histological tumor type of the metastases is difficult to distinguish. The metastasis *on the left* is contrasted with $BaSO_4$ (Micropaque, Nicholas) via the branches of the A. hepatica; the normal, noninfiltrated liver tissue *on the right* is colored black with Indian ink via the branches of the V. portae

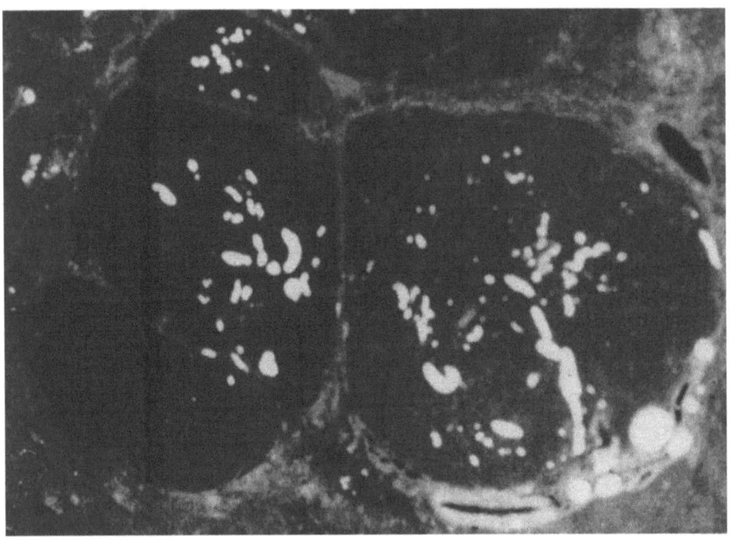

Fig. 8. Confluent metastases of a small cell carcinoma. The white contrast medium appears in many vessels. Unlike in the previous figures, they are arranged very irregularly and are quite different in size. Also this tumor is contrasted with white medium via the A. hepatica. At the edge of the metastases there are some black-colored branches of the V. portae. H & E, × 40

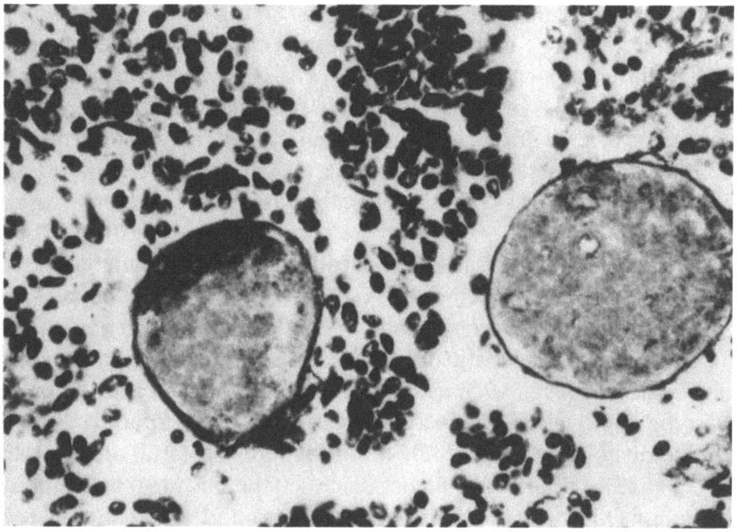

Fig. 9. Large sinusoid-like vessels in a liver metastasis of a small-cell, undifferentiated lung carcinoma. The diameter of these type of capillaries can be larger than 44 μm. Otherwise the walls of these large vessels consists only of a small layer of endothelial cells and reticular fibers. This type of tumor vessels can usually be seen in metastases of undifferentiated carcinomas. Gomorri, × 420

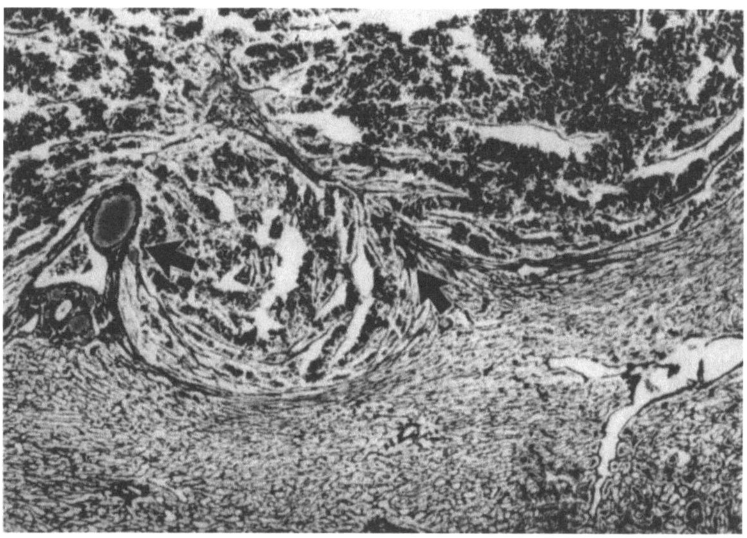

Fig. 10. Histological section of the edge of a metastasis of a small-cell carcinoma in the liver (*in the upper part* is the metastases; *in the part below* is the normal structure of the liver parenchyma). The carcinoma is growing around the portal areas *(arrows)*. Gomorri, × 220

It is very difficult, histologically at least, to distinguish the newly formed vessels in metastases or tumors, whether they are vessels of the venous or arterial type. Warren [18] has tried to differentiate the various types of vessels within tumors (Fig. 9). He was able to allocate certain types of vessels to certain tumors. The differentiation of newly formed vessels can be carried out in as far as one cannot tell them apart from the vessels of the organ from which the metastases derive. Long [13] was able to demonstrate fenestrated capillaries in brain metastases of a thyroid carcinoma, although such vessels do not normally occur in brain tissue.

The further growth of metastases leads to the integration into the metastases of preexisting vessels or organ structures (Fig. 10). Most of the local vascular system is destroyed in this process, however. On the basis of the differing collagen content, and especially of the elastic fibers, characteristic organ structures with corresponding vessels do remain in the metastases, however, such as the portal area in the liver or the bronchi in the lungs, and even sometimes glomeruli in the kidneys. Thus, using special staining techniques, it is possible to demonstrate repeatedly that rudiments of portal areas remain in liver metastases (Figs. 11-13). The artery branches disclosed thereby are mostly open and not destroyed by the tumor. Otherwise the branches of the vena portae and also other venous vessels are destroyed at an early stage by carcinoma infiltration, due to the scarcity of elastic and muscular fibers in them (Fig. 14). It happens that nearly all liver metastases are supplied arterially [1, 4].

The organ location of the metastases plays a special role, above all in the lung. Thus peripheral lung metastases are almost exclusively supplied via the branches of the A. pulmonalis, which in these sections predominate over the A. bronchiales. Central lung metastases and also central primary bronchial carcinomas are almost exclusively supplied via the branches of the A. bronchialis [5, 15, 16].

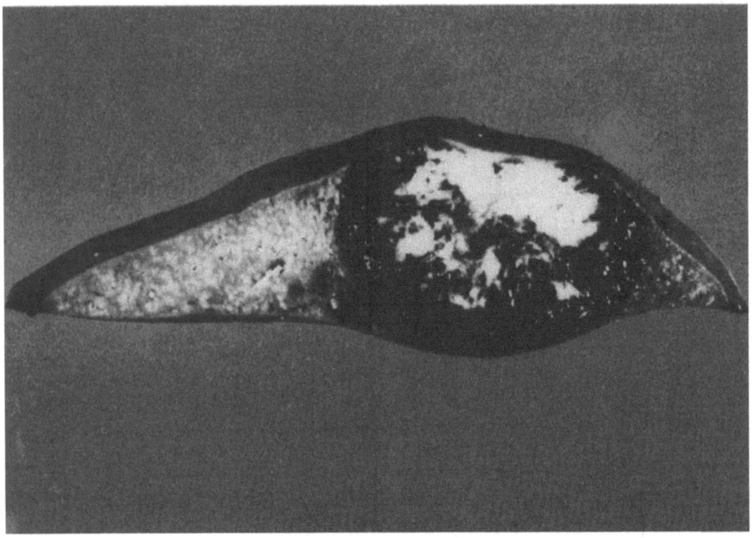

Fig. 11. Liver metastasis of a urothelial carcinoma. The metastasis is contrasted with black color (Indian ink) via the A. hepatica; the surrounding liver tissue appears partly in white after being filled via the V. portae. The *central white area* in the metastases corresponds to the avascular, not contrasted central necrosis

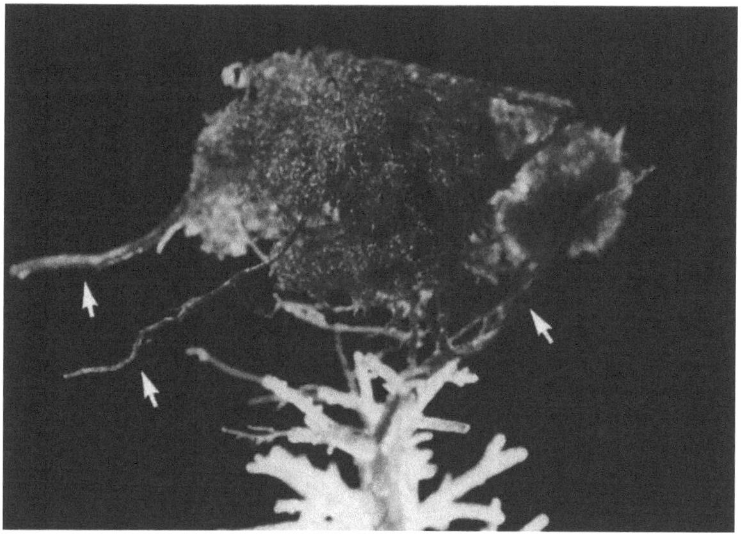

Fig. 12. Small metastases of mammary carcinoma approximately 0.5 cm in diameter. The metastases are contrasted in red (*here grey*) via the A. hepatica. The branches of the V. portae break off immediately in front of the metastases. At regular intervals, large arterial vessels are seen on the edge of the metastases *(arrows)*. The branches of the V. portae *(in white)* break off immediately before the metastases (Technovit acrylic resin, Kulzer) *in the lower part of the picture*

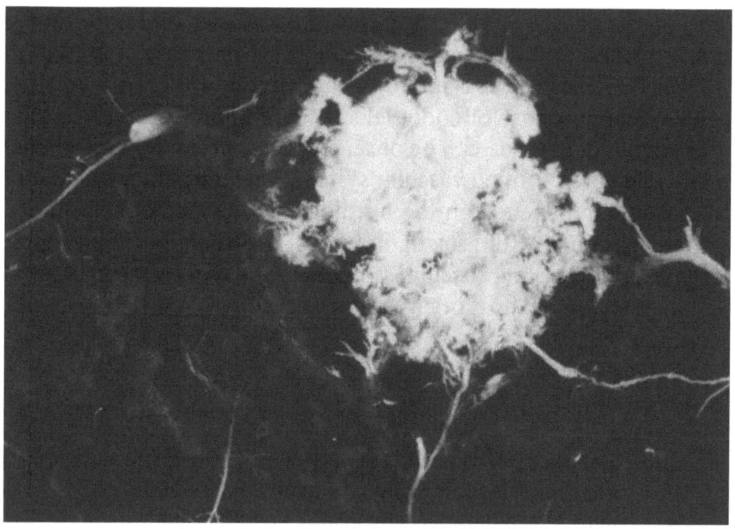

Fig. 13. Liver metastases of a fibrous malignant histiocytoma. The vascular system of the metastases is strongly contrasted with white medium by the branches of the A. hepatica. There are some big branches which seem to fill the whole metastases in the surrounding tissue. The normal, surrounding liver tissue is colored black by the V. portae with Indian ink (metastases are 1.5 cm in diameter)

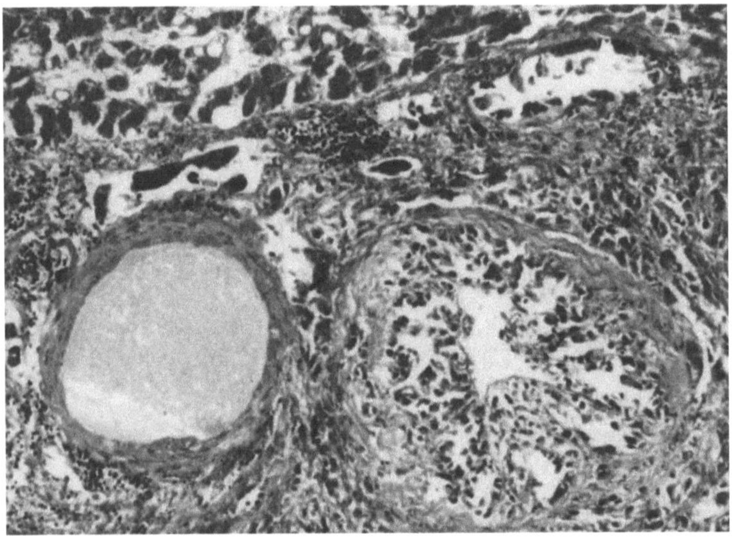

Fig. 14. Typical example of a portal area of the edge of a liver metastasis (normal liver tissue on the left side of the metastases *in the upper part*). The vein *(on the right)* is completely infiltrated by the carcinoma and destroyed; the artery (*on the left,* filled with contrast medium) is intact and also the biliary duct (over the V. portae). H & E, × 320

In summary, the vascular systems of metastases change continually with increasing growth. The change depends on certain factors in the surrounding tissue of the metastases and on the particular characteristics of the malignant tumor. The growth of metastases is inconceivable with neoangiogenesis. In the first phase of growth the micrometastases are supplied by the acquired and local capillary network. With enlargement of the metastases a significant increase of endothelial proliferation of vessels in the metastases and also in the surrounding tissue can be observed. This increasing endothelial proliferation leads finally to a newly formed vascular system. The morphological feature of this newly formed vessel system depends on the histological type of the metastases, histological degree of differentiation, rate of growth, induction of stroma, incidence of necrosis, location of the organ and preexisting vascular structures, or - as the case may be - relationship to the vascular system in the host organ.

References

1. Ackerman NB (1979) The blood supply of experimental liver metastases. IV. Changes in vascularity with increasing tumor growth. Surgery 75: 589-596
2. Bassermann R (1984) Angiogenese und Vaskularisation in Metastasen. Verh Dtsch Ges Pathol 68: 124
3. Bassermann R, Rabes HM (1983) Angiogenesis in experimentally induced metastases. Verh Dtsch Krebs Ges 4: 853
4. Breedis C, Young G (1954) The blood supply of neoplasms in the liver. Am J Pathol 30: 969-985
5. Cudkowicz L, Armstrong JB (1953) The blood supply of malignant pulmonary neoplasms. Thorax 8: 152-156
6. Denekamp J, Hobson B (1982) Endothelial-cell proliferation in experimental tumours. Br J Cancer 46: 711-720

7. Endrich B, Oda T, Messmer K, Intaglietta M (1983) Besonderheiten der Mikrozirkulation in bösartigen Tumoren. In: Vaupel P, Hammersen F (eds) Mikrozirkulation in malignen Tumoren. Karger, Basel, pp 52-68
8. Folkman J (1974) Tumor angiogenesis factor. Cancer Res 34: 2109-2113
9. Folkman J (1984) Angiogenesis: initiation and modulation. In: Nicolson GL, Milas L (eds) Cancer invasion and metastasis: biologic and therapeutic aspects. Raven, New York, pp 201-208
10. Gimbrone MA, Gullino PM (1976) Angiogenic capacitiy of preneoplastic lesions of the murine mammary gland as a marker of neoplastic transformation. Cancer Res 36: 2611-2615
11. Gunduz N (1981) Cytokinetics of tumor and endothelial cells and vascularisation of lung metastases in C_3H/He mice. Cell Tissue Kinet 14: 343-363
12. Lewis WH (1927) The vascular patterns of tumors. J Hopkins Hosp Bull 41: 156-162
13. Long DM (1979) Capillary ultrastructure in human metastatic brain tumors. J Neurosurg 51: 53-58
14. Milne ENC, Margulis C, Noonan D, Stoughton JT (1967) Histologic type-specific vascular patterns in rat tumors. Cancer 20: 1635-1646
15. Milne ENC (1967) Circulation of primary and metastatic pulmonary neoplasms. Am J Radiol 100: 603-609
16. Ogilvie WR, Blanding JD, Wood ML, Knisely WH (1964) The arterial surply to experimental metastatic VX 2 and XY tumors in rabbit lungs. Cancer Res 24: 1418-1424
17. Vaupel P, Frinak S, Bicher HI (1979) Heterogeneous PO_2 and pH distribution in C_2H mouse mammary carcinoma. (Manuskriptband) 4. Jahrestagung der Deutschen Gesellschaft für Mikrozirkulation, Mainz
18. Warren BA (1979) The vascular morphology of tumors; in Peterson (ed) Tumor blood circulation. Angiogenesis, vascular morphology and blood flow in CRC Press, Boca Raton, pp 1-47

Permanent Hepatic Artery Ligation Versus Temporary Dearterialization in the Treatment of Hepatic Tumors

S. Bengmark and B. Jeppsson

Department of Surgery, University of Lund, 22185 Lund, Sweden

The rationale for treating liver tumors by occlusion therapy is based on the derivation of the nutrition of liver tumors from the hepatic artery. Vascularity of malignant neoplasms in the liver has been investigated by many authors. Breedis and Young [10] studied the tumor circulation of experimental liver neoplasms and autopsy specimens of patients, using various dyes, gelatin, and vinyl acetate for injections into hepatic arteries and veins. Dye was demonstrated within the tumors after hepatic artery injections, but only in the periphery after the portal injection. The authors estimated that 80%-100% of the human liver tumor circulation was derived from the hepatic artery. Blanchard et al. [9] used isotope-labeled microspheres injected into the hepatic artery and portal vein in rabbits with implanted liver tumors. They found a tumor/liver ratio of 4.2 after hepatic artery injection, but only 0.3 after injection into the portal vein. Nilsson and Zettergren [22] investigated primary hepatic carcinoma induced in rats by injecting barium sulfate and formalin into hepatic vessels and used an X-ray technique to visualize vascular penetration of the tumors. In some neoplasms the contrast material from the portal vein filled vessels resembling sinusoids, although the main filling occurred from the hepatic artery. Around the periphery of the tumor a zone of vessels was filled with contrast material from the portal vein. In a series of studies, Ackerman [1] examined the blood supply of experimental liver metastases. Using isotope-labeled microspheres, he found that smaller tumors, less than 30 mg in weight, were fed by both the hepatic artery and the portal vein, while larger tumors had a predominant arterial blood supply. In an investigation of 117 patients with primary and secondary carcinoma of the liver, Suzuki et al. [27] found a highly varying vascularity of the tumor tissue. They suggested that hypovascular tumors were likely to respond better to portal vein branch ligation, while the suitable treatment for hypervascular tumors would be hepatic artery ligation. Kim et al. [16] also found a better prognosis following hepatic artery ligation and infusion chemotherapy in patients with hypervascular liver tumors.

Liver hepatic dearterialization can be performed surgically in different ways.

1. Hepatic artery ligation, with ligation of the vessel as close as possible to the liver.
2. Hepatic dearterialization. All connections to the lesser omentum and all structures, except the common duct and the portal vein, in the hepatic duodenal ligament are ligated and divided.
3. Transient hepatic dearterialization. Dearterialization is performed as above, but the hepatic artery is occluded only for a certain period.

Recent Results in Cancer Research. Vol 100

Table 1. Clinical studies on hepatic artery ligation and dearterialization in liver malignancies

	Patients	Occlusion	Drug	Survival (months)	Complication rate (%)
Bengmark et al. 1971 [6]	39 PLC	-	-	1 mean	-
Wood et al. 1976 [30]	113 Metastases, colorectal	-	-	6.6 mean	-
Bengtsson et al. 1981 [8]	25 Metastases	-	-	4.5 mean	-
Petrelli et al. 1984 [26]	97 Metastases, colorectal	HAL	-	9.5 median	10.3 †2.0
Balasegaram 1972 [4]	24 PLC	Dearterialization	-	12/18 objective response	†16.5
Almersjö et al. 1972 [2]	5 PLC 22 Metastases, various	Dearterialization	-	4.5 mean	†37.0
McDermott et al. 1978 [18]	5 Metastases, various	Dearterialization	-	14.3 mean 3.5 objective response	1
Gulessarian et al. 1972 [14]	8 Metastases, various	HAL	5-FU ia 12 mg/kg	11.6 mean	12.5
Fortner et al. 1973 [13]	6 PLC 17 Metastases, various	HAL	in 13/23 pts 5-FUdR ia 0.3 mg/kg/24 h Methotrexate 2.5-5 mg	78% subjective relief 50% objective response	22
Mokka et al. 1975 [19]	13 PLC 10 Metastases, various	HAL	5 pts 5-FU ia 15 mg/kg	8.9 mean 4.9 mean	†13 -
	15 PLC	-	-	4.1 mean	-
Tagaki et al. 1983 [28]	11 PLC 3 Metastases, colonic	HAL	Mitomycin C ia 20 mg/48 h Adriamycin ia 20 mg/48 h	7/14 pts objective response	-
Ong et al. 1975 [23]	16 PLC	Deart	-	4.2 mean	†43
	14 PLC	HAL	5-FU ip 15 mg/kg	5.2 mean	†35
	16 PLC	-	5-FU ia 15 mg/kg	5.9 mean	†44
	12PLC	-	-	5.2 mean	†42
Almersjö et al. 1976 [3]	10 PLC 30 Metastases, various	HAL 26 Dearterialization 14	5-FU ip 15 mg/kg (19/40 pts)	8 median	†17.5
Taylor 1978 [29]	6 colorectal	-	-	3.1 mean	†17
	6	HAL	-	3.0 mean	†17

Table 1 *(continued)*

	Patients	Occlusion	Drug	Survival (months)	Complication rate (%)
	7	HAL	5-FU ip 0.5 g + ia 0.5 g for 10 days	9.8 mean	†14
	5	-	5-FU ip 1 g for 10 days	4.1 mean	†20
Dahl et al. 1981 [11]	20 Metastases, various	Transient dearterialization	5-FU ia 10 mg/kg	17 mean	35 †5
El-Domeiri et al. 1978 [12]	4 PLC 9 Metastases, colorectal	Transient dearterialization	5-FUdR ia 0.6 mg/kg	8.7 mean	35.7
	6 PLC 10 Metastases, colorectal	-	5-FUdR ia 0.6 mg/kg	10 mean	25

PLC, primary liver cancer; *HAL*, hepatic artery ligation; *ia*, intraarterial; *ip*, intraperitoneal; *†*, mortality; *pts*, patients

No comparative studies have been performed of hepatic artery ligation, dearterialization, or transient dearterialization. The different techniques have developed over a 20-year-period and we will discuss results from presented series (Table 1), as well as advantages and disadvantages of the different treatment modalities. We will present the experience in our own institution with these techniques.

Hepatic Artery Ligation

The first reports of intentional ligation of the hepatic artery for the treatment of human liver tumors were published in 1966 [20, 21]. Considerable tumor regression was seen following ligation, and on microscopic examination only a few living tumor cells on the borders of the neoplasms could be observed. The hopeful influence of these initial reports has not been borne out in subsequent clinical trials. In a recent report of 97 patients with metachronous metastases from colorectal cancer, with > 50% of the liver involved in metastases, an overall survival time of 9.5 months was reported after hepatic artery ligation [26] (Table 1). Factors that adversely affected survival for hepatic artery ligation were extrahepatic metastases, poor performance status, and elevated liver function tests. In this material there was a complication rate of 10.3% and a mortality of 2.0%. It is generally considered that hepatic artery ligation alone does not significantly prolong the survival time when compared with the natural history of untreated patients [7]. The postoperative mortality after hepatic artery ligation varies in different material from 10% to 35% and the main problems are hepatic insufficiency and bleeding.

Hepatic Dearterialization

Hepatic dearterialization is a more extensive procedure with elimination of all major and minor arterial sources to the liver, including complete separation of the liver from all connections, except the portal vein, common duct, and hepatic vein. There is only one randomized study published, where dearterialization is compared with hepatic artery infusion of 5-fluorouracil (5-FU), hepatic artery ligation combined with portal vein infusion of 5-FU, and untreated controls in primary liver cancer [23]. The length of survival was almost identical in the different groups, averaging 17–21 weeks. Some palliative effects with tumor size reduction and relief of pain were noted, however, more often after hepatic dearterialization than after hepatic artery ligation. Permanent hepatic dearterialization also has a high frequency of postoperative complications and a high mortality rate, ranging from 1% to 43%. Death is usually the result of bleeding, hepatic insufficiency, infection, and abscess formation. It is obvious that this is a difficult technique, and applied alone it is of relatively small value today.

Today, most centers agree that hepatic artery ligation and dearterialization as sole procedures do not prolong survival and therefore these treatments are combined with cytotoxic drugs. In several reports, catheters are placed in the hepatic artery, distal to the area of ligation, and infusion of the chemotherapeutic agent is performed postoperatively. The different methods of complementary therapy and lack of proper control in most materials make a true comparison of results difficult. There seems to be some palliative effect with hepatic artery ligation and intraarterial infusion of 5-FU compared with untreated or historical controls. The complication and mortality rate is also low, at least in more recent series (Table 1).

Because of the apparent increase in portal perfusion to liver metastases, following hepatic artery ligation and dearterialization, theoretical benefit could result from hepatic artery ligation combined with cytotoxic infusion given by the portal vein. In 1976 we reported 40 patients with primary or metastatic liver malignancies treated with hepatic artery ligation or dearterialization, of whom 19 were given intraportal 5-FU infusion [3]. The combined treatment resulted in a somewhat prolonged survival with a median survival time of 8 months, compared with historical controls from the same group, with a mean survival of 1 month for primary liver cancer and 5.7 months for colorectal metastatic disease [5, 6].

There is a great need for randomized controlled clinical trials to assess the value of different therapies in the management of liver tumors. Only a few such studies have been published. Taylor [29] reported a trial of patients with synchronous colorectal liver metastases, comparing hepatic artery ligation with cytotoxic infusion to portal vein infusion alone. Both these therapies did not improve symptom-free survival, when compared with an untreated control group, although the group of patients undergoing both hepatic artery ligation and portal vein perfusion had an increased survival.

Transient Dearterialization

The high rate of postoperative complications and mortality mentioned above, as well as the rapid development of artery collaterals, which probably reduces the effect on the tumor, have led us to develop a method of repeated transient liver dearterialization. At laparotomy, all arterial connections to the liver except the hepatic artery are surgically divided. Strangulating slings of polyethylene are placed from the hepatic artery and pulled through a separate incision in the abdominal wall (Fig. 1). No occlusion of the main hepatic artery

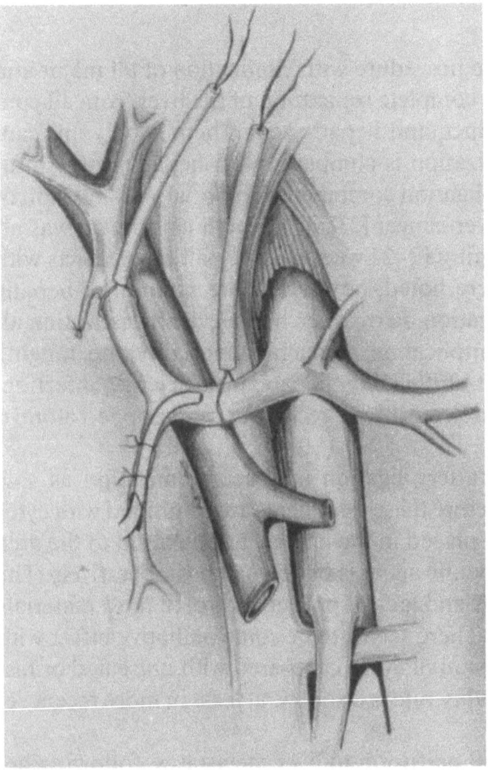

Fig. 1. Model for transient dearterialization. Two occluding strings are applied to the hepatic artery and a catheter introduced via the gastroduodenal artery

is performed during the operation, but by pulling the thin catheters an occlusion can be obtained at any time in the postoperative period. During the operation, a catheter is also placed in the hepatic artery, via the gastroduodenal artery, for control of occlusion and later infusion of cytotoxic drugs. When the patient has recovered from the immediate effects of the operative trauma, the hepatic artery is occluded for 16 h. The advantages of transient dearterialization may be manyfold. The development of arterial collaterals may not occur if the occlusion is as short as 16 h. Another advantage is that the operative trauma and the trauma of the vascular occlusion of the liver do not coincide, which may reduce the complication rate [15].

Twenty patients with liver tumors treated in this way were reported upon a few years ago [11]. Following dearterialization, 5-FU was infused for a period of at least 3 weeks. In patients with tumor localized to the liver, the mean survival was 17 months. There was an objective tumor response in 50% of the patients. One patient died of complications attributable to the procedure, giving a 5% mortality. In seven patients there were complications, but in four of the patients they were caused by the following cytotoxic infusion, while the remaining three cases of liver abscesses were probably caused by the dearterialization.

In an effort further to improve the method of repeated transient dearterialization, we have developed an implantable device, which has proven reliable in animal experiments and in a few patients in whom it has been used so far [25] (Fig. 2). This device consists of a rubber balloon, which is attached to sleeves sewn around the hepatic artery and connect-

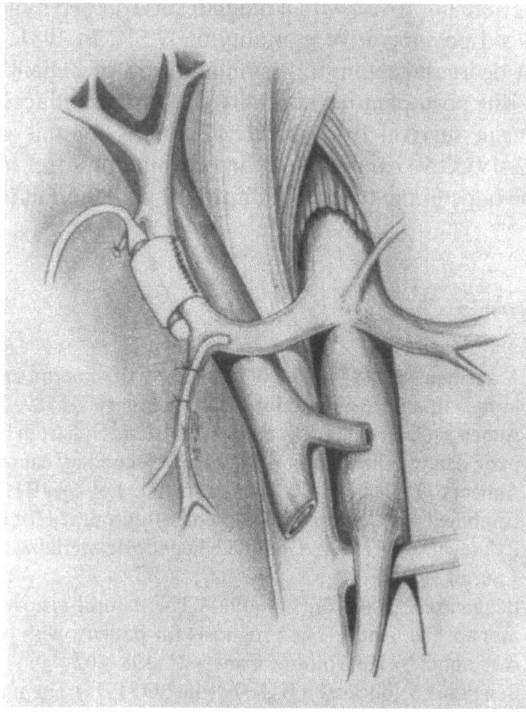

Fig. 2. An improved model for transient dearterialization. A balloon catheter attached to rubber sleeves is sewn around the hepatic artery. By injecting saline and filling the balloon, the artery is compressed. A catheter is placed via the gastroduodenal artery

ed by a small length of tubing to a chamber with a silicone rubber plug placed subcutaneously. By injecting saline, the balloon is inflated and the artery occluded. We use this for a daily occlusion of 2-4 h, followed by intraarterial infusion of 5-FU via a catheter placed in the gastroduodenal artery. Only a few patients have been treated so far. There are several theoretical advantages of performing transient hepatic dearterialization:

1. Reduced stimulus for development of arterial collaterals and a possibility for repeated hepatic arterial ischemia [25]
2. Synchronization of the cell cycle in tumor tissue after release of circulation, making the following infusion of cytotoxic drugs more effective [17]
3. Increase in NK cells (own observations)
4. Increased efficiency of cytotoxic drugs?

Thus, there is some support that repeated transient dearterialization may improve palliation in patients with unresectable liver malignancies.

No clinical trial has been performed comparing permanent and transient dearterialization. We can only judge the therapies from our own experience and from our own historical controls. The mean survival of untreated primary liver cancer is 1 month [6] and of metastases from colorectal cancers, 5.7 months. When performing dearterialization alone, the mean survival of 4.5 months was reported in 1972 [2]. This was not very different from untreated controls and the mortality was high (Table 1). By adding cytotoxic therapy, the results were improved with a median survival of 8 months, reported in 1976 [3]. There was a reduced postoperative mortality of 17.5%. In 1981, we reported our first results of transient dearterialization in a similar group of patients with a mean survival of 17 months [11]. The postoperative mortality was further reduced to 5%. By showing an improvement in mean survival from 4.5 to 17 months for this group of patients during the period 1972-1981, we cannot claim any definite proof of increase in survival. However, it gives some hope in the future for improved palliation in patients with hepatic malignancies.

References

1. Ackerman NB (1974) The blood supply of experimental liver metastases. IV. Changes in vascularity with increasing tumor growth. Surgery 75: 589-596
2. Almersjö O, Bengmark S, Rudenstam CM, Hafström LO, Nilsson LAV (1972) Evaluation of hepatic dearterialization in primary and secondary cancer of the liver. Am J Surg 124: 5-9
3. Almersjö O, Bengmark S, Hafström LO, Leissner KH (1976) Results of liver dearterialization combined with regional infusion of 5-fluorouracil for liver cancer. Acta Chir Scand 142: 131-138
4. Balasegaram M (1972) Complete hepatic dearterialization for primary carcinoma of the liver. Am J Surg 124: 340-345
5. Bengmark S, Hafström LO (1965) The natural history of primary and secondary malignant tumors of the liver. I. The prognosis for patients with hepatic metastases from colonic and rectal carcinoma by laparotomy. Cancer 23: 198-202
6. Bengmark S, Börjesson B, Hafström LO (1971) The natural history of primary carcinoma of the liver. Scand J Gastroenterol 6: 351-355
7. Bengmark S, Fredlund P, Hafström LO, Vang J (1974) Present experiences with hepatic dearterialization in liver neoplasms. Prog Surg 13: 141-166
8. Bengtsson G, Carlsson G, Hafström LO, Jönsson PE (1981) Natural history of patients with untreated liver metastases from colorectal cancer. Am J Surg 141: 586-589
9. Blanchard RJW, Grotenhuis J, La Fave JW, Perry JF Jr (1965) Blood supply to hepatic V_2 carcinoma implants as measured by radioactive microspheres. Proc Soc Exp Biol Med 118: 465-468
10. Breedis C, Young G (1954) The blood supply of neoplasms in the liver. Am J Pathol 30: 969-986
11. Dahl EP, Fredlund PE, Tylén U, Bengmark S (1981) Transient hepatic dearterialization followed by regional intra-arterial 5-fluorouracil infusion as treatment for liver tumors. Ann Surg 193: 82-88
12. El-Domeiri AA, Mojab K (1978) Intermittent occlusion of the hepatic artery and infusion chemotherapy for carcinoma of the liver. Am J Surg 135: 771-775
13. Fortner JG, Mulcare RJ, Solis A, Watson RC, Colbey RB (1973) Treatment of primary and secondary liver cancer by hepatic artery ligation and infusion chemotherapy. Ann Surg 178: 162-172
14. Gulessarian HP, Lorton RL, Condon RE (1972) Hepatic artery ligation and cytotoxic infusion in the treatment of liver metastases. Arch Surg 105: 280-285
15. Jeppsson B, Dahl EP, Fredlund PE, Stenram U, Bengmark S (1979) Hepatic necrosis in the pig produced by transient arterial occlusion. Eur Surg Res 11: 243-253
16. Kim DK, Watson RC, Pahnke LD, Fortner JG (1977) Tumor vascularity as a prognostic factor for hepatic tumors. Ann Surg 185: 31-34
17. Lieberman I, Short J (1965) Hepatic blood supply and control of deoxyribonucleic acid synthesis in liver. Am J Physiol 208: 896-902
18. McDermott WV, Paris AL, Clouse ME, Meissner WA (1978) Dearterialization of the liver for metastatic cancer. Ann Surg 187: 38-46
19. Mokka REM, Larmi TKI, Huttunen R, Kairaluoma MI (1975) Evaluation of the ligation of the hepatic artery and regional arterial chemotherapy in the treatment of primary and secondary cancer of the liver. Ann Chir Gynaecol Fenn 64: 347-352

20. Mori W, Masuda M, Miyanaga T (1966) Hepatic artery ligation and tumor necrosis in the liver. Surgery 59: 359-363
21. Nilsson LAV (1966) Therapeutic hepatic artery ligation in patients with secondary liver tumors. Rev Surg 23: 354-363
22. Nilsson LAV, Zettergren L (1967) Blood supply and vascular pattern of induced primary hepatic carcinoma in rats. Acta Pathol Microbiol Scand 71: 179-185
23. Ong GB, Chan PKW, Alagaratnam TT (1975) Clinical trials of inoperable primary carcinoma of the liver. Bull Soc Int Chir 5: 391-397
24. Persson B, Andersson L, Jeppsson B, Ekelund L, Strand SE, Bengmark S (1984 a) Development of collateral circulation after repeated transient occlusion of the hepatic artery in pigs. Eur Surg Res 16: 102 (abstr)
25. Persson B, Jeppsson B, Ekelund L, Bengmark S (1984 b) A new device for transient occlusion of the hepatic artery. J Exp Clin Cancer Res 3: 155-160
26. Petrelli NJ, Barcewicz PA, Evans JT, Ledesma EJ, Lawrence DD, Mittelman A (1984) Hepatic artery ligation for liver metastases in colorectal carcinoma. Cancer 53: 1347-1353
27. Suzuki T, Sarumaru S, Kawabe K, Honjo I (1972) Study of vascularity of tumors of the liver. Surg Gynaecol Obstet 134: 27-34
28. Takagi H, Morimotu T, Yasue M, Ochiai E, Yamada E, Ashikawa T, Kido C (1983) Ligation and catheterization of the hepatic artery for palliative treatment of malignant hepatic tumors. J Surg Oncol 23: 219-222
29. Taylor I (1978) Cytotoxic perfusion for colorectal liver metastases. Br J Surg 65: 109-114
30. Wood CB, Gillis CR, Blumgart LH (1976) A retrospective study of the natural history of patients with liver metastases from colorectal cancer. Clin Oncol 2: 285-288

Hepatic Arterial Ligation and Portal Vein Infusion: A Clinical Trial by the Gastrointestinal Tract Cancer Group of the European Organization for Research and Treatment of Cancer

A. Gerard, O. Dalesio, N. Duez, M. Lise, J. C. Pector, H. Bleiberg, D. Nitti, G. Willems, and G. Delvaux

Service de Chirurgie, Institut Jules Bordet, Centre des Tumeurs de l'Université Libre de Bruxelles, Rue Héger-Bordet 1, 1000 Bruxelles, Belgium

Liver metastases are frequently observed in the natural history of colorectal cancers. In 15% of patients they are diagnosed before or during laparotomy for surgical resection of the primary tumor [6]. If the metastatic invasion is well limited and located to one segment or to one lobe of the liver, controlled segmentectomy or hepatectomy are currently performed, with the advantage of curing approximately 10%-20% of patients [3, 6, 13, 14].

On the other hand, if liver metastases are not resectable and are diffuse and spread out in the two lobes of the liver without extra hepatic involvement, the question remains as to which treatment should be given. An association of several cytotoxic drugs administered by the systemic route does not produce better results than 5-fluorouracil(5-FU) alone. Whatever chemotherapy is used, the response rate is low and there has been no evidence of an increase in the survival rate of patients.

In 1959, Sullivan and Watkins [24] proposed the treatment of liver metastases by prolonged intraarterial liver infusions with 5-fluoro-2'-deoxyuridine (FUdR). Several authors used the same technique to administer 5-FU [4, 12, 26]. Intraarterial chemotherapy was associated with injection of *Cornynebacterium parvum* by Patt et al. in 1978 [23]. Ariel suggested the administration of Y-90 in order to obtain interstitial irradiation by microspheres [5]. Bessot et al. proposed intermittent chemotherapy combining several drugs [10] and, recently, Friedman suggested combining an infusion of 5-FU and Adriamycin with liver radiotherapy [15].

An considerable percentage of remissions has been observed in these various studies. The rate of responders is more or less 50%. However, none of the authors has produced evidence, in a rational approach, for a prolongation of survival. All these studies have used historical control groups for comparison and were not randomized clinical trials.

In 1983, Balch et al. [7, 8] reported a prospective phase II evaluation of continuous regional FUdR chemotherapy using a totally implantable drug infusion pump in patients with colorectal liver metastases. The survival results, compared with a historical control group of patients with isolated liver metastases, showed a prolongation of life of 12-18 months. These results must be confirmed by a phase III randomized prospective clinical trial. On the other hand, Kemeny et al. [18] initiated a randomized clinical trial with the aim of comparing the efficiency of intrahepatic FUDR infusion with systemic FUdR administration in colorectal carcinoma. In this study, toxicities had a relatively high rate of inflammation and ulceration of gastrointestinal mucosa and abnormalities of liver function tests. Moreover, two patients developed strictures of the bile ducts which were proven to be unrelated to tumor progression. Although this study is not yet complete,

Recent Results in Cancer Research. Vol 100

it is interesting to note that presently response rates are about the same in the intrahepatic and systemic groups. Other therapeutic approaches of liver metastases have been investigated. Most of them are the results of morphological studies on tumor vascularity.

As hepatic tumors derive their main blood supply from the hepatic artery [11, 17], it was suggested by Markowitz [21] that ligation of this artery would result in necrosis of the tumor. Experimentally, Nilsson et al. [22] produced such tumor necrosis by hepatic artery ligation and observed an increase in survival rate in the group of the treated rats compared with the control group. Gelin et al. [16] observed that the blood flow of the liver metastases decreased by 90%-95% in the tumors after hepatic artery ligation. It decreased by only 35% in the normal liver parenchyma. The remaining arterial fraction of the blood supply, after hepatic artery ligation, can be explained by the blood circulating in the arteriovenous shunts of the preportal areas, as observed by Lindell [20].

During laparotomy on a patient with liver metastases, deliberate hepatic artery ligation is followed by selective necrosis of the tumor without any damage to the liver parenchyma. In addition, the interruption of the hepatic artery produces distinct clinical improvement which reduces the pain of liver origin. Until now, there has been no evidence that hepatic artery ligation has an influence on the prolongation of life in patients with colorectal liver metastases. The explanation of such a failure of hepatic artery ligation as a radical procedure in the treatment of liver tumor seems to be complex, Within 3 weeks, a vascular supply is visible by angiography [27] through the lesser omentum, greater omentum, phrenic arteries, and celiac artery. Tumor ischemia after hepatic artery ligation is therefore temporary [9]. On the other hand, the incomplete efficiency of hepatic artery ligation in the treatment of liver metastases is also better understood thanks to anatomical studies on the vascular pattern and blood flow.

The relationship between tumor size and vascular pattern was investigated by Ackerman in 1974 [2]. Tiny tumors receive their blood supply from either arteries or veins or both. Larger tumors are supplied by new capillaries arising from arterial vessels. When the tumor grows and becomes massive, the new vascularization is insufficient and the center of the tumor necroses. Hepatic artery ligation increases the necrotic process of the tumor. Nevertheless, a rim of viable tumor cells remains. The peripheral neoplastic cells are vascularly supplied by vessels from the portal system [1, 19].

The anatomical and experimental observations mentioned above lead to the proposal of a combined procedure for the treatment of liver metastases. An occlusion of the hepatic artery will favor the necrosis of the tumor and by perfusing the liver with cytotoxic drug, via the portal vein, a higher concentration of drug will be delivered to the metastases, helping to destroy a larger volume of tumor cells.

In 1978, Taylor [25] carried out a very interesting prospective study. This clinical trial comprised three arms. In the first group, the patients were treated by hepatic artery ligation and intraarterial infusions of 5-FU. In the second group, they were treated by hepatic artery ligation with 5-FU infusions and portal infusions of 5-FU. The third group was a control group. The survival of the group treated by heaptic artery ligation and portal infusion was statistically significantly better than those of the other groups. These results are particularly promising; nevertheless, the number of patients in each group was very small.

Instead of permanent occlusion of hepatic artery with temporary ischemia, temporary occlusion by tourniquet, by an intravascular balloon catheter, or by embolization with enzymatically degradable microspheres is able to produce repeated transient ischemia. Nevertheless, no reports have yet provided evidence of its effectiveness until now. That is why the first step of a rational approach to the study of a combined therapy must include hepatic artery ligation as arterial occlusion.

In February 1981, the Gastrointestinal Group of the European Organization for Research and Treatment of Cancer (EORTC) began a randomized comparative study with the aim of evaluating the effectiveness of hepatic artery ligation and portal infusion of 5-FU versus a surgical procedure which will apparently not have an influence on the survival and will only be symptomatic as hepatic artery ligation alone. Patients with a resected colorectal primary tumor and unresectable liver metastases are stratified according to the measurability of the lesions and the presence or absence of symptoms at the time of entry in the trial. Criteria for patient selection are as follows:

1. Karnofsky performance status of 60 or more.
2. Less than 70 years old.
3. Patients in the immediate postoperative period of the primary tumor resection and patients relapsing primarily in the liver are included.

The following are criteria for tumors:

1. Pathology proven by liver biopsy
2. Unresectable disease
3. Resection of the primary tumor during a previous surgical operation

The asymptomatic group excludes patients with hepatic pain or with a loss of more than 10% of their healthy body weight. In this group, bilirubin has to be less than 2 mg%. Patients must have an involvement of less than 25% of liver parenchyma, as estimated by the surgeon during laparotomy. Symptomatic patients present hepatic pain, weight loss of over 10%, bilirubin of over 2 mg %, or an involvement of over 25% of the liver parenchyma.

A measurable tumor is defined as a known mass that can be clearly measured at the surface of the liver by a ruler or a caliper. Hepatomegaly may be accepted as a measurable disease if the liver edge is clearly defined extending at least 5 cm below the costal margin or the xyphoid process with calm respiration. Liver scan, ultrasonography, or computed tomography must be used for the evaluation of tumor invasion and as primary indicator of tumor response. The same method of measurement must be used to evaluate response to therapy. A schema of the trial is shown in Fig. 1.

Patients are randomized into two groups. In the first group, patients are treated by hepatic artery ligation and portal infusion of 5-FU for at least 10 days. Courses of 10 days are repeated every 6 weeks until progression of the disease. In the second group, patients undergo hepatic artery ligation alone.

During laparotomy, the hepatic artery and its left and right branches are dissected, double ligated with No 00 silk sutures, and sectioned as close to the liver as possible. So are any of the accessory hepatic arteries which may have been demonstrated by preoperative angiography. The lesser omentum, triangular ligaments, and falciform ligaments are transected in an attempt to retard the development of collateral arterial circulation to the liver. The middle colic vein is identified and tied distally. A catheter is threaded cephalad until its tip lies in the portal vein. The efficacy of the perfusion is checked by fluorescin peroperatively. To avoid infection of the catheter and to provide repeated access to the vascular system without trauma or complications, an Infuse-a-port or Port-a-cath is placed subcutaneously. This device is totally implantable. Patients are not subject to frequent heparin flushes of dressing changes, nor are their normal activities restricted. Continuous infusions are connected through a pump system to provide an adequate pressure in the portal system. During surgery, a rough estimation of the percentage of liver parenchyma invaded should be given. Also, an evaluation of the volume and the number of the

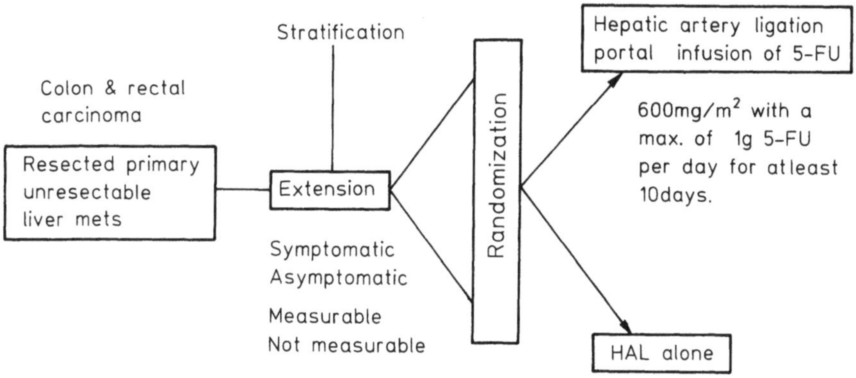

Fig. 1. The aim of the trial is to compare, in a prospective randomized trial, the effect of hepatic artery ligation and portal infusion of 5-FU in patients with biopsy-proven liver metastases, with respect to: (1) survival, (2) rate of response, (3) time to progression, (4) duration of objective response, and (5) quality of live

metastases must be reported with the greatest accuracy possible. The size of the larger metastases must be measured with a caliper.

The patients treated by hepatic artery ligation and portal infusion receive 600 mg/m^2 5-FU/day for 10 days per course. These courses of infusion will be repeated every 6 weeks. The 5-FU is given as a continuous infusion in 5% dextrose. Heparin can be added to this solution. Portograms are performed by injecting contrast medium into the catheter before the 1st day of infusion. A liver function test and full hematological investigation are performed daily during the first course of infusion. The 5-FU infusion should be stopped in the case of patient progression, catheter complications (displacement, obstruction, infection), severe hematological toxicity, i.e., leukocytes count of less than 2000 and platelet count of less than 100000, and other severe toxicities, such as diarrhea or acute mucositis.

Until now 40 patients have been registered. One patient has been found to be ineligible and six patients are unevaluable, three for insufficient data and three for protocol violation. For 19 patients, it is to early for a complete evaluation. The patient characteristics are well distributed in both arms, with a median age of 58 years and a median performance status of 90%. Most of the liver metastases are diagnosed before or during surgery for the primary tumor. Hepatic artery ligation is a surgical procedure without postoperative mortality. Few local and general complications are observed and they were never life threatening. Toxicity due to chemotherapy is very low and no chemical hepatitis has been reported. No sclerosing cholangitis has been noted. At the beginning of the clinical trial, we used an external catheter without beats. This technique presented the complication of catheter displacement in four patients. Since we perform the liver infusion through an Infuse-a-port or a Port-a-cath with beats, no more displacements were observed. Two partial portal thromboses were shown by angiography and resulted in the stopping of the liver infusion, after the third and fifth courses of 5-FU respectively. The quality of life of the patients was definitely improved when compared with the quality of survival of the patients who presented immediate progression.

A formal comparison of the two treatments cannot be carried out with respect to response rate, time to progression, or duration of survival because of the small number of patients registered. Moreover, half of the patients cannot yet be evaluated since they have been recently entered on study. Median time to progression in the whole group of patients registered for whom follow-up is available is approximately 5½ months. Median duration of survival in the same group of patients is 11 months.

In conclusion, among the various treatment possibilites for liver metastases of colorectal cancer, an occlusion of the hepatic artery, combined with a portal infusion of cytotoxic drug, seems the most rational approach. Experimental data show that hepatic artery ligation increases the necrosis of the tumor and that most of the remaining viable neoplastic cells receive their blood supply from the portal system. The preliminary results of this clinical trial are promising. Hepatic artery ligation and 5-FU portal infusion have a very low toxicity, without clinical hepatitis and without gastrointestinal bleeding, as they were observed after cytotoxic drug infusion by the arterial route. We need more clinical trials with new drugs to improve this procedure of liver metastases treatment. In fact, hepatic artery ligation is followed by revascularization and, until now, cytotoxic drugs available are not very efficient against colorectal cancer.

References

1. Ackerman NB (1972) Experimental studies of the circulatory dynamics of intrahepatic tumor blood supply. Cancer 29: 435-439
2. Ackerman NB (1974) The blood supply of experimental liver metastases. IV. Changes in vascularity with increasing tumor growth. Surgery 75: 589-596
3. Adson MA, Van Heerden JA (1980) Major hepatic resections for metastatic colorectal cancer. Ann. Surg. 191: 576-583
4. Ansfield FJ, Ramirez G, Skibba JL, Bryan GT, Davis HL Jr, Wirtanen GW (1971) Intrahepatic arterial infusion with 5-fluorouracil. Cancer 28: 1147-1151
5. Ariel IM (1965) Treatment of inoperable primary pancreatic and liver cancer by the intra-arterial administration of radioactive isotopes (Y90 radiating microspheres). Ann Surg 162: 267-278
6. Attiyeh FF, Wanebo HJ, Stearns MW (1978) Hepatic resection for metastasis from colorectal cancer. Dis Colon Rectum 21: 160-162
7. Balch CM, Urist MM, Soong S-J, McGregor M (1983a) A prospective phase II clinical trial of continuous FUDR regional chemotherapy for colorectal metastases to the liver using a totally implantable drug infusion pump. Ann Surg 198, 5: 567-573
8. Balch CM, Urist MM, McGregor M (1983b) Continuous regional chemotherapy for metastatic colorectal cancer using a totally implantable infusion pump. Am J Surg 145: 285-290
9. Bengmark S, Rosengren K (1970) Angiographic study of the collateral circulation to the liver after ligation of the hepatic artery in man. Am J Surg 119: 620-624
10. Bessot M, Mauuary G, Lorenzini C, Fays J, Duprez A (1977) Technique and results of locoregional and sequential chemotherapy of advanced cases of cancer of the rectum. Ann Gastroenterol Hepatol (Paris) 13: 119-126
11. Breedis C, Young G (1954) The blood supply of neoplasms in the liver. Am J Pathol 90: 969-985
12. Cady B, Oberfield A (1974) Regional infusion chemotherapy of hepatic metastases from carcinoma of the colon. Am J Surg 127 (2): 220-227
13. Fortner JG, Kim BJ, Maclean MK, Barrett S, Iwatsuki AD, Turnbull WS, Howland EJ, Beattie Jr (1978) Major hepatic resection for neoplasia: personal experience in 108 patients. Ann Surg 186: 363-371
14. Foster JH (1970) Survival after liver resection for cancer. Cancer 26: 493-502
15. Friedman M, Cassidy M, Levine M, Philipps T, Spivack S, Resser KJ (1979) Combined modality therapy of hepatic metastasis. Cancer 44: 906-913
16. Gelin LE, Lewis DH, Nilsson L (1968) Liver blood flow in man during abdominal surgery. II. The effect of hepatic artery occlusion on the blood flow through metastatic tumor nodules. Acta Hepatosplenol (Stuttg) 15: 21-24

17. Healey JE Jr (1965) Vascular patterns in human metastatic liver tumors. Surg Gynecol Obstet 120: 1187-1193
18. Kemeny N, Daly J, Oderman P, Schun H, Petroni G, Geller N (1984) Randomized study of intrahepatic versus systemic infusion of fluorodeoxyuridine in patients with liver metastases from colorectal carcinoma. Proc ASCO 3: 141
19. Lien WM, Ackerman NB (1970) The blood supply of experimental liver metastases. II. A microcirculatory study of normal and tumor vessels of the liver with the use of perfused silicone rubber. Surgery 68: 334-340
20. Lindell B (1977) Transient liver ischemia by intra-arterial injection of degradable microspheres. (Paper issued by the Experimental Department, the Department of Surgery, and the Department of Nuclear Medicine, Malmö General Hospital) University of Lund, Malmö
21. Markowitz J, Rappaport A, Scott AC (1949) Prevention of liver necrosis following ligation of hepatic artery. Proc Soc Exp Biol Med 70: 305
22. Nilsson L, Zettergren L (1967) Effect of hepatic artery ligation on induced primary liver carcinoma in rats. Acta Pathol Microbiol Scand 71: 187-193
23. Patt YZ, Wallace S, Hersh EM, Hall SW, Menachem YB, Granmayeh M, McBride CM, Benjamin RS, Mavligit GM (1978) Hepatic arterial infusion of *Corynebacterium parvum* and chemotherapy. Surg Gynecol Obstet 147: 897-902
24. Sullivan RD, Watkins E Jr, Rodriguez FR, Miller E, Norcross JW (1963) Continuous arterial infusion chemotherapy of human liver cancer using 5-fluoro-2′-deoxyuridine: autodetoxification studies and clinical effects. Proc Am Assoc Cancer Res 4: 66
25. Taylor I (1978) Cytotoxic perfusion for colorectal liver metastases. Br J Surg 65: 109-114
26. Watkins E Jr, Khazei AM, Nahra KS (1970) Surgical basis for arterial infusion chemotherapy of disseminated carcinoma of the liver. Surg Gynecol Obstet 130: 580-605
27. Wright RD (1937) The blood supply of newly developed epithelial tissue in the liver. J Pathol Bacterol 45: 405-414

Indications and Therapeutic Possibilities Using Degradable Microspheres in Liver Malignancies

K. F. Aronsen, H. Teder, and B. Lindberg

Department of Surgery, Malmö General Hospital, 21401 Malmö, Sweden

The treatment of inoperable primary and metastatic liver malignancies is still unsatisfactory. Systemic chemotherapy is often associated with toxic effects, resulting in considerable discomfort to patients, which limits a more aggressive therapeutic approach. To avoid these side effects, regional liver infusions of cytostatic drugs have been widely employed [3, 4].

Hepatic dearterialization has also been used in the treatment of liver malignancies [1, 8].

To avoid revascularization, temporary occlusion of the hepatic artery has been tried [2]. Hepatic artery administration of degradable starch microspheres (DSM) was suggested by Rothman et al. [9] as a method for temporarily interrupting the hepatic artery blood flow. In the treatment of liver malignancies, concurrent administration of cytostatic drugs and degradable starch microspheres has been suggested as a method of increasing drug concentration in tumor tissue and of decreasing systemic toxicity [7].

Degradable Microspheres; Physical and Chemical Properties

Degradable starch microspheres consist of cross-linked starch and are degraded by amylase. Under the microscope at amylase concentrations similar to that in human serum, the microspheres maintain their diameters for a considerable time, after which they rather abruptly disappear. However, when agitated with a large amount of amylase, microspheres are degraded from the periphery with a continuous decrease in the diameter. The degradation time in vitro depends on the amylase activity, the degree of cross-linking, the size of the microspheres, and the amount to be degraded. However, in vivo, the blocking effect on circulation depends not only on degradation time, but varies with other factors such as the speed of injection and the occurrence of arteriovenous shunts within the target organ.

When injected intraarterially into the target organ, microspheres of suitable size are trapped in the arterioles of the organ. If a drug is dissolved in the microsphere suspension, it will be retained in the blood vessels of the target organ as long as the blood flow is blocked or considerably reduced. If the drug can cross the capillary walls and enter the target organ during the period of circulatory arrest, effective targeting would be achieved and the systemic concentration of the drug reduced. This would be expected to induce a better local therapeutic effect and reduce undesirable systemic drug effects.

Recent Results in Cancer Research. Vol 100

In our experimental and clinical studies we selected the liver as the first target organ for the following reasons: (1) the treatment of inoperable primary and secondary liver cancer is at present unsatisfactory and (2) the liver has a blood supply accessible for arterial infusion.

Experimental Studies

The blocking effect of the microspheres on hepatic arterial blood flow was first studied in dogs [9]. After injection of degradable microspheres into the hepatic artery, the effect on the liver blood flow was evaluated using a ^{133}-Xenon wash-out method. As can be seen in Fig. 1, when xenon is injected together with the microspheres the elimination of Xenon is prolonged, as compared with the injection of only xenon. Figure 2 shows that the xenon elimination curves gradually return to normal when repeated injections of Xenon only are made after an initial injection of xenon together with microspheres. This indicates a reversible blocking effect of the hepatic arterial blood flow.

The ability of degradable microspheres to modify drug distribution and drug response has been shown in the following studies on rats: Lindell et al. [7] injected ^{14}C-inulin together with microspheres into the rat liver artery. This resulted in increased inulin concentration in the liver, as compared with values found with inulin alone (Fig. 3). The concentration of inulin in peripheral blood (Fig. 4, upper panel) was reduced in the presence of microspheres, and the renal excretion of inulin (Fig. 4, lower panel) was delayed. Injection of ^{14}C-5-fluorouracil (5-FU) together with DSM into the liver artery in rats [10] resulted in increased total ^{14}C activity in the liver compared with the activities found with 5-FU injected alone into the hepatic artery or intravenously (Fig. 5). With microspheres there was also a reduction in the initial ^{14}C activities found in peripheral blood (Fig. 6). Similar results have also been obtained using Adriamycin as test substance (Teder H. et al., preliminary results). In another experiment in the rat, Lindell et al. [7] studied the tolerance of 5-FU (300 mg/kg body weight), which was injected into the hepatic artery with and with-

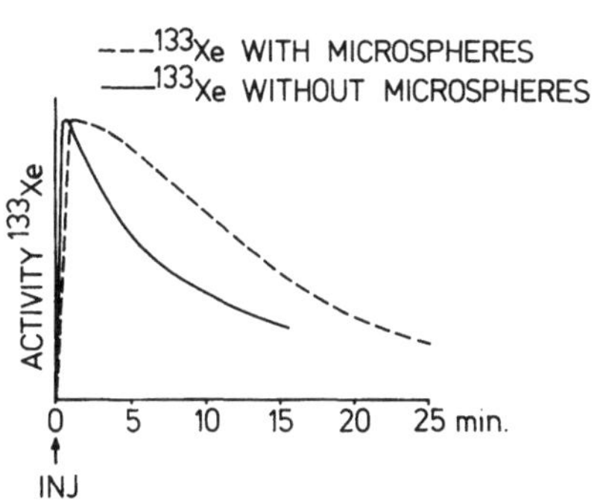

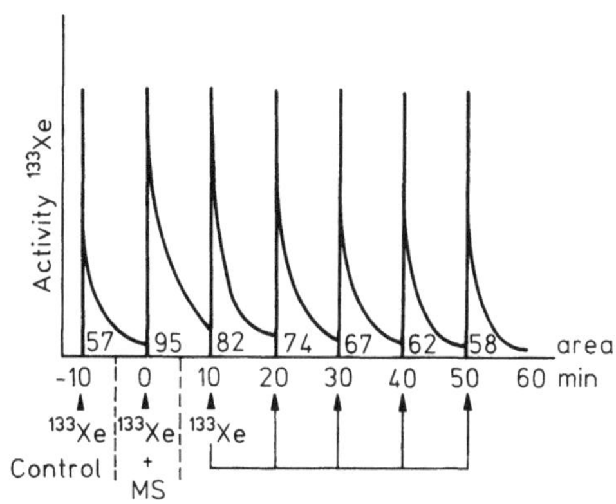

Fig. 1 *(Left).* Disappearance rate of ^{133}Xenon from dog liver after hepatic artery administration of ^{133}-Xenon with or without degradable microspheres

Fig. 2 *(Right).* Repeated hepatic artery injections of ^{133}Xenon after an initial infusion of ^{133}-Xenon with degradable microspheres (MS) into the hepatic artery. Elimination rates are represented by the areas under the curves

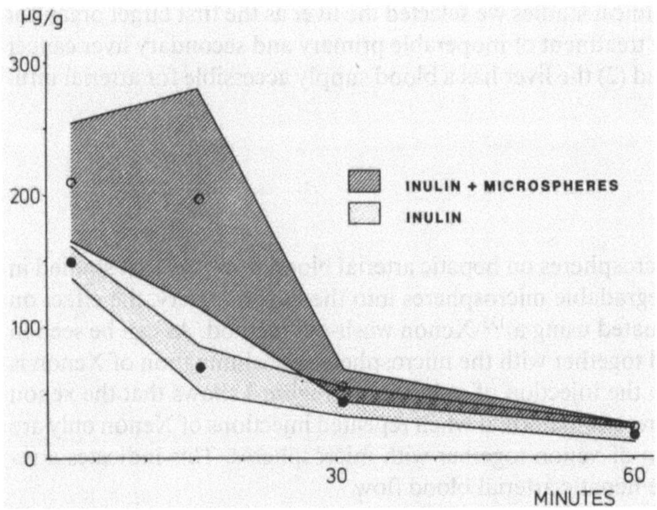

Fig. 3. ^{14}C-inulin in rat liver parenchyma after hepatic artery injection of ^{14}C-inulin with or without degradable microspheres. Individual variations within *shaded areas*, mean values indicated [7]

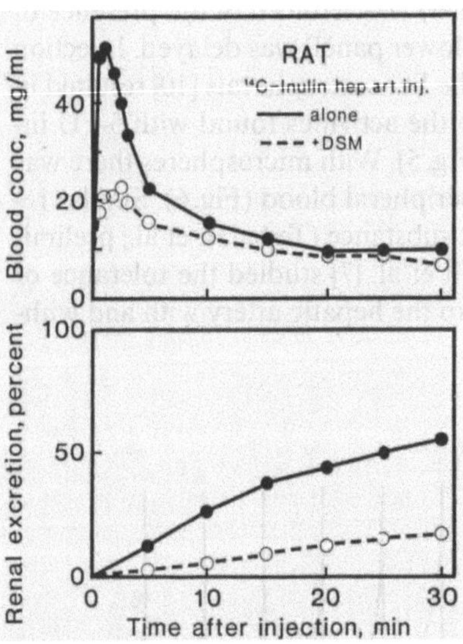

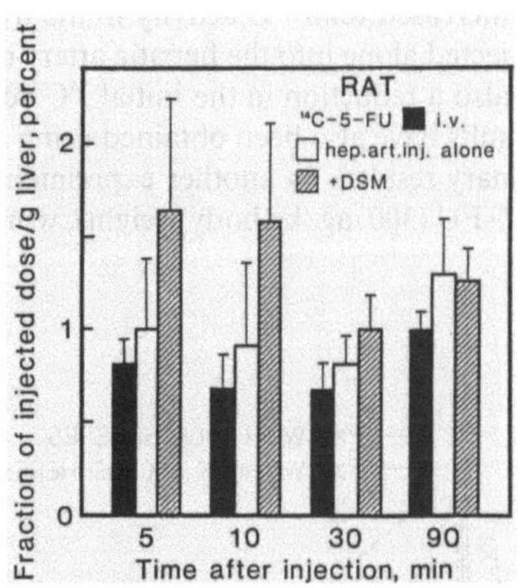

Fig. 4 *(Left).* Administration into the rat liver artery of ^{14}C-inulin ($n=5$) or ^{14}C-inulin together with degradable microspheres (DSM) ($n=5$). *Upper panel,* mean ^{14}C-inulin concentrations in peripheral blood; *lower panel,* renal inulin excretion as percentage of administered inulin dose [7]

Fig. 5 *(Right).* ^{14}C-activity in rat liver tissue after hepatic artery administration of ^{13}C-5-FU with or without degradable microspheres and peripheral venous injection of ^{14}C-5-FU. Mean values, percentage of injection ^{14}C-labeled 5-FU dose/g liver tissue ($\pm$SD) [10]

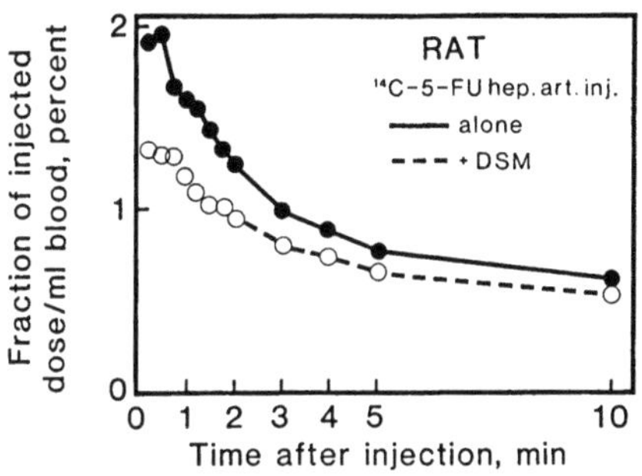

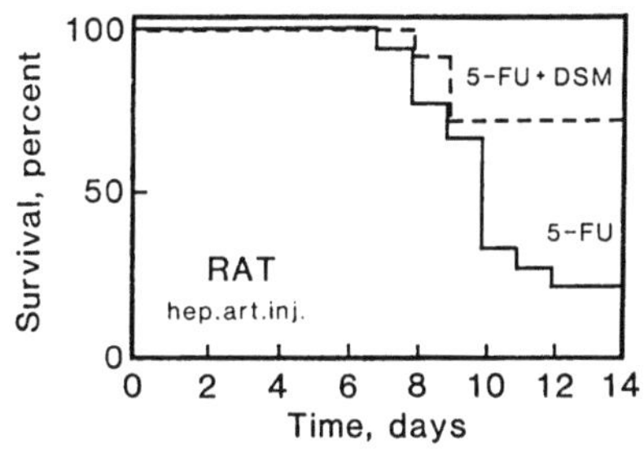

Fig. 6 *(Left).* ^{14}C-activity in peripheral blood after injection into the hepatic artery of ^{14}C-labeled 5-FU alone ($n = 8$) or mixed with degradable microspheres ($n = 8$). Mean values, percentage of injected ^{14}C-labeled 5-FU dose/ml blood [10]

Fig. 7 *(Right).* Survival after injection into the rat liver artery of 5-FU (300 mg/kg body weight), injection of 5-FU alone ($n = 18$), or injection of 5-FU mixed with degradable microspheres ($n = 16$) [7]

out DSM. The experiments with microspheres resulted in increased survival, compared with injection of 5-FU alone (Fig. 7). This suggests that when using microspheres, there is an increased liver metabolism of 5-FU and hence a decreased systemic toxicity.

Clinical Studies

Modification of drug distribution by means of DSM has been applied clinically to administrate anticancer drugs to patients with liver malignancies. In five patients with primary and secondary liver cancer, hepatic artery injections were made with Adriamycin and DSM [11]. In each patient two pharmacokinetic studies were made. Firstly, the patients were given Adriamycin alone (10 mg/m^2 body surface) into the hepatic artery. One week later, the patients were given the same dose of Adriamycin mixed with 900 mg microspheres (Spherex, mean diameter 40 μm). The injection time was 10 s and the injection volume 20 ml. After being extracted with chloroform, Adriamycin in plasma was analyzed by high pressure liquid chromatography (HPLC) with fluorescence detection. The upper part of Fig. 8 illustrates hepatic venous Adriamycin concentration versus time in one typical patient after injection of Adriamycin alone and Adriamycin mixed with microspheres. As can be seen there is a marked reduction in both the peak value and the area under the curve using microspheres. The lower panel of Fig. 8 shows the peripheral blood concentration in the same patient when Adriamycin is given either alone or mixed with microspheres. In this case too, the peak value and the area under the curve are reduced with microspheres.

The effect of microspheres on the peak value for all five cases is shown in Table 1. In four of the patients the hepatic venous peak was reduced by 75%–92% using microspheres. In peripheral blood, the maximum values were reduced by 41%–69%. In case number 4, the reduction of the hepatic venous peak was less pronounced and the maximum concentration in peripheral blood was higher with microspheres. Table 2 shows the effect on the areas under the curves during the observation period. In the same four patients, when microspheres were added there was a 31%–72% reduction in the hepatic venous Adriamycin exposure and a 21%–42% reduction in the systemic Adriamycin expo-

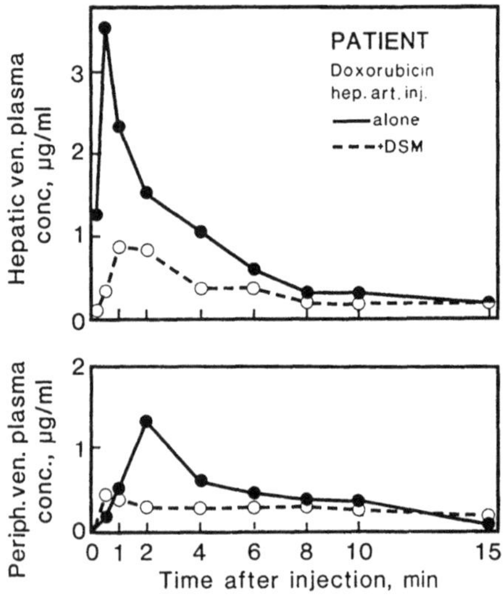

Fig. 8. Injection of Adriamycin alone or mixed with degradable starch microspheres. *Upper panel,* hepatic venous plasma concentrations of Adriamycin. *Lower panel,* peripheral venous plasma concentrations of Adriamycin [10]

Table 1. Reduction in initial peak values of Adriamycin in hepatic and peripheral veins with degradable starch microspheres

Patient	Hepatic vein	Peripheral vein
1	−76%	−46%
2	−76%	−69%
3	−92%	−42%
4	−46%	+16%
5	−75%	−41%

Table 2. Reduction in the area under the curve of Adriamycin plasma concentrations with degradable microspheres

Patient	Hepatic vein	Peripheral vein
1	−60%	−38%
2	−56%	−40%
3	−72%	−42%
4	−14%	+42%
5	−31%	−21%

sure. Case number 4 had a large hepatic tumor with marked arteriovenous shunting, which may account for the different results with an increased systemic Adriamycin exposure when the microspheres were added.

Similar results have been reported by Dakhil et al. [5], who studied the effect of microspheres on plasma concentration of BCNU (carmustine) and Gyves et al. [6], who used mitomycin together with microspheres.

In a multicenter study the microspheres were used together with mitomycin C to study the effect on drug toxicity and pharmacokinetics. Twenty-three patients with liver malignancies were given only mitomycin C (15 mg/m^2 body surface) or mitomycin C together with the microspheres (Spherex, 360 mg) as a hepatic artery injection over 4 min. The concentration of mitomycin C was analyzed in peripheral blood by HPLC. With the microspheres added, in 16 patients out of 23 there was a reduction of the area under the curve (AUC) by a mean value of 44%. In seven patients, no reduction of the AUC was found. The difference between pretreatment and nadir values of platelets and leukocytes was less pronounced in the patients where the addition of microspheres to the mitomycin C injection resulted in a reduction of the systemic exposure of mitomycin C (16 patients out of 23). From this study, no conclusions can be drawn concerning tumor response. The experience from the participating centers shows that the hepatic artery injections of mitomycin C together with the degradable microspheres are well tolerated and in several cases a remarkable tumor response was observed. This autumn a new multicenter study will start at four Scandinavian hospitals. In this study the mitomycin dose will be increased to 25 mg/m^2.

Conclusions

The results from the studies summarized above show that drugs injected into the hepatic artery together with degradable microspheres were retained longer in the target organ. This might result in an increased extraction ratio for the drug in the liver with an increased therapeutic effect and/or increased metabolism of the drug and reduced systemic toxicity.

References

1. Almersjö O, Bengmark S, Rudenstam CM, Hafström LO, Nilsson LAV (1972) Evaluation of hepatic dearterialization in primary and secondary cancer of the liver. Am J Surg 124: 5-9
2. Bengmark S, Fredlund P, Hafström LO, Vang J (1974) Present experiences with hepatic dearterialization in liver neoplasm. Prog Surg 13: 141-166
3. Brennan MJ, Talley RW, Drake EH, Vaitkevicius VK, Poznanski AK, Brush BE (1963) 5-Fluorouracil treatment of the liver metastases by continuous hepatic artery via Cournand catheter. Ann Surg 158: 405-419
4. Clarkson B, Young C, Dierick W, Kuehn P, Kim M, Berrett A, Clapp P, Lawrence W (1962) Effects of continuous hepatic artery infusion of antimetabolites on primary and metastatic cancer of the liver. Cancer 15: 472-488
5. Dakhil S, Ensminger W, Cho K, Niederhuber J, Doan K, Wheeler R (1982) Improved regional selectivity of hepatic arterial BCNU with degradable microspheres. Cancer 50: 631-635
6. Gyves JW, Ensminger WD, Van Harken D, Niederhuber J, Stetson P, Walker S (1983) Improved regional selectivity of hepatic arterial mitomycin by starch microspheres. Clin Pharmacol Ther 34: 259-265
7. Lindell B, Aronsen KF, Nosslin B, Rothman U (1978) Studies in pharmacokinetics and tolerance of substances temporarily retained in the liver by microsphere embolization. Ann Surg 187: 95-99
8. Nilsson LAV (1966) Therapeutic hepatic artery ligation in patients with secondary liver tumors. Rev Surg 23: 374-376
9. Rothman U, Arfors KE, Aronsen KF, Lindell B, Nylander G (1976) Enzymatically degradable microspheres for experimental and clinical use. Microvasc Res 11: 421

10. Teder H, Aronsen KF, Lindell B, Rothman U (1978) Studies in pharmacokinetics of 5-fluorouracil temporarily retained in the rat liver by degradable microsphere embolization. Acta Chir Scand 144 (Suppl 487): 71
11. Teder H, Nilsson B, Jonsson K, Hellekant C, Aspegren K, Aronsen KF (1983) Hepatic arterial administration of doxorubicin (Adriamycin) with or without degradable starch microspheres: a pharmacokinetic study in man. In: Hansen HH (ed) Anthracyclines and cancer therapy. Excerpta Medica, Amsterdam, pp 166-176

Radiotherapy and Additional Locoregional Treatment Modalities

Therapeutic Strategies in Primary and Metastatic Liver Cancer: Indication and Results of External Radiation Therapy

K. zum Winkel, C. Wieland, and U. Weischedel

Abteilung Allgemeine Radiologie mit Poliklinik, Zentrum Radiologie, Strahlenklinik, Klinikum der Universität Heidelberg, Vosstrasse 3, 6900 Heidelberg, FRG

Introduction

Locally applied external radiotherapy, either alone or in combination with chemotherapy, frequently leads to significant improvement in primary and metastatic cancer of the liver. Mostly it has a palliative effect in metastatic disease and may play an equally palliative role in unresectable primary liver tumors [11, 19]. Radiotherapy and chemotherapy may also palliate the symptoms of patients with unresectable gallbladder cancer but certainly does not produce long-term survival.

Radiation Sequelae

The major limiting factor is the total-organ radiation dose; also of great importance is the fraction course (Table 1). Doses of more than 30 Gy given at a rate of 10 Gy/week may cause radiation hepatitis. After higher doses the risk of fibrosis also increases. Generally, hepatitis occurs within 1-3 months after irradiation. It is accompanied by ascites and a Budd-Chiari-like syndrome associated with injury to the central vein region leading to obstruction and portal hypertension. Whole-organ radiation tolerance concomitant with or preceded by chemotherapy is calculated by Sherman et al. [20] to be 18-30 Gy, by Webber et al. [24] to be 25 Gy, and by Friedman et al. [7] to be 15-24 Gy.

Radiation Planning

In primary cancer the target volume should include the tumor bed of the unresected tumor and the lymph nodes along the porta hepatis, the pancreaticoduodenal system, and the celiac axis. In metastatic disease frequently the target volume must cover the whole organ.

Table 1. Approximate whole liver irradiation tolerance [5]

18 - 24 Gy	at 3 Gy/fraction
25 Gy	at 2.5 Gy/fraction
30 Gy	at 1.5-1.8 Gy/fraction

Recent Results in Cancer Research. Vol 100

In hepatocellular cancer as well as in circumscribed metastases sophisticated diagnostic techniques are necessary for radiation planning. To define the target volume we carefully perform computed tomography, giving unique information about the size and the inner structure of the tumors, the relationship between tumor and surrounding tissue, the size of the liver, and the neighbouring organs. Ultrasound is less suitable for radiation planning.

According to Macdonald et al. [11] the potential of long-term palliation and cure increases with shrinking field techniques, sparing as much normal tissue in liver, duodenum, stomach, and spinal cord as possible. For this reason we frequently use rotating irradiation in primary cancer (Fig. 1).

Due to the fact that one-half to two-thirds of the right kidney is included, the function of both kidneys is tested by sequential scintigraphy before radiotherapy.

In the individual case it has to be decided whether to irradiate the total liver with 20–30 Gy in 1.5 Gy-fractions initially followed by an additional 20–30 Gy boost to the solitary lesion or to irradiate the target volume exclusively (Fig. 1). Many metastatic lesions are not sensitive to less than 25 Gy.

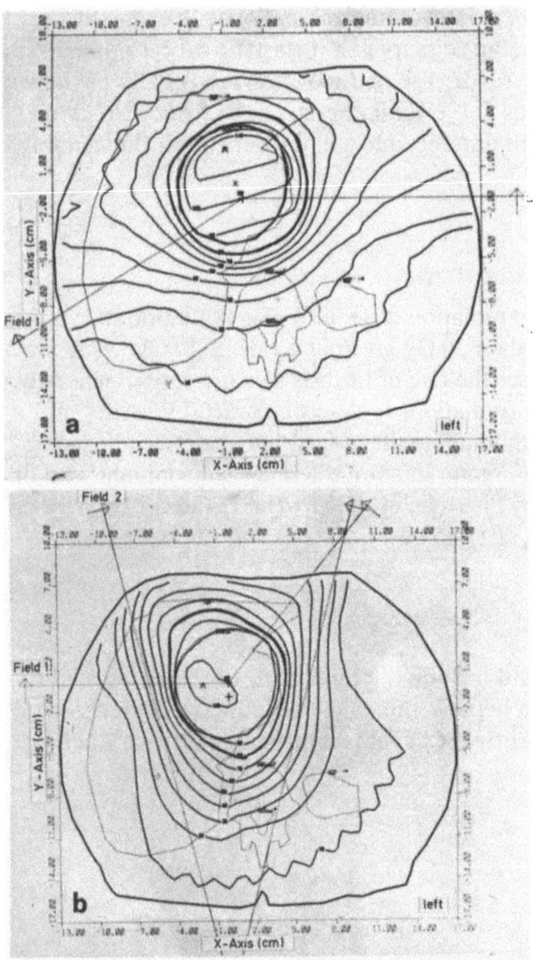

Fig. 1 a, b. Dose distribution of rotating irradiation on the basis of computed tomography in a supine patient with metastases of gastric cancer in the porta hepatis. **a** Cobalt-60 gamma rays, field size 10 × 8 cm, rotation angle −120° to +90°, target volume in the 80% isodose, 20% dose to the spinal cord and the kidneys. **b** 42-MV X-rays, field size 10 × 8 cm, rotation angle −90° to +40° combined with 35 MeV electrons, 12 × 3-cm field size in telecentric rotation from −15° to +15°. The dose to the liver outside the target volume is less than with cobalt-60 therapy

Fast neutron therapy was useful in nine patients with liver cancer as reported by Nagashima et al. [13]. With special beams like protons or heavy ions even higher doses can be applied due to the protection of the surrounding tissues. Besides, regional hyperthermia is helpful in combination with radiation and chemotherapy.

During and after radiation therapy we control the bilirubin and the enzymes in serum, the ultrasound, the CT findings (Fig. 2), and sometimes the liver scan (Fig. 3).

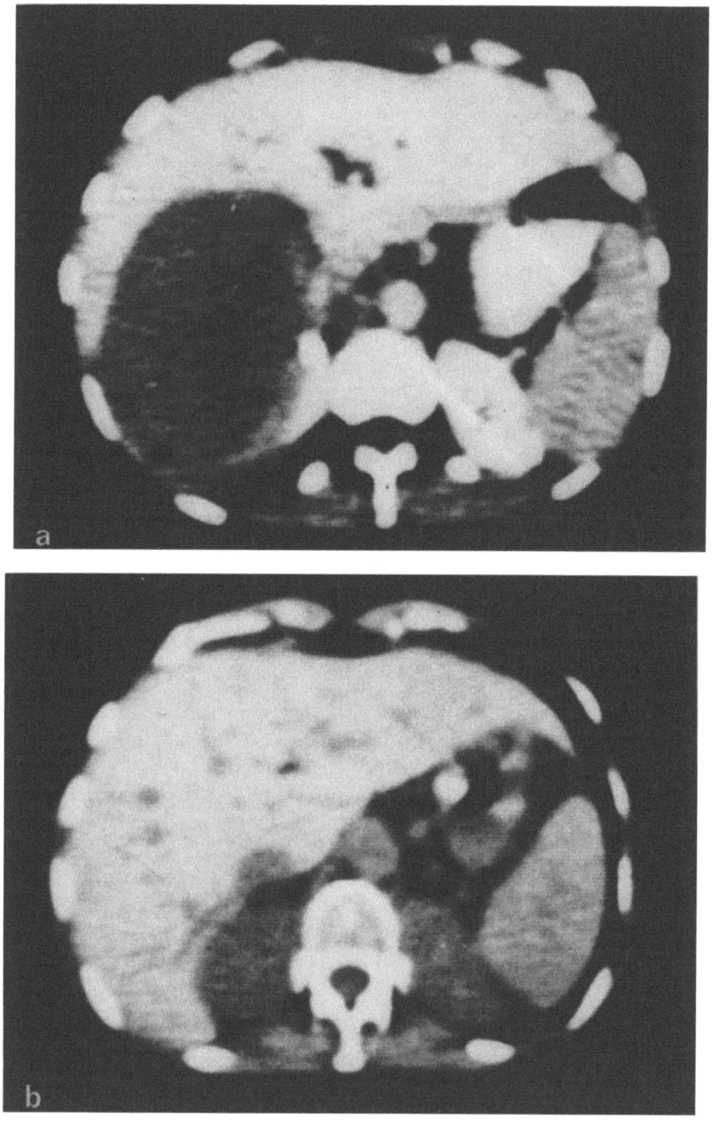

Fig. 2 a, b. Computed tomography in a patient with non-Hodgkin's lymphoma. **a** Big lesion in the posterior part of the liver without uptake of contrast medium. **b** Good response after 25-Gy whole liver irradiation

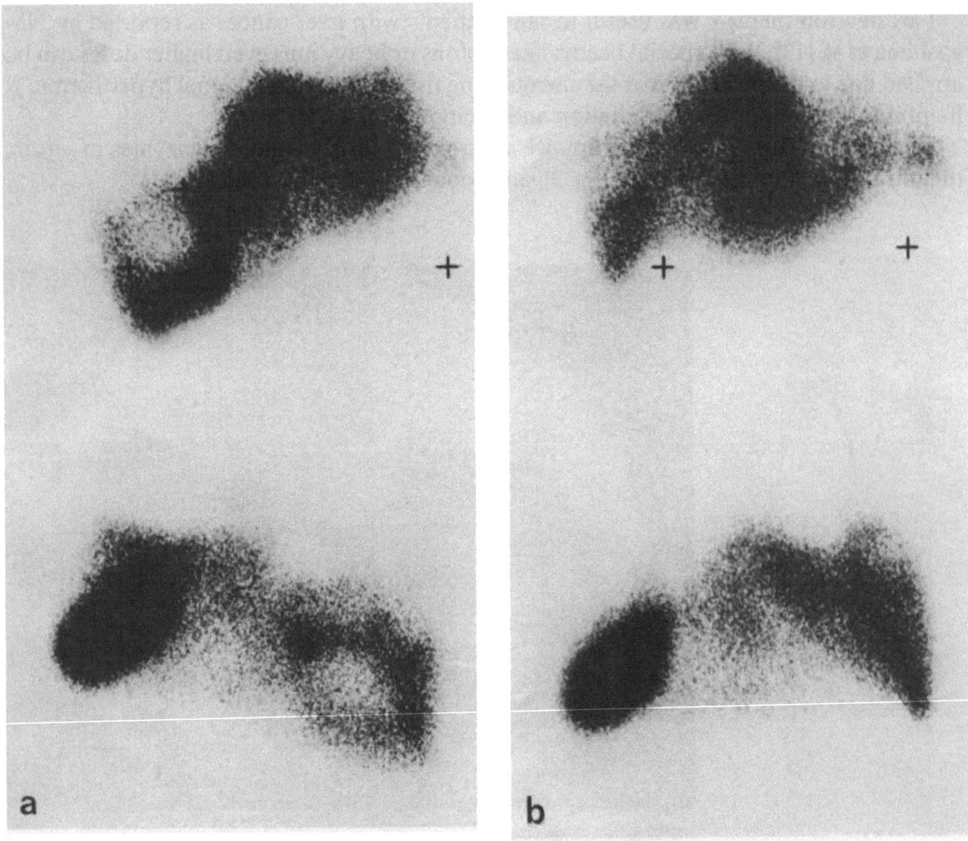

Fig. 3 a, b. Liver scan in ventral *(upper part)* and dorsal *(lower part)* view in a patient with liver metastases of a lipomyxosarcoma in the left gluteal region. **a** Multiple defects; **b** improvement after 25-Gy whole liver irradiation

Table 2. Results of radiation therapy in 26 patients with primary liver cancer [15]

Twenty-two patients evaluated	
Average dose about 30 Gy	
Marked regression	9 cases
Additional measurable regression	5 cases
Excellent symptomatic relief	11 cases
Some relief	5 cases

Primary Tumors

Phillips and Murikami [15] analyzed 26 patients with primary malignant tumors and reported notable results (Table 2). Friedman et al. [7] combined intraarterial Adriamycin and 5-fluorouracil (5-FU) with 15–24 Gy whole liver radiation therapy (5–8 fractions) in 13 patients. They observed regression for 4 to more than 15 months in 6 patients and stable disease for more than 1 to 7 months in an additional 5 patients. Symptomatic improvement could be seen in 11 patients with hepatocellular carcinoma.

Due to the fact that the combination of radiotherapy and chemotherapy yielded better results than either method alone, the results of Kopelson et al. [9] in 13 patients with extrahepatic bile duct carcinoma may be informative. Survival in the unresectable or recurrent group was: radiation group alone, 2 of 7 patients for more than 7 months, but none at 12 months; radiation and chemotherapy (5-FU), 4 of 5 patients for mor than 7 months and 2 of 5 for mor than 12 months (no evidence of disease at 12 and 16 months in 2 patients).

As induction therapy Order et al. [14] used external beam radiation with 21 Gy, 3 Gy per fraction, together with doxorubicin and 5-FU in hepatoma. This was followed by ^{131}I-radiolabeled antiferritin IgG.

Vaittinen [23] reported better survival rates (63 months, 7 patients) after postoperative radiation in gallbladder cancer compared with curative surgery alone (19 months, 24 patients). Due to the very advanced stage of most tumors of the gallbladder and the extrahepatic bile ducts connected with an unfavorable prognosis, Koester and Scherer [8] suggest postoperative radiotherapy either percutaneously or intraoperatively or with afterloading technique.

According to Ryu et al. [18] irradiation is recommended as one of the multidisciplinary treatments of hepatoma.

Metastatic Tumors

Dalluege et al. [4], Turek-Maischeder and Kazem [22], and Ramming et al. [17] published the results of radiation therapy to the total organ, with 25 Gy given slowly over a 4-week period in smaller groups of patients with liver metastases. In each case the serum alkaline phosphatase, the serum glutamic pyruvic transaminase (SGPT), and the serum glutamine oxaloacetic transaminase (SGOT) were improved. No serious complications were observed. Eight of 11 patients had a good respose [22].

Mantyla and Nordman [12] found good responses after 20-46 Gy in 8 out of 19 patients with primary liver carcinoma (5 patients), biliary duct carcinoma (4 patients), or liver metastases (10 patients). Spencer et al. [21] saw relief of massive splenomegaly after irradiation of the liver involved by Wilms' tumor.

Prasad et al. [16], reported symptomatic improvevments in 19 out of 27 paitents (70%) after doses averaging 25 Gy within 3-3.5 weeks. Whereas ascites and bilirubin were improved no significant change in survival was noted compared with nontreated patients. The results of the pilot study by the Radiation Therapy Oncology Group (RTOG) in 109 patients with metastases of solid tumors are reported by Borgelt et al. [1]. Average 30 Gy/15 fractions total liver radiation followed by 20 Gy/10 fractions boost to residual disease were applied. Seventy-four percent completed the planned course of treatment. There were no documented cases of radiation-induced hepatitis, nephritis, or pneumonitis. The degree of symptom improvement ranged from 19% (weakness, fatigue) to 55% (pain). Improvement of liver function chemistry values (e.g., bilirubin, serum enzymes) occurred in 40%. The results of the study indicate that whole liver irradiation is well tolerated, with good therapeutic benefit in patients with symptomatic liver metastases. However, the overall median survival of patients who died was only 11 weeks.

Sherman et al. [20] applied 21-24 Gy during 2 weeks in 3 Gy/fraction to 55 patients with liver metastases, 92% from adenocarcinomas. Eighty-nine percent of the patients responded, with 44% showing excellent pain relief, decreased liver size, and improved liver function. No correlation could be found between palliative response and prior (14 patients) or concomitant (31 patients) chemotherapy. The 1-year survival rate was 21%. Due to the good tolerance a radiation dose of 30 Gy within 3 weeks to the whole organ is now recommended.

Foster [5] too recommends 3 Gy daily for 7 treatments.

Attempts have been made recently to enhance response to radiation by the addition of intraarterial [6, 24] or intravenous chemotherapy. Frequently good palliation can be obtained. However, the median survival time of 4-5 months is nearly unchanged even after radiotherapy combined with misonidazole [10].

In Heidelberg, Wieland et al. [25] performed radiation of total liver with chemotherapy in seven patients with primary breast cancer (four patients), sarcoma, and prostatic and gastric carcinoma. Complete regression was registered in two cases, partial regression in an additional two cases, no change in one case, and progression in two cases. The mean survival time in 6 deceased patients was 10 months.

Recent Results in Heidelberg

Wieland and Weischedel evaluated 66 out of 75 patients with primary tumors (5 patients) or liver metastases (61 patients) who had undergone radiation therapy in Heidelberg during 1969-1984. In 13 patients the primary tumor was colorectal carcinoma, in 11 patients breast cancer, and in 7 patients bronchogenic carcinoma (Table 5). In 21 patients radiotherapy was used exclusively; 28 patients had prior and 17 patients concomitant chemotherapy.

Mostly radiotherapy was performed with the cobalt-60 unit. One ventral or two opposing fields were used. A favorable dose distribution was achieved with biaxial rotating irradiation (Fig. 1). The total doses were 24-30 Gy, 1.5 Gy/fraction, 5 fractions/week. In four

Table 3. Primary tumors in 61 patients with liver metastases (Universitäts-Strahlenklinik Heidelberg 1969-1984)

No. patients	Primary site
13	Colorectal
11	Breast
7	Bronchial (5 small cell)
4 each	Gallbladder, biliary tract, unknown
3 each	Upper digestive tract, Non-Hodgkin's lymphoma, gynecological tumors
2 each	Morbus Hodgkin, testicular (seminoma), sarcoma
1 each	Pancreas, otorhinolaryngological, prostate, testicular (teratoma), kidney, cutis (melanoma), CNS (neuroblastoma)
61 patients	

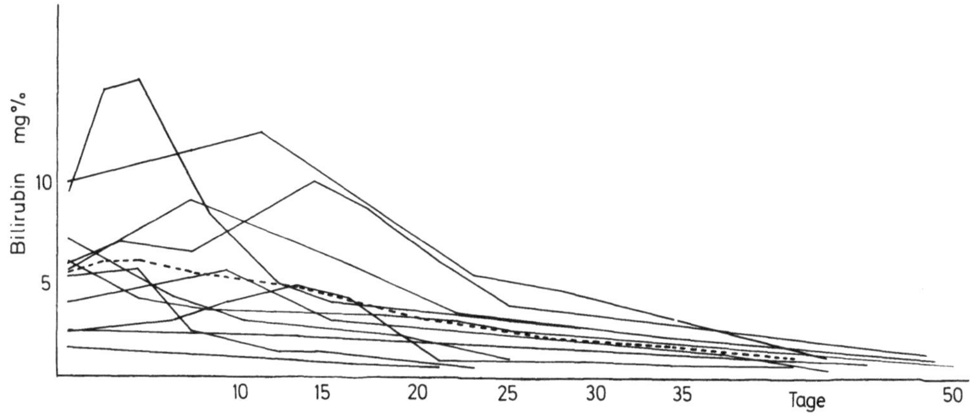

Fig. 4. Bilirubin values in 11 patients with liver metastases and obstructive jaundice during and after radiotherapy

patients radiation therapy was used with infrared hyperthermia. The liver was heated first during 20 min up to 42 °C; afterward radiation was performed. The procedure was well tolerated.

Indications were: obstructive jaundice, reduced liver function, enlarged organ, and pain.

In 11 of 26 patients with obstructive jaundice the bilirubin values went to normal, sometimes after an initial progression within the first week (Fig. 4). In 6 of 26 patients with obstructive jaundice partial improvement was seen. Nine patients gave no response. A 34-year-old patient with high-risk non-Hodgkin's lymphoma showed a good regression after 25 Gy with opposing fields (Fig. 2).

Sixty-three of the 66 patients have died. The mean survival time of the deceased patients was 5 months. Twenty-nine of these patients (54%) had metastases also in other organs. In 9 patients survival was 1 year and more; the mean survival time in these patients was 17 months. The survival rate was not or nearly not influenced by chemotherapy. The patients without jaundice had mean survival times of 7 months corresponding to what Brady and Borgelt [2] reported. The 3 living patients have survival times of 1 year and 4 months after 40 Gy (colorectal adenocarcinoma), 7 years after 60 Gy and chemotherapy because of liver metastases and recurrence of gastric carcinoma, and 5.5 years after 30 Gy and chemotherapy because of reticulosarcoma. One patient with primary adenocarcinoma had hemihepatectomy and postoperative radiotherapy with 54 Gy because of residual tumor. The survival time was 2.5 years.

Following suggestions by Herrmann (personal communication) patients with liver metastases now receive 5-FU (800 mg/24 h) and 1.5 Gy total liver radiation daily for 5 days. After 3 weeks the combination of radiation with chemotherapy is continued. According to Byfield et al. [3] in this pilot study the interaction of 5-FU with radiotherapy is used.

Discussion

Corresponding to the statements of several authors and to our own observations radiation is an efficient therapy in primary and metastatic liver tumors. It is of special value in obstructive jaundice. The radiation dose must be at least 24 Gy, 1.5–2.0 Gy/fraction. After more than 30 Gy total liver dose, side effects can occur; therefore the radiation field must be reduced.

Friedman et al. [6] did not notice increased liver toxicity during radiotherapy combined with chemotherapy. Because we have the same experience, the combination of radiation and chemotherapy can be recommended. The radiosensitizer misonidazole does not improve the results [2, 10].

Postoperative radiation therapy can improve the survival time as well as the living quality in patients with primary tumors or solitary metastases.

Conclusion

The role of radiotherapy in the treatment of hepatic tumors is growing. There is opportunity to combine localized irradiation with intraarterial or systemic chemotherapy or isotopic therapy and - in some situations - with surgery. Optimum combinations of the therapeutic modalities may eventually lead to the control of hepatic metastases. Fundamentals of radiation must be considered such as the effects on liver tissue as well as on primary and on secondary liver tumors. Before starting radiation careful planning including dose distribution and fractionation is necessary.

References

1. Borgelt BB, Gelber R, Brady LW, Griffin T, Hendrickson FR (1981) The palliation of hepatic metastases: results of the radiation therapy oncology group pilot study. Radiat Oncol Biol Phys 7: 587-591
2. Brady LW, Borgelt BB (1983) The palliation of metastatic disease of the liver using radiation therapy. Rays (Roma) 8: 135-140
3. Byfield JE, Sharp TR, Frankel SS, Tang SG, Callipari FB (1984) Phase I and II trial of five-day infused 5-fluorouracil and radiation in advanced cancer of the head and neck. J Clin Oncol 2: 406-413
4. Dalluege KH, Eichhorn HJ, Scholz P, Huettner J (1972) Zur Strahlentherapie von Lebermetastasen. Strahlentherapie 144: 522-532
5. Foster JW (1982) Treatment of metastatic cancer to the liver. In: DeVita VT, Hellman S, Rosenberg SA (eds) Cancer. Principles and practice of oncology. Lippincott, Philadelphia
6. Friedman MA, Cassidy MJ, Levine M, Philips T, Spivack S, Kessler KJ (1979a) Combined modality therapy of hepatic metastases. Cancer 44: 906
7. Friedman MA, Volberding PA, Cassidy MJ, Resser KJ, Wasserman TH, Phillips TL (1979b) Therapy for hepatocellular cancer with intrahepatic arterial adriamycin and 5-fluorouracil combined with whole liver radiation: an NCOG study. Cancer Treat Rep 63: 1885
8. Koester R, Scherer E (1984) Gegenwärtiger Stand und Möglichkeiten der Strahlentherapie bei der interdisziplinären Behandlung der Malignome des Magens, des Pankreas und der Gallenwege. III. Extrahepatische Gallenwege und Gallenblase. Strahlentherapie 160: 403-410
9. Kopelson G, Harisiadis L, Tretter P (1977) The role of radiation therapy in cancer of the extrahepatic biliary system: an analysis of thirteen patients and a review of the literature of the effectiveness of surgery, chemotherapy and radiotherapy. Int J Radiat Oncol Biol Phys 2: 883
10. Leibel SA, Order SE, Rominger CJ, Asbell SO (1981) Palliation of liver metastases with combined hepatic irradiation and misonidazole. Results of a Radiation Therapy Oncology Group Phase I-II study. Cancer 4: 285
11. Macdonald JS, Gunderson LL, Adson MA (1982) Cancer of the hepatobiliary system. In: DeVita VT, Hellman S, Rosenberg SA: Cancer. Principles and practice of oncology. Lippincott, Philadelphia

12. Mantyla M, Nordman E (1978) Radiation treatment of liver metastases. Strahlentherapie 154: 182-184
13. Nagashima T, Ryu M, Watanabe Y, Yamamoto H, Ariga T, Yamamoto Y, Koide Y, Odaka M, Sato H, Ishikawa T, Tsunemoto H (1984) Experiences of fast neutron irradiation therapy in liver and biliary tract cancers. J Jpn Soc Cancer Ther 19: 354
14. Order SE, Ettinger DS, Leibel SA, Klein JL, Leichner PK (1983) Cyclic radiolabeled 131-I Antiferritin in multimodality therapy of hepatocellular carcinoma. (Abstract Proc Am Soc Clin Oncol C-464
15. Phillips R, Murikami K (1960) Primary neoplasms of the liver: results of radiation therapy. Cancer 13: 714
16. Prasad B, Lee MS, Hendrickson FR (1977) Irradiation of hepatic metastases. Int J Radiat Oncol Biol Phys 2: 129-132
17. Ramming KP, Sparks FC, Eilber FR, Morton DL (1977) Management of hepatic metastases. Semin Oncol 4: 71-80
18. Ryu M, Watanabe Y, Yamamoto H, Nagashima T, Ariga T, Ishikawa T, Kawana M, Odaka M, Sato H (1984) The role of irradiation in multi-disciplinary treatments of primary hepatoma. J Jpn Soc Cancer Ther 19: 353
19. Scherer E (1980) Leber, Gallenwege und Pankreas. In: Scherer E (ed) Strahlentherapie. Radiologische Onkologie. 2 ed Springer, Berlin Heidelberg New York
20. Sherman DM, Weichselbaum R, Order SE, Choud L, Trey C, Piro AJ (1978) Palliation of hepatic metastases. Cancer 41: 2013-2017
21. Spencer RP, Antar MA, Touloukian RJ, Knowlon AH (1973) Relief of massive splenomegaly after irradiation of liver involved by Wilms' tumor. J Nucl Med 14: 939
22. Turek-Maischeder M, Kazem I (1975) Palliative irradiation for liver metastases. JAMA 232: 625
23. Vaittinen E (1970) Carcinoma of the gallbladder: a study of 390 cases diagnosed in Finland 1953-1967. Ann Chir Gynaecol Fenn 29, 168: 7
24. Webber BM, Soderberg CH, Leone LA, Rege VB, Glicksman AS (1978) A combined treatment approach to management of hepatic metastases. Cancer 42: 1087
25. Wieland C, Kleibel F, Weischedel U (1980) Kombination von Chemo- und Teilkörperstrahlentherapie bei Lungen- und Lebermetastasen. Strahlentherapie 156: 409-413

Combined Use of Drugs and Radiation in the Treatment of Liver Metastases

J. E. Byfield

Department of Radiation Oncology, Daniel Freeman Memorial Hospital, 333 North Prairie Avenue, Inglewood, CA 90301, USA

Introduction

The liver presents a unique opportunity to study the potential benefits of drug and X-ray combinations in a complete organ system. The entire liver can be radiated without delivering an excessive dose to nearby organ systems since they are either less radiosensitive (gut) or can be screened or even partially sacrificed (kidney). On the other hand the liver itself is extremely radiosensitive and cannot tolerate the dose of radiation required to sterilize other than subclinical epithelial tumor burdens. This chapter is devoted to a survey of means by which radiation and drugs can be combined in order to overcome this severe limitation. Recently developed techniques which promise a more quantitative evaluation of drug X-ray interactions as they affect hepatocyte survival are also included.

Classification of Potentially Useful Drugs

There are three types of drugs that may be of use with radiation in hepatic treatment: (1) conventional chemotherapeutic agents; (2) radiosensitizers, either hypoxic or oxic; and (3) radioprotectors. Initial clinical studies have been completed for the first two classes and promising preclinical studies have now been published for the third group. Since these classes overlap to a significant degree they are discussed in order of progressive current usefulness.

Radiation Sensitivity of the Liver

It is well known that the liver is among the most radiosensitive of the visceral organs. The liver cannot withstand much over 3000 rads (30 gray) X-irradiation with conventional fractionation [8, 25] and it remains to be seen whether or not hyperfractionation (multiple daily treatments with small radiation doses) will have any added benefit. Perhaps the most important recent advance in furthering our understanding of hepatic radiosensitivity has been the development of quantitative hepatic cell cloning techniques by Jirtle and colleagues [18]. These assays will now permit comprehensive studies of the effects of drug and radiation combinations on hepatic cell functioning and survival.

Recent Results in Cancer Research. Vol 100

Clonogenic Assays of Hepatocytes

The techniques developed by Jirtle's group involve isolation of in situ hepatic cells using a perfusion technique that enzymatically liberates clonogenic hepatocytes. The hepatocytes are then studied by quantitative cloning in recipient animals that have just undergone partial hepatectomy. Hepatectomy induces the necessary (but as yet poorly understood) circulating hepatic growth factors needed to stimulate the liver cells to clone [18]. These studies have clearly shown that in situ hepatocytes are quite radiosensitive with the approximate X-ray surviving fractions shown in Table 1 (R. Jirtle, personal communication). Most noteworthy has been the demonstration by Jirtle et al. that hepatocyte survival is *enhanced* by harvesting the cells 24 h *after* radiation [19]. This indicates that the resting liver has the capacity to recover from or to repair some of the damage induced by ionizing radiation. Similar results have recently been obtained by Fisher and Hendry, who found a further increase in clonogenicity in the months following the initial radiation insult [14].

Repopulation of Radiated Liver

Since there is no evidence for a significant repopulation by liver cells during or immediately after hepatic radiation it is apparent that a dose of 3000 rads delivered in 15 fractions of 200 rads each would reduce hepatic cell clonogenic survival (normally about 10^9 hepatocytes/g) to about 2.4×10^7, i. e., about a 50-fold reduction. Viewed as a "partial hepatectomy" this would be the equivalent of removing almost all visible liver! Clearly, the failure of the liver to repopulate *during* a radiation series [14, 18] seems a potentially important aspect of eventual liver failure and a prime area for future investigation.

Radioprotection of Normal Liver: WR-2721

One of the first contributions made by these new hepatocyte cloning procedures has been the demonstration that it is possible to protect hepatocyte growth (repopulation) potential with an added radioprotecter. Thus the compound called WR-2721 (which has been proposed [29] to protect normal tissues but not tumor cells) has been shown significantly to reduce X-ray killing of hepatocytes [20]. To what extent this will be applicable clinically is not as yet known but this is an active area of current investigation. It can be anticipated that important new information will be forthcoming in the next few years as a result of further elaboration and use of these ingenious cloning techniques.

Table 1. Clonogenic X-ray survival of in situ rat hepatocytes after clinical levels of radiation. (R. L. Jirtle, unpublished data)

Dose (rads)	Immediate cloning	Cloning after 24 h
200	0.48	0.78
250	0.40	0.69
300	0.33	0.60

Clinical Liver Injury by Drugs and X-Rays

These observations raise the other important unresolved problem, viz., what is the relationship between hepatocyte killing (by drugs and X-rays) and the development of clinical radiation hepatitis. It seems clear that other components in the liver (e.g., blood vessels) contribute to the pathophysiology of this syndrome [25]. Whether these are primary events or are secondary changes induced by slow hepatocyte failure remains to be established. The recent observation that a high drug infusion rate can itself induce damage to the biliary tree [17] is another example of how unexpected problems may develop. The importance of quantitative preclinical models such as cited above can scarcely be overestimated.

Patient Selection in Clinical Hepatic Radiation Studies

Prior to consideration of existing studies looking at drugs added to X-rays for metastatic liver cancer it is worthwhile reviewing the data now available for quantitatively evaluating this patient group. In this context the extensive data from Pajak et al. are noteworthy [23]. Based on an analysis of results of two large randomized trials, they concluded that the important pretreatment characteristics affecting patient *survival* were performance status, existence of malignant disease outside the liver, and the source of the primary tumor. Patients with a high performance status, disease limited to the liver, and a colon primary were likely to survive longer than any other categories. Elevated bilirubin (> 1.5 mg%) adversely affected survival in all groups. On the other hand with a large enough patient population (e.g., with 200 patients or more in aggregate treatment arms) they found virtually superimposable survival curves for two distinct treatments (i.e., the single variable under study had no effect). This kind of analysis shows clearly that patient selection will greatly influence even as objective a parameter as survival. However, their data also show that if a population is sufficiently large and heterogeneous, the overall survival pattern is quite reproducible (i.e., identical survival in a two-arm study). Therefore large series can give rapid results for events early in a study (e.g., toxic deaths) while small series, *if carefully stratified,* can probably detect important improvements in treatment results.

Hypoxic Radiosensitizers

It is generally believed that hypoxia, a feature of some but not all tumors, contributes to radioresistance. The Radiation Therapy Oncology Group (RTOG) has been involved in the study of hypoxic radiosensitizers for a considerable period [24]. The first RTOG studies [5] examined the effects of radiation alone while a more recent protocol (80-03) has studied the effect of added misonidazole on pain relief. While the final results of the latter study have not yet been published, preliminary analysis has failed to show any significant benefit from misonidazole. This is in agreement with other related investigations which showed the drug unlikely to benefit patients because of its inherent pharmacologic limitations [24]. The fact that over 5000 patients received this drug before these conclusions were reached [12] offers food for thought for the more vigorous supporters of cooperative, randomized trials as the sole source of useful scientific information.

Conventional Chemotherapeutic Agents: Choice of Drugs

There have now been several reports of the combination of conventional drugs with radiation used for metastatic liver cancer (cf. review by Kinsella). In general the drugs used have been selected from those agents thought be useful per se against the specific cancer. As such they have necessarily been limited by the modest response rates seen with the drug(s) alone. Since most patients eligible for locoregional treatment are patients with colorectal cancer, studies of patients with that disorder predominate. 5-Fluoro-2'-deoxyuridine (5-FUdR) has been the most commonly used intraarterial agent but various other agents have also been added.

FUdR and Radiation

As an example of this approach we have recently reported our own experience with such a regimen, but with added whole liver radiation [4, 9]. Our study employed continuously infused 5-FUdR at 0.2 gm/kg per day (to systemic toxicity) along with cyclical fractionated radiation (250 rads/fraction with 4 treatments or 1000 rads/week, given every other week). This fractionation was adapted from our developing experience in the use of fluorinated pyrimidines as radiosensitizers (see below). 5-FUdR (which is *not* a radiosensitizer) was chosen because of what initially appeared to be its favorable intraarterial pharmacology [13]. The total radiation dose, given in the three cycles over 5 weeks, was 3000 rads. This was clearly a tolerance dose with this X-ray fractionation. The details of these studies are available elsewhere [4, 6] but the general survival pattern is shown in Fig. 1. The most salient points are: patients who are entered with significant abnormalities in liver tests (i.e., elevations of either their bilirubin or alkaline phosphatase to twice or more the level considered upper limits of normal) do very poorly. All such patients die without real evidence of treatment benefit. This is to be expected from a therapy whose complete response rate to drug alone is certainly 20% or less (cf. ref 3 and this volume) and where a maximum radiation dose of only 3000 rads can be used. Such an X-ray dose can *maximally* reduce epithelial tumor cell deposits by a factor of about only four logs and can therefore sterilize only microscopic tumor metastases (since solid tumor deposits contain about 10^9 cells/g). In this patient group the disease is simply too advanced for much to be achieved by therapy.

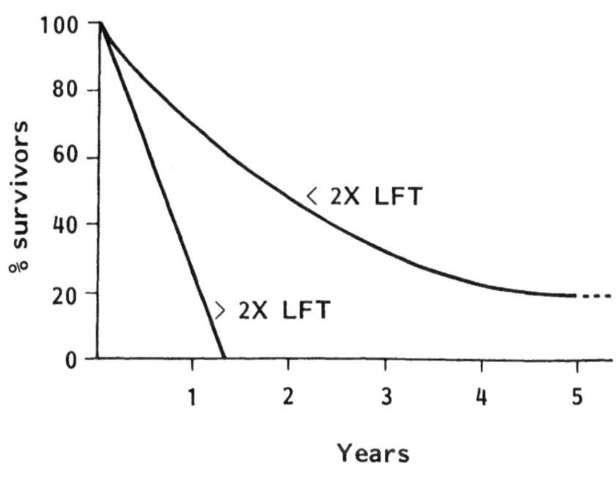

Fig. 1. General survival pattern of patients given FUdR and radiation. *LFT*, liver function test

Potential of Local Control for Cure

On the other hand patients who enter with measurable disease volume but no major liver impairment do considerably better. In our small series over 60% of such patients lived 1 year and 20% of such patients survived over 3 years [6]. In our retrospective analysis of the results of this pilot study it was apparent that virtually all the 1-year+survivors had normal or close to normal bilirubin levels when initially treated. All of the 2-year survivors had, in addition, no evidence of extrahepatic tumor at entry at the time of treatment. In these latter long-term survivors disease *outside* the liver becomes as great a problem as the metastatic liver cancer. For example, in our series those patients treated under "ideal" conditions (no known extrahepatic disease and normal or minimally abnormal liver function tests) nevertheless *all* eventually developed disease outside the liver if the liver metastases were controlled well enough to permit such long-term survival. The single 5-year survivor required two pulmonary resections for metastatic disease [6]. Thus while we believe that perhaps 50% of such "early" patients can have their liver sterilized of cancer with this approach almost all such patients will still not be cured without additional measures effective against extrahepatic metastases.

Impact of Methods of Arterial Infusion

It is worth pointing out that we could not find evidence that the use of implanted constant infusion pumps were "better" than older extracorporeal methods in terms of survival [6]. Indeed, the only patient in our first series who developed fatal treatment-related hepatitis had a "new" permanently implanted pump. The central benefit of such devices in this patient group lies in their convenience to the patient, which we believe is considerable. However, it should be remembered that the lack of "problems" associated with such "new" infusions also implies a truly continuous drug dose; such treatment may therefore lack the (artificial) "rests" that were always associated with external catheter and pump problems and technical infusion failures.

Drug and Radiation Doses: Possible Reciprocity

In our series 5-FUdR was administered continuously at a lower dose - 0.2 mg/kg per day - i. e., less than the 0.3 mg/kg that has been used in most series in which radiation was not given. Our overall survival (Fig. 1) is about the same as others using drug alone as reviewed extensively at this meeting. One cannot therefore be certain to what extent the radiation component contributed although the survival curve for our small series now has reached 5 years (with only one 5-year survivor). What is most clearly apparent is the observation that extrahepatic disease comes to dominate the picture when hepatic tumor control has been improved and that therefore a reevaluation of drug selection and scheduling (see below) is important. Extrahepatic disease *must also* be controlled if any further progress is to be made in terms of survival. Infusions with 5-FUdR, with or without radiation, do not accomplish this despite clearly toxic drug infusion rates [6].

Halopyrimidine Oxic Radiosensitizers: Introduction

As noted above biophysical radiation resistance can appear as a result of hypoxia in many cancers. However, must cancers are also resistant to radiation sterilization either as an intrinsic growth property of their cells or because the tumor burden within the treatment region is simply too large for control by a tolerable X-ray dose. These latter two sources lead to "oxic" radioresistance and are, in the author's opinion, more important than hypoxia. Moreover, *if* sufficent oxygenated cells are killed during treatment, then hypoxia will (by definition) vanish since it stems from an imbalance of tumor cells to tumor blood vessels. These observations suggest that drugs that sensitize oxygenated tumor cells to radiation may have clinical usefulness if properly applied. The reader is referred to recent work on this topic for a fuller explanation and examples [7, 8].

Bromodeoxyuridine and 5-Fluorouracil

There are two oxic radiosensitizers with potential applications in liver tumors. These are 5-bromodeoxyuridine (BUdR) and 5-fluorouracil (5-FU). Like 5-FUdR these compounds were invented by Heidelberger's group as rationally synthesized analogues of thymidine and uracil respectively [16]. Their modes of action are quite different, however, and their single common feature (apart from radiosensitization) is catabolism by the liver. The latter gives them both a potential advantage for use in arterial infusions against hepatic cancers. Experience with BUdR is limited [21] and there are as yet no studies of selective liver infusion with BUdR combined with radiation.

Radiosensitization by 5-Fluorouracil

There have been many studies of the combination of 5-FU with radiation (cf. citations in ref. [6-10]). These were based on the very early demonstration by Bagshaw that 5-FU could radiosensitize tumor cells [2]. However, it was only recently recognized that *clinical* radiosensitization could only be achieved in vivo in man through continuous infusions of 24 h or more [6]. Since radiosensitization requires about 24 h *postradiation* 5-FU exposure to develop bolus 5-FU cannot sensitize since the half-life of the drug is only 10-15 min [22].

Pharmacology of 5-FU as a Radiosensitizer

We have completed several studies of infused 5-FU as a radiosensitizer including one phase I study in which the upper abdomen and liver were treated in some patients [10]. We found no evidence that radiation of the patients influenced the pharmacokinetics of 5-FU metabolism [10]. However, the pharmacokinetics of 5-FU are unusual in being nonlinear [15, 22] and showing what appears to be a first saturation point at a daily dose rate (constant rate infusion) of about 15 mg/kg per 24 h [10]. Above that level one sees a linear relationship between the daily dose rate and the mean serum 5-FU level [10]. However, the fact that a major source of 5-FU catabolism has been saturated leads to accumulation of the drug with time at all dose rates above 15 mg/kg per day [11]. Moreover, this is accentuated by the presence of large liver metastases [15]. All of these features must be taken into account in the use of 5-FU as a clinical radiosensitizer. However, for the reasons described below we feel such an application is worthy of consideration. In at least one gastrointestinal cancer (squamous anal carcinoma) infused 5-FU used alone as a radiosensitizer has been shown to be capable of controlling even very large cancers [7] and there is existing evidence suggesting infused 5-FU (alone) has an increased response rate on colorectal cancer [26].

Conclusions and Future Prospects

It seems clear that the use of more aggressive measures such as arterial infusions, and possibly liver radiation, has somewhat improved the prognosis of patients with colonic cancer when treated early in its metastatic course in the liver. There is as yet insufficient data on the precise role that liver radiation plays. When FUdR is used as the main chemotherapeutic agent it appears possible that a lower drug infusion rate can be employed with added X-rays, which in turn *may* reduce the incidence of biliary stenosis caused by the drug. However, the data are still too sparse to be certain. To date no combination has really been successful in patients with advanced liver disease or those with coincident extrahepatic cancer.

These observations call into question the choice of drugs now being used. No series gives convincing evidence that any drug other than the arterially infused 5-FUdR plays a significant role in inducing responses. On the other hand 5-FUdR is clearly an ineffective *systemic* drug in colorectal cancer patients since most such patients who respond in the liver still fail systemically [3, 4, 9, 28]. 5-FUdR is a very toxic drug when given as a systemic infusion, the daily tolerable dose of drug being 1/30 to 1/60 of an equitoxic, equitherapeutic bolus exposure [27].

In this light it seems reasonable to suggest that other intraarterial drugs, possibly 5-FU, might be more useful. 5-FU has the pharmacologic advantages of 5-FUdR but is a much more acceptable drug for systemic, long-term infusions [26]. Moreover, it is a radiosensitizer, which 5-FUdR is not. Intraarterial hepatic infusions with 5-FU have been attempted with some success [1]. A rather low infusion dose was employed which nevertheless achieved a 55% objective response rate. Interestingly, marrow suppression was very modest and only about 5% of patients developed stomatitis [1]. The latter confirms that much higher 5-FU doses could propably be given with modern catheter techniques. Accordingly, infusion of the heaptic artery with 5-FU combined with liver radiation appears to offer some theoretical advantages over 5-FUdR. Recent preoccupation with mechanical advances in infusion technique should not prevent researchers from exploring alternative drugs and schedules in the search for combinations effective at both the local and systemic levels.

References

1. Ansfield FJ, Ramirez G, Davis HL, Wirtanen GW, Johnson RO, Bryan GT, Manalo FP, Borden EC, Davis TE, Esmaili M (1975) Further clinical studies with intrahepatic arterial infusions with 5-Fluorouracil. Cancer 36: 2413-2417
2. Bagshaw M (1961) Possible role of potentiators in radiation therapy. AJR 85: 822-833
3. Balch CM, Urist MM, Soong S-J, McGregor M (1983) A prospective phase II clinical trial of continuous FUDR regional chemotherapy for colorectal metastases to the liver using a totally implantable drug infuson pump. Ann Surg 198: 567-573

4. Barone RM, Byfield JE, Goldfarb P, Frankel SS, Ginn C, Greer S, Callipari FB (1982) Intra-arterial chemotherapy using an implantable infusion pump and liver irradiation for the treatment of hepatic metastases. Cancer 50: 850-862
5. Borgelt BB, Gelber R, Brady LW, Griffin T, Hendrickson FR (1981) The palliation of hepatic metastases: results of the Radiation Therapy Oncology Group pilot study. Int J Radiat Oncol Biol Phys 7: 587-591
6. Byfield JE, Calabro-Jones PM, Klisak I, Kulhanian F (1982) Pharmacologic requirements for obtaining sensitization of human tumor cells in vitro to combined 5-Fluorouracil or Ftorafur and radiation. Int J Radiat Oncol Biol Phys 8: 1923-1933
7. Byfield JE, Barone RM, Sharp TR, Frankel SS (1983) Conservative management of squamous anal cancer by cyclical 5-Fluorouracil infusion alone and x-rays. Cancer Treat Rep 67: 709-712
8. Byfield JE, Sharp TR, Tang SS, Frankel SS, Callipari FB (1984) Phase I and II trial of cyclical 5-day infused 5-Fluorouracil and coincident radiation in advanced cancer of the head and neck. J Clin Oncol 2: 406-413
9. Byfield JE, Barone RM, Frankel S, Sharp TR (1984) Treatment with combined intra-arterial 5-FUDR infusion and whole-liver radiation for colon carcinoma metastatic to the liver: preliminary results. Am J Clin Oncol 7 (4): 319-325
10. Byfield JE, Frankel SS, Sharp TR, Hornbeck CL, Callipari FB (1985) Phase I and pharmacologic trial of 72-hour infused 5-Fluorouracil and hyperfractionated cyclical radiation. Int J Radiat Oncol Biol Phys 11 (4): 791-800
11. Calabro-Jones PM, Byfield JE, Ward JF, Sharp TR (1982) Time-dose relationships for 5-Fluorouracil cytotoxicity against human epithelial cancer cells in vitro. Cancer Res 42: 4413-4420
12. Dische S (1984) Misonidazole - results of randomized controlled clinical trials - an evaluation. Int J Radiat Oncol Biol Phys 10 (9): 1811-1814
13. Emsminger WD, Rosowski A, Raso V, Levin DC, Glode M, Come S, Steele G, Frei E III (1978) A clinical pharmacological evaluation of hepatic arterial infusions of 5'-Fluoro-2'-deoxyuridine and 5-Fluorouracil. Cancer Res 38: 3784-3792
14. Fisher DR, Hendry JH (1984) Clonogenicity of x-irradiated hepatocytes *in vivo* assayed both early and late. Int J Radiat Biol (abstract) 46 (5): 644
15. Floyd RA, Hornbeck CL, Byfield JE, Griffiths JC, Frankel SS (1982) Clearance of continuously infused 5-Fluorouracil in adults having lung or gastrointestinal carcinoma with or without hepatic metastases. Drug Intell Clin Pharm 16: 665-667
16. Heidelberger C (1975) Fluorinated pyrimidines and their nucleosides. In: Sartorelli AC, Johns DG (eds) New antineoplastic and immunosuppressive agents, Pt 2. Springer, New York Heidelberg Berlin, pp 193-231
17. Hohn D, Stagg R, Ignoffo R, Friedman M, Melnick J, Altman D, Lewis B (1984) Incidence and prevention of complications of cyclic hepatic artery infusions (HAI) of floxuridine (FUDR): severe biliary sclerosis, gastritis, and ulcer. Proc Am Soc Clin Oncol 3: (abs) 148
18. Jirtle RL, Michalopoulos G, McLain JR, Corwley J (1981) Transplantation system for determining the clonogenic survival of parenchymal hepatocytes exposed to ionizing radiation. Cancer Res 41: 3512-3518
19. Jirtle RL, McLain JR, Strom SC, Michalopolous G (1982) Repair of radiation damage in noncycling parenchymal hepatocytes. Br J Radiol 55: 847-851
20. Jirtle RL, Michalopolous G, Strom SC, DeLuca PM, Gould MN (1984) The survival of parenchymal hepatocytes irradiated with low and high LET radiation. Br J Cancer 49: (Suppl 6) 197-201
21. Kinsella TJ (1983) The role of radiation therapy alone and combined with infusion chemotherapy for treating liver metastases. Semin Oncol 10: 215-222
22. Myers CE, Diasio R, Eliot HM, Chabner BA (1976) Pharmacokinetics of the fluoropyrimidines: implications for their clinical use. Cancer Treat Rev 3: 175-183
23. Pajak TF, Davis DR, Leibel SA, Russell AH (1984) Selection of an optimal population for future liver metastases studies Proc Am Assoc Cancer Res 25: (abs) 199
24. Phillips TL, Wasserman TH (1984) Promise of radiosensitizers and radioprotectors in the treatment of human cancers. Cancer Treat Rep 68: 297-302

25. Reed GB, Cox AJ (1966) The human liver after radiation injury. Am J Pathol 46: 597–611
26. Seifert P, Baker LH, Reed ML, Vaitkevicius VK (1975) Comparison of continuously infused 5-Fluorouracil with bolus injection in treatment of patients with colorectal adenocarcinoma. Cancer 36: 123–128
27. Sullivan RD, Miller E (1965) The clinical effects of prolonged intravenous infusion of 5-Fluoro-2'-deoxyuridine. Cancer Res 25: 1025–1034
28. Weiss GR, Garnick MB, Osteen RT, Steele GD Jr, Wilson RE, Schade D, Kaplan WD, Boxt LM, Kandarpa K, Mayer RJ, Frei E-T III. (1983) Long-term hepatic arterial infusion of 5-Fluorodeoxyruidine for liver metastases using an implantable infusion pump. J Clin Oncol 1: 337–344
29. Yuhas JM, Spellman JM, Culo F (1980) The role of WR-2721 in radiotherapy and/or chemotherapy. Cancer Clin Trials 3: 211–216

Radiolabeled Antibody in the Treatment of Primary and Metastatic Liver Malignancies

S. E. Order, J. L. Klein, P. K. Leichner, D. S. Ettinger, K. Kopher, K. Finney, M. Surdyke, and S. A. Leibel

The Johns Hopkins Hospital, Radiation Oncology, 600 North Wolfe Street, Baltimore, MD 21205, USA

Primary hepatic malignancy is the present dominant cancer in the world [1]. Often silent in its early manifestations, by the time of clinical presentation it may be ten times larger than a T3 carcinoma of the head and neck (1500 cm^3 vs. 125 cm^3). Chemotherapy, hepatic artery ligation, and external radiation with or without chemotherapy have led to brief palliation [2-4]. A series of etiologic agents including viral hepatitis [5], carcinogenic chemicals [6], and hormones [7] may also lead to varied tumor aggressiveness. In our own experience, the presence or absence of alpha-fetoprotein also indicated tumor aggressiveness, with alpha-fetoprotein positive expressing a more primitive and undifferentiated tumor [8]. A second and less common intrahepatic cancer, intrahepatic biliary cancer, remains equally as lethal, with a 3- to 4-month median survival [9].

The most common liver malignancy in the United States is metastatic disease, in particular colorectal carcinoma. Clearly the median survival of such patients regardless of method of treatment has been profoundly influenced by the physiologic status of the patient (Karnofsky score), the duration of time between primary and metastatic disease expression, and the tumor burden carcinoembryonic antigen (CEA) titer, number of metastatic sites, magnitude of organ replacement] [10, 11]. Standard methods of treatment for multiple liver metastases include intravenous chemotherapy [12], intraarterial continuous infusion chemotherapy [13], external radiation, and external radiation and chemotherapy (both intravenous and intraarterial) [10, 11, 14, 15]. The median remissions have been 3-4 months with some survival up to 1 year, and clearly patient selection has played a role. The results further indicate a high local failure rate of 70% or greater and the need for more effective agents [11].

In this review a discussion of radiolabeled antibodies as a new modality in the treatment of these malignancies, the antigens as targets for radiolabeled antibodies, the criteria of effectiveness of therapy, and the cascade of new technologies and methods of analysis as well as future therapeutic developments are discussed.

Hepatoma

Experimental

The H4IIE rat hepatoma has been used in our laboratory and ferritin, a tumor-associated antigen, which was synthesized and secreted by the tumor, was used to study ^{131}I-antiferritin antibody. Initially comparison of ^{131}I normal IgG with ^{131}I-antiferritin demonstrated a

Recent Results in Cancer Research. Vol 100

threefold increase in tumor deposition with the ^{131}I-antiferritin. Normal tissues did not differentially concentrate ^{131}I normal IgG or ^{131}I-antiferritin [16]. In later experiments the correlation of tumor size, ferritin synthesis and secretion, and vascularity were shown to explain the "biologic window," that is, the factors causing selective tumor localization of the immunospecific radiolabeled antibody [17, 18].

It is particularly important to point out that if in vitro criteria for antigen biodistribution were used as the determinant for the potential value of this antigenic target (ferritin) both the experimential and clinical trials would not have been undertaken. The ferritin antigen has demonstrated the fallacy of the supposed necessity of singular tumor antigenic uniqueness and absence of cross-reactivity as important criteria, and underlines the need for in vivo evaluation as a prerequisite to clinical trials rather than solely in vitro evaluation. Active tumor synthesis and stromal accumulation of ferritin acts as a repository of high antigen concentration which is exposed by tumor neovasculature for selective radiolabeled antibody deposition.

It has not always been appreciated that for radiolabeled antibody to be used in therapeutic applications it is total dose deposited in malignant and normal tissue that determines therapeutic efficacy and not ratio at a moment in time between these sites. Radiation dose consits of tumor saturation (μCi/g) and tumor-effective half-life (composite of physical and biologic half-lives) until full decay of the radiolabeled antibody at the tumor. In our experimential hepatoma, the ratio between tumor and normal tissue continually expands until full decay. Thus larger tumor-to-normal tissue ratios are achieved with increasing time following infusion. This does not reflect total tumor dose. In contrast, in the science of nuclear scanning such foreground (tumor) to background (normal tissue) ratios determine scanning potential. Similarly a Fab fragment will yield superior scanning qualities due to rapid passage out of the host and greater ratios of difference between tumor and normal tissue, but will be inferior as a vehicle for ^{131}I, which requires prolonged tumor deposition to achieve significant radiation dose [19, 20].

Clinical Hepatoma

In our early experience with ^{131}I-antiferritin the research was designed to determine toxicity and dose of radiolabeled antibody for potential response. Due to the 3- to 4-month median survival associated with conventional treatment of hepatoma, we elected initially to carry out induction therapy with external radiation and chemotherapy, seeking tumor reduction prior to two cycles of chemotherapy and the experimental radiolabeled antibody. Therefore 2100 rad (300 rad fractions) and concomitant Adriamycin, 15 mg, and 5-FU, 500 mg (chemotherapy on alternate days), were given 4 times a week for 1½ weeks (7 treatments). Previous clinical experience indicated that remission if it occurred would take no longer than 1 month after external radiation and then conventional chemotherapy could be given and finally the experimential radiolabeled antibody [21, 22].

Experience with this protocol rapidly indicated that many patients were failing during the two cycles of chemotherapy. Therefore the induction therapy of external radiation and chemotherapy was maintained but followed in 1 month by the radiolabeled antibody. Dose escalation of ^{131}I-antiferritin (50, 100, and 150 mCi) demonstrated that 30 mCi was sufficient for tumor saturation and doses as high as 150 mCi represented no advantage for the patients, for they increased free circulating radiolabeled antibody and not tumor dose [22]. Several developments rapidly followed and included the description of thrombocytopenia as the major toxicity, determination of tumor dosimetry, and a schedule of 30 mCi on day 0 and 20 mCi on day 5, later followed by integration of Adriamycin, 15 mg, and 5-FU, 500 mg [23, 24]. Cyclic therapy was next introduced and consisted of alternating the species from which antibody was derived, rabbit, pig, monkey, and bovine antiferritins [25]. These latter antiferritins had significant tumor effective half-lives between 3 and 4.5 days, whereas sheep and goat were intermediate and chicken and turkey antiferritin immunoglobulin had even shorter tumor effective half-lives and were of no value.

Studies of ^{131}I-anti-AFP (alpha-fetoprotein) were compared with those of ^{131}I-antiferritin and demonstrated significant differences in tumor saturation: 2.7 μCi/g for anti-AFP compared with 8.4 μCi/g for antiferritin [26]. The obvious dosimetric advantage of antiferritin was further amplified by the associated remissions (50%), which will be discussed. Affinity purification of antiferritin was studied and resulted in reduced tumor effective half-life as was also seen with Fab fragments of the IgG molecule. The dehalogenation of ^{131}I monoclonal antiferritin was noted when ^{131}I was used as the radiolabel [27].

Future progress will lie in new radiolabels for monoclonal and polyclonal antibodies while studies of cyclic polyclonal antibody are being completed.

Cyclic Therapy

Cyclic therapy was the next protocol examined with initial external radiation and chemotherapy followed 1 month later by Adriamycin, 15 mg, and 5-FU 500 mg (day −1), and 30 mCi ^{131}I-antiferritin (day 0) and 20 mCi ^{131}I-antiferritin (day 5). Cycling radiolabeled

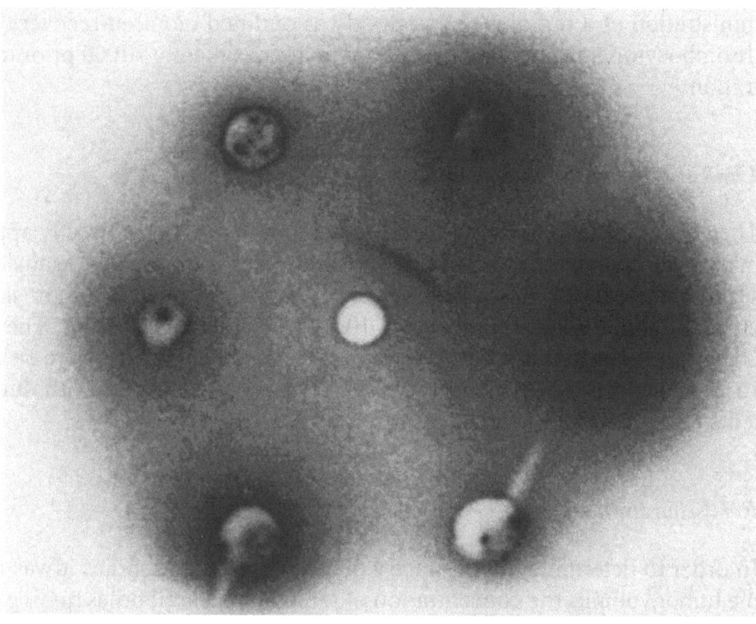

Fig. 1. Center well of an Ouchterlony plate with patient's serum. Peripheral wells contain rabbit (positive), pig, monkey, bovine, baboon, and African green monkey antibodies. The precipitin line is developed by autoradiography since the peripheral wells contain radiolabeled antibodies. This patient has human anti-rabbit antibodies. Recycling with rabbit antibodies will lead to rapid degradation and will not be associated with significant tumor targeting

antibody derived from rabbit, pig, monkey, and bovine sources every 2 months was based on the known hematologic toxicity with recovery. Other species that were examined have been eliminated since species of antibody derivation had a direct correlation with tumor effective half-life. Those species no longer in clinical use include sheep, goat, chicken, and turkey antibodies.

As patients improved, and remitted patients lived longer, the necessity of examining recycling original antibodies which led to clinical remission became necessary. In the preliminary experience of seven recycled patients, a new method of clinical evaluation using Ouchterlony plates was developed by Jerry L. Klein of our faculty. The absence of precipiting lines, i. e., no anti-antibody in these gels, was correlated with successful recycling in three of seven patients in whom recycling was successful. Tumor targeting and retention of tumor effective half-life occurred when the patient did not produce anti-antibody. In the remaining four patients, who had positive precipiting lines between their sera and the radiolabeled antibodies, all patients hat tumor effective half-lives under 12 h and such rapid degradation of the radiolabeled antibodies that tumor targeting was not documented (Fig. 1). The methods of this analysis and its sensitivity will re reported by Klein et al. (unpublished data).

Modification for Hematologic Toxicity

Modification of radiolabeled antibody used in a given cycle of therapy was due to toxicity, usually grade III thrombocytopenia from a previous treatment cycle, and included a change to 20 mCi ^{131}I-antiferritin on day 0 and 10 mCi on day 5. The modification and administration of a radiolabeled antibody as outlined required recovery from the grade III thrombocytopenia and a platelet count of approximately 70000 prior to the next administration.

Clinical Intrahepatic Biliary Cancer

The general principles as outlined for hepatoma have been directly applicable to this primary liver malignancy except that the antibodies were derived against CEA. Among the several differences in application in ^{131}I-anti-CEA was a tumor saturation requiring 20 mCi ^{131}I-anti-CEA following by 10 mCi to achieve 4.7 μCi/g. The absence of a high CEA titer in the blood stream contrasts to ferritin titers, which were elevated in hepatoma. In a smaller series of patients (20), 50% have remitted to date with duration in some patients beyond 1 and 2 years.

Remission Evaluation

In order to determine the dosimetry of radiolabeled antibodies it was necessary to assess the tumor volume, the concentration of radiolabeled antibodies (μCi/g), and the tumor effective half-life. The tumor volume was determined by reconstruction of CT scans every 8 mm on a secondary computer [26]. These tumor volumes then became available as sequential evaluations of tumor progression (25% increase in volume), tumor stability, or tumor remission (30% or greater reduction in tumor volume). To date there have been five complete remissions. One patient was disease free at 3 years, one had recurrent disease at 5 years, and three were without primary disease but with metastases at 1-2 years.

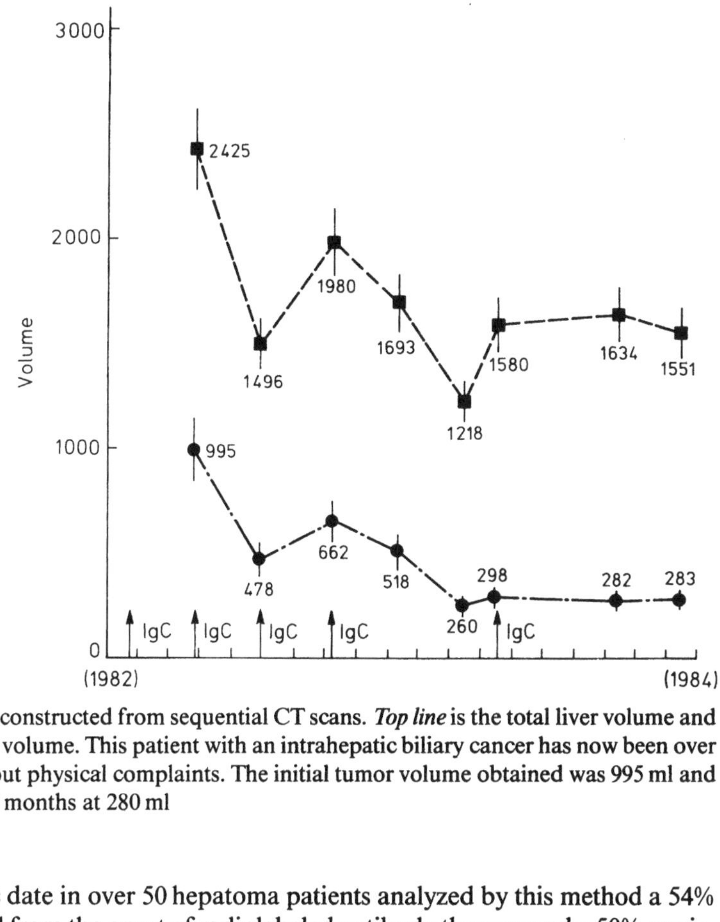

Fig. 2. Volumetric data reconstructed from sequential CT scans. *Top line* is the total liver volume and the *bottom line*, the tumor volume. This patient with an intrahepatic biliary cancer has now been over 2 years in remission without physical complaints. The initial tumor volume obtained was 995 ml and has been stable for over 9 months at 280 ml

Based on volumetric date in over 50 hepatoma patients analyzed by this method a 54% remission was recorded from the onset of radiolabeled antibody therapy and a 50% remission rate was recorded in 20 patients with intrahepatic biliary cancer (Fig. 2).

Metastatic Colorectal Cancer

More efforts have been directed toward identification of colorectal metastasis and the varied tumor normal tissue ratios with ^{131}I-affinity-purified polyclonal anti-CEA and ^{131}I, ^{111}In, and ^{99}Tc monoclonal antibodies [28–30]. Unequivocally, scanning with radiolabeled anti-CEA may be achieved [28, 30].

Using polyclonal ^{131}I anti-CEA we found that intrahepatic biliary cancers would saturate at 4.7 μCi/g, whereas the same radiolabeled antibody in colorectal metastases achieved little more than the normal liver concentration of 2 μCi/g. ^{131}I-anti-CEA was not therapeutic in colorectal metastases to the liver.

Why was this anti-CEA not of value? The neovasculature of primary tumors could be different than the blood vessels induced by metastatic disease. The antigen (CEA) may extrude from the cell surface rapidly into the blood stream and does not bind, and has a shortened tumor effective half-life much as alpha-fetoprotein. The antigens which are in high concentration may not be CEA and may be cross-reactive and therefore not studied for immunologic specificity. The lack of focus on "concentration in vivo at tumor" as a primary requirement for radiolabeled therapy may lead to studies not pertinent to therapeutic goals. Until there is reorientation to tumor concentration in μCi/g and tumor effective half-life in conjunction with a variety of specificities studied in regard to therapeutic application the appropriateness of the present radiolabeled antibodies remains doubtful.

New Modalities, Isotopes, and Radiolabeled Antibodies

In the 1960s conventional radiotherapeutic approaches to liver metastases were not accepted. However, studies carried out at Harvard revealed that external radiation giving 300-rad fractions 4 times a week to 2100 rad led to 60%-70% remission of liver metastases and improvement in quality of life [10]. This study was followed by a group wide program carried out by the Radiation Therapy Oncology Group (RTOG) and demonstrated similar results.

More recently, there has been increasing interest in hyperfractionation of radiation giving one course twice a day. The RTOG will investigate 150 rad-4 h-150 rad given daily with dose escalation to see if radiation tolerance (3000 rad at 150-rad fractions) may be extended and increase the success of palliation, particularly local control.

Isotopes with beta disintegration remain promising for radiolabeled antibody applications; however, significant problems exist. First, the isotopes must be available on a commercial basis. Secondly, impurities that exist must be removed. For example, ^{90}Strontium decays to^{90}Yttrium, the latter having a half-life of 64.6 h and a mean energy of 0.93 Mev/distintegration. If either the parent isotope exists as a contaminant or the daughter product as a free isotope, bone marrow fatality could follow therapeutic application. Purification and permanent chemical isolation of the free isotope is necessary. In radiolabeled antibody applications chemical linkage of stable isotope combinations must be achieved in the laboratory prior to clinical testing. Preliminary results with Hybritech, Inc. (La Jolla, California) indicate the viability of such an approach.

Other isotopes, although attractive and mentioned in the literature, remain unavailable, or without purification and linkage chemistry.

If priority was to be given to the most needed requirements for rapid progress they consist of automated dosimetry and a new beta isotope label. The former would allow treatment planning for radiolabeled antibodies and the latter outpatient therapy. Based on present-day results, there is much to anticipate from this newly developing therapeutic modality.

Acknowledgements. This study was supported by grant Nos. ACS PPD 227, NIH NCI CA 06973-22, and NIH NCI CA 29536-04 and by Hybritech Inc.

References

1. Shafritz DA, Shouval D, Sherman HI, Hadziyannis SJ, Kew MC (1981) Integration of hepatitis B virus DNA into the genome of liver cells in chronic liver disease and hepatocellular carcinoma. Studies in percutaneous liver biopsies and post mortem tissue specimens. N Engl J Med 305: 1067-1073
2. Olweny CL, Katongole-Mbdidde E, Bahendeka S, Otim D, Mugerwa J, Kyalwazi SK (1980) Further experience in treating patients with hepatocellular carcinoma in Uganda. Cancer 46: 2717-2722

3. Yamada R, Nakatsuka H, Nakamura K, Sato M, Tamacoka K, Takemoto K, Munakuchi K, Yamaguchi S, Tamaki M, Monna T, Yamamoto S (1979) Transcatheter arterial embolization therapy in unresectable hepatomas: experience in 15 cases. Kazeo 20: 595-603
4. Friedman MA, Volberding PA, Cassidy MJ, Resser KS, Wasserman TH, Phillips TL (1971) Therapy for hepatocellular cancer with intrahepatic arterial Adriamycin and 5-fluorouracil combined with whole liver irradiation. Northern California Oncology Group Study. Cancer Treat Rep 63: 1885-1888
5. Larouze B, Londdon WT, Weiner BG, Lustbader ED, Sainot G, Payet M, Blumberg BS (1979) Studies on the prevention of primary hepatic carcinoma, parental influence on the transmission of, and host responses to, hepatitis B virus. Cancer Detect Prev 2: 65-74
6. Lusell CA (1979) Environmental chemical carcinogens and liver cancer. J Toxicol Environ Health 5: 173-181
7. Newberger J, Nunnerly HB, Davis M, Portmann B, Laws JW, Williams R (1980) Oral contraceptive associated liver tumors: occurrence of malignancy and difficulties in diagnosis. Lancet 1: 273-276
8. Order SE, Klein JL, Leichner PK, Wharam MD, Chambers J, Kopher K, Ettinger DS, Siegelma SS (1984) Radiolabeled antibodies in the treatment of primary liver malignancies. In: Levin B, Riddell R (eds) Gastrointestinal cancer. Elsevier North Holland, New York, pp 222-232
9. Ravory MJ (1980) Combination chemotherapy of hepatocellular and biliary tract carcinoma with adriamycin plus bleomycin. Proc Am Assoc Cancer Res 21: 366
10. Sherman D, Weichselbaum R, Order SE, Cloud L, Trey C, Piro A (1978) Palliation of hepatic metastasis. Cancer 41: 2013-2017
11. Leibel SA, Order SE, Rominger CJ, Asbell SO (1981) Palliation of liver metastases with combined hepatic irradiation and misonidazole. Results of a Radiation Therapy Oncology Group, Phase I-II Study. Cancer Clin Trials 4: 285-293
12. Ansfield FJ (1964) A less toxic fluorouracil dosage schedule. JAMA 190: 686-688
13. Reed ML, Vaitkevicius VK, Al-Sarraf M, Vaughn CB, Singhakowinta I, Sexon-Porte M, Izbicki R, Baker L, Straatsma GW (1981) The practicability of clinic hepatic artery infusion therapy of primary and metastatic hepatic malignancies: ten year results of 124 patients in a prospective protocol. Cancer 47: 402-409
14. Order SE, Leibel S (1981) The treatment of hepatic metastases. In: Weiss L (ed) Combined hepatic irradiation and misonidazole for palliation of liver metastases, chap 21. Hall, Boston, pp 629-636
15. Friedman M (1979) Combined modality therapy of hepatic metastases. Cancer 44: 906-913
16. Rostock RA, Klein JL, Leichner PK, Kopher KA, Order SE (1983) Selective tumor localization in experimental hepatoma by radiolabeled antiferritin antibody. Int J Radiat Oncol Bio Phys 9: 1345-1350
17. Rostock RA, Klein JL, Kopher KA, Order SE (1984) Variables affecting the tumor localization of I-131 antiferritin in experimental hepatoma. Am J Clin Oncol 6: 9-18
18. Rostock RA, Klein JL, Leichner PK, Order SE (1984) Distribution of and physiologic factors that affect I-131 antiferritin tumor localization in experimental hepatoma. Int J Radial Oncol Biol Phys 10: 1135-1141
19. Leichner PK, Klein JL, Garrison JB, Jenkins RE, Nickloff EL, Ettinger DS, Order SE (1981) Dosimetry of I-131 labeled antiferritin in hepatoma: a model for radioimmunoglobulin dosimetry. Int J Radiat Oncol Biol Phys 7: 323-333
20. Leichner PK, Klein JL, Siegelman SS, Ettinger DS, Order SE (1983) Dosimetry of I-131 labeled antiferritin in hepatoma: specific activities in the tumor and liver. Cancer Treat Rep 6: 647-657
21. Order SE, Klein JL, Ettinger DS, Alderson P, Siegelman SS, Leichner PK (1980) Phase I-II study of radiolabeled antibody integrated in the treatment of primary hepatic malignancies. Int J Radiat Oncol Biol Phys 6: 703-710
22. Ettinger DS, Order SE, Wharam MD, Parker MK, Klein JL, Leichner PK (1982) Phase I-II study of isotopic immunoglobulin therapy for primary liver cancer. Cancer Treat Rep 66: 289-297
23. Order SE (1985) Newer radiotherapeutic approaches to hepatoma. Dekker, New York

24. Order SE (1985) The use of radiolabeled antibody in cancer chemotherapy. In: Wolff KB (ed) Kluwer-Nijhoff, Boston (in press)
25. Order SE, Klein JL, Leichner PK, Self S, Leibel S, Ettinger D (1984) I-131 radiolabelled antibody (antiferritin) in the treatment of hepatoma - an update. Proc Am Soc Clin Oncol 3: 138
26. Leichner PK, Klein JL, Fishman EK, Siegelman SS, Ettinger DS, Order SE (1984) Comparative tumor dose from I-131 labeled polycyclonal antiferritin, anti-AFP, and anti-CEA in primary liver cancer. Cancer Drug Delivery 1 (4): 321-328
27. Order SE (1982) Monoclonal antibodies potential in radiation therapy and oncology. Int J Radiat Oncol Biol Phys 8: 1193-1201
28. Goldenberg DM, Deland F, Kim E, Bennet S, Primus FJ, VanNagell GR, Estes N, DeSimone P, Rayburn P (1978) Use of radiolabeled antibodies to carcinoembryonic antigen for the detection and localization of diverse cancers by external photoscanning. N Engl J Med 25: 1384-1388
29. Halpern SE, Hagen PL, Graves PR, Koziol JA, Cheu AWN, Frincke JM, Bartholomew RM, Bird GS, Adams TH (1983) Stability, characterization and kinetics of In-111 labeled monoclonal anti-tumor antibodies in normal animals and nude mouse-human tumor models. Cancer Res 43: 5347-5355
30. Morrison RT, Lyster DM, Alcorn LN, Rhodes BA, Breslow K, Burchiel SW (1984) Gamma scintigraphy using Tc-99m labeled antibody to human chorionic gonadotropin. Clin Nucl Med 9: 20-24

Thermochemotherapy for Unresectable Hepatic Cancer

R. E. Falk, L. Newhook, F. L. Moffat, W. B. Lopatin, J. A. Heine, L. Makowka, V. Howard, D. Laing, D. Venturi, and J. A. Falk

1-046 Mulock Larkin Wing, Toronto General Hospital, 101 College Street, Toronto, Ontario, M5G 1L7, Canada

Introduction

The prognosis of unresectable neoplastic disease of the liver, whether primary or metastatic, remains poor. Current methods of treatment are unsatisfactory. The use of standard systemic chemotherapy has resulted in objective tumor responses to 7%-45% of patients so treated [1, 2]. Hepatic artery infusion of chemotherapeutic drugs has allowed for higher response rates of 30%-60% [3-5] but this is an invasive technique and its effect on survival is unclear. Regional radiofrequency hyperthermia (RFHT) has been used to treat deep tumors of the chest, abdomen, and pelvis [6-8] and has been used in combination with hepatic arterial obliteration and intratumor injection of cytotoxic drugs [9] and in combination with internal radiation [10].

A phase II clinical study of regional capacitive RFHT with cytotoxic chemotherapy has been in progress at the Toronto General Hospital since August 1981. Locally and regionally applied RFHT produces only infrequent adverse effects in man when employed in combination with chemotherapy [11-17]. Our preliminary results with combined RFHT and chemotherapy have been published previously [8]. Our experience with RFHT and cytotoxic chemotherapy in patients with unresectable liver malignancies is updated in this report.

Methods

To date, 847 patients with various tumors have been treated with RFHT and chemotherapy in this center, 291 for hepatic malignancies, 113 patients of the hepatic group have been excluded from this analysis. Fifty-nine patients were moribund when initially seen (anticipated survival less than 2 weeks), 35 patients have been lost to follow-up, and 19 patients did not complete even a single treatment course. The remaining 178 patients form the substance of this report and include 99 men and 79 women ranging in age from 28 to 80 years (median 57 years). The primary malignancies in these patients are described in Table 1.

The IIMS-100 model capacitive RFHT machines in use at this center were produced by the International Institute of Medical Science, New York. These machines generate RF energy at 13.56 MHz through three channels of 500 W power capacity each. The output of one or all channels is delivered to the patients through two flexible planar copper-lead electrodes embedded in silicon rubber. The positioning of the electrodes and treatment

Recent Results in Cancer Research. Vol 100

Table 1. Site of origin of hepatic neoplasms in 178 patients

Site	No. of patients
Secondary tumors	
Colon and rectum	137
Breast	6
Pancreas	5
Gallbladder	5
Stomach	4
Lung	2
Esophagus	1
Ovary	1
Duodenum	1
Pancreatic (gastrinoma)	1
Jejunum (carcinoid)	1
Melanoma	5
Unknown	4
Primary tumors	5
Total	178

protocols have been described in detail elsewhere [8]. Informed consent was obtained from all patients participating in this therapeutic program and treatment was given on an outpatient basis except for patients undergoing concomitant transfemoral hepatic artery infusional chemotherapy (HAI) or requiring hospital admission for other reasons.

Patients received 1 to 25 treatment courses (median 6 courses) of RFHT and chemotherapy. Treatment courses consisted of 1-5 consecutive daily sessions of 75-120 min thermotherapy, each course comprising 80-565 min (median 271 min) RFHT. Machine power was set at the maximum level compatible with patient comfort, ranging from 58 to 360 W (median 145 W).

To evaluate the efficiency of deep heating, tumor core temperatures were initially monitored in 27 of the 178 patients in this study. Eleven patients among those excluded from this analysis also underwent tumor temperature monitoring. Two electronic thermometry systems were used, both of which require the percutaneous insertion of a wire thermistor or fiber-optic heat-sensitive probe into the tumor mass being treated. Systemic temperatures were measured orally or rectally at the beginning and conclusion of each RFHT treatment.

Medication administered during treatment included mild sedatives or analgetics as necessary, metronidazole (1500 mg i.v./p.o) [18] and cytotoxic chemotherapy. Systemic chemotherapeutic agents used included 5-fluorouracil, methotrexate, mitomycin-C, *cis*-chloronitrosourea, vincristine, vinblastine, procarbazine, and doxorubicin, alone or in conventional combinations for the tumor type involved. Chemotherapy was administered concomitantly to all but three patients. Eighty-three patients received conventional regimens of systemic i. v. chemotherapy, 49 patients received HAI chemotherapy following a standard protocol [3], and the remaining 43 patients received cytotoxic agents by both routes during different courses of RFHT. Twenty-two of the patients receiving HAI chemotherapy had indwelling silastic hepatic artery catheters (Port-A-Cath, Pharmacia, Piscataway, NJ) placed at laparotomy for various unrelated indications. These patients were injected through a subcutaneous port on an outpatient basis.

Results

As of April 1984, 92 patients (52%) have survived, with follow-up of 3–107 weeks (median 36.5 weeks) from the date of initial treatment. Eighty-six patients (48%) who received combined RFHT and chemotherapy have died, having survived 3–76 weeks (median 26 weeks). For purposes of analysis the patients have been retrospectively stratified into four groups by extent of disease and previous chemotherapy.

Group I: 51 patients with advanced disease whose expected survival was less than 8 weeks
Group II: 69 patients whose expected survival was greater than 8 weeks and who had failed to respond to the best available chemotherapy for their tumors prior to treatment by RFHT
Group III: 58 patients with newly diagnosed hepatic metastases with or without extrahepatic metastatic disease
Group IV: 37 patients from group III whose metastatic disease was from colorectal adenocarcinoma and was limited to the liver

Cumulative survival data for all groups are given in Table 2. Objective response using conventional criteria as outlined by Moertel [18] was assessed by hepatic angiography, CT scan, abdominal ultrasound, and/or scintigraphic liver scan. Response rates and duration of response are given for each group in Table 3. In groups III and IV partial tumor regression was seen in 67.2% and 78.4% of patients respectively, with a median duration of response of 32 weeks. Partial tumor regression in patients who had failed previous attempts at therapy was seen in 43.5%, group II, (median duration 26 weeks). It is apparent that patients with previously untreated hepatic neoplasms (group III and IV) have fared substantially better with RFHT than those who had failed previous conventional therapy (group I).

There were no differences in survival or objective tumor response between patients receiving systemic chemotherapy and those receiving chemotherapy by hepatic arterial infusion.

Temperature Monitoring

The results of tumor core temperature measurements in the 38 monitored patients have been published previously [13]. Systemic temperatures in all 178 patients increased by only 0.6°–0.3 °C during RFHT, a clinically negligible increment.

Table 2. Cumulative survival of patients treated with RFHT and chemotherapy for hepatic malignancies

	26 weeks % (No. of patients followed)	52 weeks % (No. of patients followed)	78 weeks % (No. of patients followed)
Group ($n=51$) I	20% (11)	0%	0%
Group ($n=69$) II	83% (4)	26% (8)	-
Group ($n=58$) III	93% (42)	60% (12)	33% (4)
Group ($n=37$) IV	93% (28)	80.5% (11)	67% (3)

Table 3. Objective partial tumor response to RFHT and chemotherapy in 178 patients with hepatic tumors

		No. of patients (%)	Duration of response in weeks (median, range)
Group ($n=51$)	I	8 (15.7%)	15, 12-28
Group ($n=69$)	II	30 (43.5%)	26, 12-45
Group ($n=58$)	III	39 (67.2%)	32, 14-90
Group ($n=37$)	IV	29 (78.4%)	32, 14-90

Toxicity

There has been no systemic toxicity or mortality associated with RFHT in this series. Local RFHT toxicity was seen infrequently. Significant partial thickness skin burns occurred in 6 patients (3.4%) and subcutaneous fat necrosis was seen in 18 patients (10.1%). All thermal injuries healed quickly and uneventfully. Two patients became febrile and another patient became septicemic while receiving HAI chemotherapy. These patients promptly recovered following removal of their catheters and coverage with broad-spectrum antibiotics [13]. Thrombocytopenia (less than 20000 platelets/mm^3) was seen in three patients receiving systemic chemotherapy. Their platelet counts returned to normal when the drugs were withheld.

The adverse effects related to tumor core temperature monitoring have been reported previously [13]. Briefly, two patients developed local peritonitis and in one patient a thermistor probe broke off and was retained in the liver without ill effect. These complications were managed successfully by conservative treatment.

Discussion

The liver is involved with secondary deposits in one-third to one-half of fatal cases of colorectal malignancy [19]. Once liver metastases have developed the prognosis is bleak. Data from a number of reviews [19-23] show that the mean survival after discovery of hepatic metastases ranges from 6 to 9 months, independent of the mode of therapy used. Tumor response to systemic chemotherapy ranges from 7% to 21% of patients treated with single-drug therapy and from 30% to 43% with combination chemotherapy [1]. Hepatic arterial infusional chemotherapy produces tumor regression in 30%-60% of treated patients [3]. We have shown that when RFHT is combined with chemotherapy by either route, the 1-year cumulative survival in our series of patients with previously untreated colorectal metastases confined to the liver was 80.5%. Partial tumor regression was seen in 43.5% of patients failing previous attempts at conventional chemotherapy and in 78.4% of patients as yet untreated for colorectal metastatic disease confined to the liver.

The quality of life in patients who respond to therapy is excellent. Dramatic reduction in pain and fatigability was reported by all patients responding to treatment. In patients whose tumors did not respond to RFHT, quality of life was not compromised by the treatment protocol. It is apparent that RFHT when applied to hepatic tumors has little inherent toxicity, but major morbidity is a real possibility with invasive tumor core temperature monitoring. We have stopped inserting probes or thermistors into deeply situated tumors for the purposes of monitoring temperature because we feel that the risk of serious misadventure resulting from these procedures outweighs the value of the often spurious data obtained. We await the development of noninvasive methods of monitoring tumor core temperature in patients and the animal laboratory.

In conclusion, we feel that RFHT in combination with selective chemotherapy provides good palliation for patients with incurable hepatic cancer, particularly patients with newly diagnosed hepatic metastases of colorectal origin.

References

1. Taylor I (1982) A critical review of the treatment of colorectal liver metastases. Clin Oncol 8: 149-158
2. Lightdale CJ, Sherlock P (1982) Management of metastatic liver disease. Prog Liver Dis 7: 649-662
3. Falk RE, Greig P, Makowka L, Ambus U, Ropchan G, Larratt L, Langer B, Taylor BR, Hobbs BB, Colapinto RF, Bugala R, Gollish C, Calman P (1982) Intermittent percutaneous infusion into the hepatic artery of cytotoxic drugs for hepatic tumors. Can J Surg 25: 47-50
4. Sundqvist K, Hafström LO, Jonsson PE, Ryden S, Forsberg L, Lunderquist A (1978) Treatment of liver cancer with regional intra-arterial 5-FU infusion. Am J Surg 136: 328-31
5. Patt YZ, Wallace S, Freireich EJ, Hersh EM, Chuang VP, Mavligit GM (1981) The palliative role of hepatic arterial infusion and arterial occlusion in colorectal carcinoma metastatic to the liver. Lancet 1: 349-351
6. Babu HW, Saedeor PA, Goss JC, Gale WP, Galliver JT, Horowitz IJ, Dugan K (1982) Regional hyperthermia for cancer. Am J Surg 143: 586
7. LeVeen HH, Waprick S, Pricone V, Falk G, Ahmid N (1976) Tumor eradication by radiofrequency therapy. JAMA 235: 2198
8. Moffat FL, Falk RE, Calhoun F, Langer JC, Dreznik A, Makowka L, Rotstein LE, Ambus A, Howard V, Campbell A, Laing D, Venturi D, Falk JA (1983) The effect of radiofrequency hyperthermia and chemotherapy on primary and secondary hepatic malignancies when used with metronidazole. Surgery 94 (4): 536-542
9. LeVeen HH, Rajajopalan PR, Vryui I, Gobies RP, O'Brien PH, Hutto R, Pontiygian P, d'Ovidio N, Pethig R, Armitage D (1984) Radiofrequency thermotherapy, local thermotherapy, and arterial occlusion in the treatment of nonresectable cancer. Am Surg 59 (2): 61-65
10. Grady ED, McLaren J, Auda SP, McGinley PH (1983) Combination of internal radiation therapy and hyperthermia to treat liver cancer. South Med J 76 (9): 1101
11. Storm FK, Kaiser LR, Goodnight JE, Harrison WH, Elliott RS, Gomes AS, Morton DL (1982) Thermochemotherapy for melanoma metastases in liver. Cancer 49: 1243-1248
12. Falk RE, Moffat FL, Calhoun K, Dreznik Z, Makowka L, Ambus U, Langer JC, Howard V Rotstein LE, Falk JA (1983) The effect of radiofrequency hyperthermia on human neoplasms when used with metronidazole. Surg Gynecol Obstet 157: 505-512
13. Moffat FL, Falk RE, Calhoun K, Langer JC, Dreznik Z, Makowka L, Rotstein LE, Ambus U, Howard V, Campbell A (1983) The effect of radiofrequency hyperthermia and chemotherapy on primary and secondary liver neoplasms when used with adjuvant metronidazole. Surgery 94: 536-542

14. Moffat FL, Rotstein LE, Calhoun K, Langer JC, Makowka L, Ambus U, Palmer JA, Campbell A, Howard V, Mikkelsaar R (1984) Palliation of advanced head and neck cancer with radiofrequency hyperthermia and cytotoxic chemotherapy. Can J Surg 27: 38-41
15. Kowal CD, Bertino JR (1979) Possible benefits of hyperthermia to chemotherapy. Cancer Res 39: 2285-2289
16. Hahn GM (1979) Potential for therapy for drugs and hyperthermia. Cancer Res 39: 2264-2268
17. Marmor JB (1979) Interactions of hyperthermia and chemotherapy in animals. Cancer Res 39: 2269-2276
18. Moertel CG (1978) Chemotherapy of colorectal cancer. In: Grundmann E (ed) Colon cancer. Fischer, New York, pp 207-216
19. Bengrah S, Hobstion L (1969) The natural history of primary and secondary malignant tumors of the liver: I: the program for patients with hepatic metastases from colon and rectal carcinoma by laparotomy. Cancer 192-202
20. Pestana C, Beitemeur RJ, Moertel CC (1964) The natural history of carcinoma of the colon and rectum. Am J Surg 108: 826-829
21. Swinton NW, Samaan S, Rosenthal D (1967) Cancer of the rectum and sigmoid. Surg Clin North Am 47: 657-662
22. Bengtsson G, Carlsson G, Hafström L, Jonsson PE (1981) Natural history of patients with untreated liver metastases from colorectal cancer. Am J Surg 141: 586-589
23. Taylor I, Rawling J, Went C (1979) Adjuvant cytotoxic liver perfusion for colorectal cancer. Br J Surg 66: 833-837

Monoclonal Antibody Infusion in Gastrointestinal Cancer Patients

Z. Steplewski, H. F. Sears, and H. Koprowski

The Wistar Institute, 36th at Spruce Street, Philadelphia, PA 19104, USA

Monoclonal antibody 1083-17-1A (CO 17-1A) was selected in 1978 for its in vitro binding specificity [1]. The antibody is of IgG2a isotype and is active in antibody-dependent cell-mediated cytotoxicity (ADCC) in the murine system [2]. Furthermore, Co 17-1A antibody inhibits colorectal carcinoma (CRC) tumor growth in nude mice [3]. This antibody, together with other IgG2a antibodies, was found to be destructive to tumor cells in vitro and in vivo through macrophage activation [4, 5]. The hypothesis was recently presented that macrophages are effector cells for tumor cell destruction by monoclonal antibodies in man [6]. Antibody CO 17-1A was thus included in the series of experiments in which we have shown that human macrophages isolated from cancer patients and cultured human monocytes express Fc receptors (FcR) that cross-react strongly with murine immunoglobulins of the IgG2a subclass. FcR-expressing macrophages in the presence of CO 17-1A antibody also mediated the killing of tumor cells in vitro [7].

In the ex vivo perfusion experiments we have shown specific localization of 17-1A antibody at the tumor site [8]. The tumor localization of CO 17-1A antibody was also confirmed by radiolabeled antibody imaging in nude mice [9, 10] and in man [11-13].

All tests described above indicated that CO 17-1A is a good candidate for its application in clinical immunotherapy trials.

A phase I study of administration of mouse monoclonal antibody CO 17-1A has been conducted to identify in vivo tumor binding, antibody distribution, kinetics, and immunogenicity. Four patients with advanced gastrointestinal tumors have been entered into this study. Three have received a single injection of purified sterile, pyrogen free antibody (30-150 mg). One patient with widespread hepatic, retroperitoneal, and bony metastasis received five injections (365 mg total) of an ultracentrifuged antibody given every 2-3 days in an attempt to induce tolerance. During this trial, the techniques of immunoperoxidase detection of antigen became available to us and the primary tumor in the last patient was shwon to contain the CO 17-1A-recognized antigen prior to the administration of antibody. No immediate allergic reactions were observed [14]. Circulating mouse antibody could be detected up to 2 weeks postinfusion in these patients receiving doses given at greater than 15 mg antibody, and the day after administration in the urine of one patient given 100 mg antibody.

Three of these patients, in whom an immune response might be expected, developed human antimouse antibodies 9-12 days after administration. Rising titers or concentrations corresponded with decreasing circulating levels of whole antibody CO 17-1A. There were no urinary function changes or symptoms of serum sickness in this group.

Recent Results in Cancer Research. Vol 100

The second stage of clinical trials has also been finalized. Of the 20 patients treated with antibody CO 17-1A between December 1980 and January 1983, all had metastatic gastrointestinal malignancies, refractory to all conventional therapies [15]. Patients received increasing doses of CO 17-1A antibody up to 1000 mg in a single intravenous infusion, with the following exceptions: one patient received five separate infusions over 11 days, and another received a second infusion 350 days after the first infusion. In three patients who had only liver metastases, CO 17-1A antibody was infused through a percutaneously placed hepatic artery catheter using a volumetric infusion pump [15]. There were no toxic or adverse reactions observed. Murine Ig was detectable in patients circulation for 2-50 days, depending on the dose of antibody injected. The antibody was detectable in tumor tissue up to 1 week after administration. Of the nine patients who received 366-1000 mg CO 17-1A, eight did not develop anti-mouse antibodies. Eight of nine patients who received less than 200 mg CO 17-1A developed anti-mouse antibody. Four of those patients who developed anti-murine antibodies produced immunoglobulins with anti-idiotypic specificities that reacted with binding site on the monoclonal antibody CO 17-1A molecule [16]. This reaction was hapten inhibited, suggesting the presence of internal image of the antigen in the anti-idiotypic response. Patients who developed anti-idiotype antibodies also improved clinically [16, 17]. Since in some of these patients there are indications of the presence of Ab3 [17], such internal image of cancer antigen on the human immunoglobulin may be responsible for the change in the patients' immune responses and may be considered as one of the mechanisms responsible for the control of tumor growth.

Of the total group of 55 patients treated to date, in 10 cases a significant improvement was documented [14-17]. Four patients of this group are without evidence of disease for 29, 23, 15, and 13 months, respectively [17]. Two patients had nonresectable metastatic pancreatic adenocarcinomas and two others had metastatic colon adenocarcinomas.

References

1. Herlyn M, Steplewski Z, Herlyn D, Koprowski H (1979) Colorectal carcinoma specific antigen: detection by means of monoclonal antibodies. Proc Natl Acad Sci USA 76: 1438-1442
2. Herlyn D, Herlyn M, Steplewski Z, Koprowski H (1979) Monoclonal antibodies in cell mediated cytotoxicity against human melanoma and colorectal carcinoma. Eur J Immunol 9: 654-659
3. Herlyn D, Steplewski Z, Herlyn M, Koprowski H (1980) Inhibition of colorectal carcinoma tumor growth in nude mice by monoclonal antibody. Cancer Res 40: 717-721
4. Herlyn D, Koprowski H (1982) IgG2a monoclonal antibodies inhibit human tumor growth through interaction with effector cells. Proc Natl Acad Sci USA 79: 4761-4765
5. Adams DO, Hall T, Steplewski Z, Koprowski H (1984) Tumors undergoing rejection induced by monoclonal antibodies of IgG2a isotype contain increased numbers of macrophages activated for a destructive form of antibody-dependent lysis. Proc Natl Acad Sci USA 81: 3506-3510
6. Steplewski Z, Herlyn D, Maul G, Koprowski H (1983) Hypothesis: macrophages as effector cells for human tumor destruction mediated by monoclonal antibody. Hybridoma 2: 1-5
7. Steplewski Z, Lubeck MD, Koprowski H (1983) Human macrophages armed with murine IgG2a antibodies to tumors destroy human cancer cells. Science 221: 865-867
8. Sears HF, Herlyn D, Herlyn M, Steplewski Z, Grotzinger P, Koprowski H (1982) Ex vivo perfusion of human colon with monoclonal anti-colorectal cancer antibodies. Cancer 49: 1231-1235
9. Herlyn D, Powe J, Alavi A, Mattis JA, Herlyn M, Ernst C, Vahm R, Koprowski H (1983) Radioimmunodetection of human tumor xenografts by monoclonal antibodies. Cancer Res 43: 2731-2735

10. Powe J, Pak KY, Paik CH, Steplewski Z, Ebbert MA, Herlyn D, Ernst C, Alavi A, Eckelman WC, Reba RC, Koprowski H (1984) Labeling monoclonal antibodies and $F(ab')_2$ fragments with (^{111}I) Indium using cyclic DTPA anhydride and their in vivo behavior in mice bearing human tumor xenografts. Cancer Drug Delivery 1: 125-135
11. Mach J-P, Chatal J-F, Lumbroso J-D, Buchegger F, Forni M, Ritschard J, Berche C, Douillard JY, Carrel S, Herlyn M, Steplewski Z, Koprowski H (1983) Tumor localization in patients by radiolabeled monoclonal antibodies against colon cancer. Cancer Res 43: 5593-5600
12. Moldofsky PJ, Powe J, Mulhern CB, Hammond N, Sears HF, Gatenby RA, Steplewski Z, Koprowski H (1983) Metastatic colon carcinoma detected with radiolabeled $F(ab')_2$ monoclonal antibody fragment. Radiology 149: 549-555
13. Moldofsky PJ, Sears HF, Mulhern CB, Hammond N, Powe J, Gatenby RA, Steplewski Z, Koprowski H (1984) Detection of metastatic tumor in normal-sized retroperitoneal lymph nodes by monoclonal antibody imaging. N Engl J Med 311: 106-107
14. Sears HF, Atkinson B, Mattis J, Ernst C, Herlyn D, Steplewski Z, Hayry P, Koprowski H (1982) Phase I clinical trial of monoclonal antibody in the treatment of gastrointestinal tumours. Lancet 1: 762-765
15. Sears HF, Herlyn D, Steplewski Z, Koprowski H (1984) Effects of monoclonal antibody immunotherapy on patients with gastrointestinal adenocarcinoma. J Biol Response Mod 3: 138-150
16. Koprowski H, Herlyn D, Lubeck M, DeFreitas E, Sears HF (1984) Human anti-idiotype antibodies in cancer patients: is the modulation of the immune response beneficial for the patient? Proc Natl Acad Sci USA 81: 216-219
17. Koprowski H (1984) Mouse monoclonal antibodies in vivo. In: Monoclonal Antibodies and Cancer. Eds Boss, BD et al Academic Press, NY pp 17-38

Subject Index

MIX
Papier aus verantwortungsvollen Quellen
Paper from responsible sources
FSC® C105338

If you have any concerns about our products,
you can contact us on
ProductSafety@springernature.com

In case Publisher is established outside the EU,
the EU authorized representative is:
Springer Nature Customer Service Center GmbH
Europaplatz 3, 69115 Heidelberg, Germany

Printed by Libri Plureos GmbH
in Hamburg, Germany